HAVING TWINS — and More

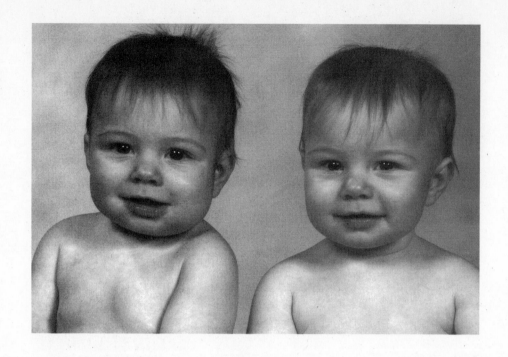

Books by Elizabeth Noble

Having Twins

Essential Exercises for the Childbearing Year, 4th edition, revised

The Joy of Being a Boy

*Primal Connections: How Our Experiences from Conception to Birth Influence
Our Emotions, Behavior, and Health*

Childbirth with Insight

Marie Osmond's Exercises for Mothers-to-Be

Marie Osmond's Exercises for Mothers and Babies

Having Your Baby by Donor Insemination

HAVING TWINS — and More

A Parent's Guide to Multiple Pregnancy, Birth, and Early Childhood

Third Edition

Elizabeth Noble

with Leo Sorger, M.D., F.A.C.O.G., Medical Consultant
Foreword by Louis Keith, M.D., F.A.C.O.G.

Houghton Mifflin Company   Boston New York 2003

To Julia and Carsten

For information about permission to reproduce selections from this book, write to Permissions, Houghton Mifflin Company, 215 Park Avenue South, New York, New York 10003. Visit our Web site: www.houghtonmifflinbooks.com.

Library of Congress Cataloging-in-Publication Data

Noble, Elizabeth, date.
    Having twins — and more : a parent's guide to multiple pregnancy, birth, and early childhood / Elizabeth Noble with Leo Sorger ; foreword by Louis Keith. — 3rd ed.
      p. cm.
    Previous ed. published with title: Having twins
    Includes bibliographical references and index.
    ISBN 0-618-13873-0 (pbk.)
    ISBN 978-0-618-13873-9 (pbk.)
    1. Twins—Care. 2. Multiple pregnancy. 3. Multiple birth. 4. Infants—Care. 5. Parenting. 6. Child rearing. 7. Pregnancy. I. Noble, Elizabeth. Having twins. II. Sorger, Leo.
III. Title.
RG567.N62 2002
618.2'5—dc21   2002191944

THIS PUBLICATION IS MEANT TO SERVE AS A GUIDE FOR ACHIEVING THE MAXIMUM COMFORT AND HEALTH FOR WOMEN HAVING MULTIPLES — FROM CONCEPTION THROUGH EARLY CHILDHOOD. BECAUSE EACH INDIVIDUAL HAS HER OWN PARTICULAR MEDICAL HISTORY, THE READER SHOULD CONSULT HER PHYSICIAN BEFORE BEGINNING ANY REGIMEN DESCRIBED IN THIS BOOK AND BEFORE DISCONTINUING ANY REGIMEN PRESCRIBED BY HER PHYSICIAN. THE AUTHOR AND PUBLISHER DISCLAIM ANY RESPONSIBILITY FOR ANY ADVERSE EFFECTS RESULTING DIRECTLY OR INDIRECTLY FROM INFORMATION CONTAINED IN THIS BOOK.

For photo credits see page 546.
Printed in the United States of America
DOC 10

Contents

Foreword

More than a decade ago, Elizabeth Noble asked me to prepare the foreword for what was a revised and expanded version of her earlier book. Little did I imagine that the explosion of multiples that I suggested was about to become a reality would occur, not only in the United States but in much of the developed and developing world. The nature of this explosion has been so important that twins, once representing one in approximately one hundred conceptions, now represent one in less than forty conceptions in the United States. More importantly, it is now clearly recognized that the result has been enormous medical and social consequences. The major complications of twin pregnancies, preterm labor, and low-birth-weight infants have overwhelmed the capacity of many neonatal intensive care units with preterm and often dangerously low-birth-weight infants whose survival is problematic. The medical community also clearly realizes that these low-birth-weight, preterm infants contribute to at least a 10 percent increase in the number of survivors with cerebral palsy, whose lifetime care costs represent an enormous burden to individual families and all of society. These circumstances confirm the comments written by Aristotle in the fourth century B.C. when he noted that twins were "Praeter naturam" — outside nature's course.

Although much has changed in physicians' perceptions of twin pregnancies in the past decade, certain principles remain valid. First and foremost, all twin pregnancies represent high-risk pregnancies despite the fact that the patient may obtain what is considered optimal prenatal care. Second, preterm delivery and the resulting low-birth-weight infants remain the most important and expected complications. This book provides a wealth of information generally not available in traditional medical textbooks or in the lay publications and Internet citations used by patients. Several chapters here remain unique and are extraordinarily insightful. All chapters represent a point of view developed over a period of decades of interacting with patients, physicians, and worldwide medical research. In this regard, Elizabeth's ability to draw on quotations from a wide variety of sources offers the reader a crash course in diverse opinions. Indeed, I know of no author who is as skilled in connecting medical literature, lay commentary, and personal quotations as Elizabeth Noble.

Readers should prepare themselves for a full immersion in the world of multiples. Regardless of educational background, the reader cannot help but learn and appreciate things that have never been understood before. Some reviewers might suggest that the book should be re-titled "A Short Course for Making Your Pregnancy and Life Thereafter as Wonderful as Possible," and they would be entirely correct. The book is a tour de force for expectant parents, as well as parents of twins and grandparents. It is easy to read and understand — a wonderful primer, extraordinarily comprehensive in its scope, paying due respect to old ground and the latest concepts, as well as giving proper attention to the medical, psychological, and social aspects of parenting.

Practical hints abound, as do personal vignettes and marvelous guidelines for obtaining optimal prenatal conditions. The discussion and description surrounding the intrauterine bonding process should be read with care, even by those who do not believe that such behavior exists. The chapter on nontraditional therapy, including the ingestion of essential fatty acids to reduce the incidence of toxemia of pregnancy, should be considered by patients as well as their physicians in view of the heightened incidence of this condition in multiple pregnancies. There is a thorough description of what to expect during labor and when the moment of delivery arrives, regardless of whether delivery is vaginal or abdominal. And this is not all. The other chapters are equally informative.

Elizabeth Noble firmly believes that when a patient is fully informed she is in a better position to make a rational decision, even under difficult circumstances. Because of this belief, she is always frank and never hesitates to inform the reader if she thinks traditional medicine has lost its way. Her discussion of the controversy surrounding elective infant circumcision is a perfect example of what I mean.

All in all, this book represents a valuable contribution to the resources that parents of multiples have available to them. The publication of a third edition attests to the fact that the public has endorsed Noble's work — and for almost three decades. As president of the Center for Study of

Multiple Birth and co-president of the International Society for Twin Studies, I will be happy to see this volume on my shelf and even happier to take it off the shelf and recommend it to my patients.

Louis Keith, M.D., Ph.D.
Professor of Obstetrics and Gynecology
The Feinberg School of Medicine of Northwestern University

Acknowledgments

Countless parents, multiples, physicians, psychologists, psychiatrists, teachers, nurses, researchers and others shared their insights, experiences, and photographs. It has been a long project to bring my book up to date and I hope that I have listed all contributors to this third edition. My thanks to: Katri Ahlgrén, Brandy Alexandre, Abigail Alves, Kelly Bailey, Jeannine Parvati Baker, Sherry Bechtel, Nils Bergman, Karen Berner, Carmen Mariscal Blackburn, Janet and Jeffrey Bleyl of The Triplet Connection, Elizabeth Boa, Patrice Bobier, Charles Boklage, Meg Bost, Maureen Boyle of M.O.S.T., Tanya Breese, Tom Brewer, Bernadine Brook, Elizabeth Bryan and the Multiple Births Foundation, Ashley Brunson, Amy Bustamante, Terry Callaghan, Heather Cardon, Freeda Cathcart, Vito Cardone and the Fertility Center of New England, Shari Cawley, David Chamberlain, Nancy Christy, Meribeth Cipriano, Lea Cohen, Robert Cohen, Susanrachel Condon, Linda Cooper, Alison Coppock, Don Creevy, Alison Curtis, Laura Dana and the Orlando Mothers of Multiples Club, Hubert de la Motte, Lee Deschler, Laura Gail Diamond, Nancy Donaldson, Becky Dodds, Darcie Donegan, Elise F. Drake, Hannah Elliot, William Emerson, Jessica Ercoli, Heather Ewer, Katrina Folkwell, Kittie Frantz, Elainie Gagne, Debbie and Lisa Ganz of Twinsworld, Henci Goer, Kim Goodger, Mark and Nancy Graver, Stephanie Gross, Linda Guillem, David Hay, Barbara Havey, Amy Hickey, Kay Hoover, Alessdandra Hubbell, Yoko Imaizumi, Carol Ann M. Inbomone, Nancy Jamison, the Jeffrey family, Cindy Joers, Sharon Johnson, Janet Kalhally, Louis Keith, Elizabeth Key, Nicolette and George King, Helen Kirk, Jean Kollantai, Hannah Elliott, Aimee and Jim Krauss Gail S. Krebs, Judith Lasater, Stacy Levine, the Lewis family, Rosie Lowey, Barbara Luke, Kimberly Lusk, Karen Mahon, Davini and David Malcolm, Pat Malmstrom, Kathleen Mattozzi, Leilah McCracken, Bill McKeller, Bob McFarland, Anne McLean, Conner Middlemann, Terri Moore, the Myers family, Carol A. Nadeau, NOCIRC, Dorothy Nunemaker, Michel Odent, the O'Kane family, Mariellen O'Hara, Melissa

Park and the National Center for Health Statistics, Tami Petersen, Melanie Pieterse of AMBA, Pamela Prindle and aboutmultiples.com, Sarah Proud, Rachana, Patti Ramos, Ashley Reimiller, Chris Ridge, Marilyn Riese and the Louisville Twin Study, Ocean Robbins, Veronica Robertson, Stephanie Rubio, Kathleen Sanders, Jennifer Schmaedke, Debbie Scott, Lynnet Scully, Julie Seely, Nancy Segal, Esther Singley, Anita Showalter, Kimberley Smith, Jim Sprott, Corey Steinman, Clinton Stoneking, Tami Strong, Triplets, Quads and Quints Association, Melanie E. Thompson, Peggy Toman, Michelle Unger, Susan Van Lierup, Jim Sprott, Debbie Sumalpong, TwinsList at USC, Kimberly Vollweiler, Maya Rushing Walker, Marcia Weaver, Emma Weiler, Jill M.D. Werner, Cody White, Kristin Winspear, Diony Young, and Jasmine Zelaya.

I wish to express my appreciation to Louis Keith for his support of my work and kind comments in his foreword. Susan Canavan at Houghton Mifflin slaved over the illustrations and I thank her for the line art. Anita McClellan, my former editor at Houghton Mifflin, brought the first edition to fruition and has remained a good friend and wise counsel ever since. My tireless assistant Judy Cunniff helped coordinate many aspects of the project and was a wizard at turning raw data from the National Center for Health Statistics into important graphs—information not available elsewhere. I am grateful to Janet Stone, Lee Shenkman, Arny Spielberg, Katherine Anderson, and Victory Productions for their boundless patience with the finishing touches.

Special thanks to Leo, who shared his experiences and commitment to natural birth and helped in many ways through the two years of this project.

Introduction

Thanks to the ongoing interest and support of you, my readers, this book has been published in multiple editions! Almost a quarter-century has passed since I was first asked questions about twins I couldn't answer, and I promised I would research the topic for those couples. In the late 1970s, I found not a *single* book for parents expecting multiples; and back then triplets and higher-order multiples were infrequent. What a huge difference today with a daunting array of resources, especially on the Internet!

The research I undertook in the 1970s for the first edition of this book convinced me that many problems can be prevented or alleviated by *optimal* prenatal care; that is, by the mother's commitment to a vigilant program of nutrition, hydration, exercise, rest, and education. In the decades since the first edition, evidence has continued to mount in support of this view. The focus of *Having Twins — and More*, then and now, is on the physiological and psychological dimensions of the experience. Learning how mothers successfully carried normal-birth-weight babies to term empowers other women to do the same. Such mothers can still be found despite the preoccupation with pathology that has occurred with the medicalization of childbearing in general, and of multiple pregnancies in particular.

This ever-increasing medicalization is a direct result of the focus on potential problems in litigious societies and has undermined women's confidence in their ability to give birth. Blood plasma volume expansion (causing low hemoglobin levels), hypertension (increasing arterial blood flow), and altered glucose tolerance (making more carbohydrate available for the babies) should be interpreted as signs of successful placental activity, not disease processes! Yet expectant mothers (especially of multiples) are aggressively treated for anemia, high blood pressure, and gestational diabetes!*

*The U.S. Preventive Services Task Force (Obstetrics and Gynecology, February, 2003) concluded that current evidence is insufficient to recommend for or against routine screening for gestational diabetes.

Prevention Is the Key: Health Care Is Self-Care

The privilege of working with childbearing couples for more than thirty years has helped me to clarify what is important. In this book I tackle, rather than avoid, controversies, without the usual suggestion that readers consult their doctors. As an independent observer, I am not obliged to be politically correct in order to obtain grant money or to keep an academic or clinical position.

Being pregnant today, especially if "high risk," is full of challenges that our grandmothers never considered. More than ever, parents need to be *thoroughly* informed and empowered to make choices and take responsibility for their decisions. They need guidance right from the start to face confidently the months and years ahead.

One of the drawbacks of gaining knowledge and insight is that feelings of reproach and guilt can emerge over prior events. "If only . . ." is a natural, though not a constructive, reaction. When natural childbirth, breast-feeding, and genital integrity, for example, are endorsed, mothers who did otherwise may become regretful. Therefore, many health care professionals, in the well-intentioned attempt to spare women such feelings, fail to recommend unequivocally the practices that are clearly best for mother and babies. I call this the "white bread" philosophy. To explain with an example: whole grain bread is healthier than white bread, but it is not widely available. Therefore, let us reassure the people who get the inevitable white bread in the store, restaurant, hospital, airplane, and school that it is just as good. This type of philosophy promotes mistaken ideas about pregnancy and birth: bottle-feeding is the equivalent of breast-feeding, the "abdominal birth canal" (Caesarean section) is just another way to give birth, and bed rest, like white bread, must be acceptable if so many people partake of it! Such reassurances have backfired; outcomes have worsened as interventions in pregnancies and births have increased, and breast-feeding remains a low priority in our society. Mothers end up feeling guiltier than ever!

It helps to explore all possible facets of any health challenge and to resist suggestions that a problem is "all in the mind," when the evidence is clearly in the body! Such exploration may include the study of complementary holistic therapies that address physical, mental, and emotional aspects of childbearing. In her book *Molecules of Emotion*, research scientist Candace Pert showed how a single thought can set off a chain of reactions throughout the body. Evidence has convinced me of the value of natural remedies such as homeopathy and herbal supplements along with visualization and affirmations for treating both the emotional and physical aspects of some medical problems.

According to the Food and Drug Administration (FDA), during the five years spanning 1993 to 1998, federal, state, and local agencies reported a total of only 184 deaths from using herbs and supplements (most of which were associated with weight loss formulas). Contrast this with the figures for pharmaceuticals, discussed below, which are responsible for almost 100 times more deaths annually!

Nutrition remains paramount. A builder cannot construct a house without all the supplies, right down to specific screws and nails. If extra rooms are added, more supplies are needed. A multiple pregnancy is the same. A contractor hires subcontractors; parents of multiples need to assemble a team of helpers who will optimize the outcome.

> The most powerful remedy is not always the most appropriate; surgery is the treatment of choice for appendicitis, but not for diarrhea. A brain tumor may cause a headache but not every headache indicates a brain tumor.

The Nocebo Effect: The "Evil Twin" of the Placebo Effect

The attitude of a health care provider that something is wrong and needs to be fixed leads to anxiety and stress. *Nocebo* effects refer to symptoms that occur when the suggestions, instructions, and expectations are negative, in contrast with *placebo* effects that occur when intent and expectations are positive.

Stress affects women in all walks of life, especially those who are poor, hungry, beaten, or isolated, for example. However, anxieties about the pregnancy, and especially an unplanned one, have been shown to be more serious stressors for the unborn babies. We must realize the role of stress as a *cause* as well as an effect in pregnancy complications.

Affluent expectant mothers may be exposed to more prenatal anxiety because they can afford perinatologists and the latest fetal surveillance technology. They receive a heavy dose of the nocebo effect when maternity care providers anticipate problems. One woman felt as though she had contracted a rare disease when her family doctor referred her to an obstetrician.

Countless women can attest to the nocebo effect from the disclosure of the multiple pregnancy or the genders of their multiples. For example, triplets are seen on an ultrasound scan and the doctor enters the room to talk about selective fetocide. Or the technician announces, "I'm sorry to say, *four* boys." Many couples have felt their panic thermostat rise because of an unclear test result, even when everything turns out to be fine.

New research in genetics has turned some of our theories around. First, the Human Genome Project showed that we have only 34,000 genes (experts had anticipated three times as many!). Also surprising was the discovery that cells cannot program themselves: influences that switch them on or off come from the *environment*. Ninety-five percent of us come into the world with an intact genome permitting a healthy life. The causes of disease in this majority have not been studied as intensely as have the defective genes in the other 5 percent.

Furthermore, scientist Bruce Lipton's research ("uncovering the biology of belief") has shown that it is not just the environment that has an impact on genes but a person's *perception* of that environment that determines the kind of change that unfolds. The mother is the mediator of the world outside and transmits her perceptions to the unborn babies. Her perceptions, of course, are learned behaviors due to perceptions and beliefs programmed at the beginning of *her* life by her mother and others.

Perceptions experienced by unborn babies affect their development and function. The babies are awash in the biochemical brew of their mother's emotions. These regulators cross the placenta and affect the same target systems in each baby as in the mother. The development of the fetal tissues and organs depends on the amount of blood received. A mother experiencing chronic stress will impair her unborn babies' growth and immunity. The hormone cortisol, secreted by the adrenal glands under stress, is known to inhibit fetal growth.

Expectant parents of multiples need the facts on which to base their decisions. By discussing complications and the associated medical interventions to help parents make an informed decision, I do not necessarily imply endorsement. I have played devil's advocate wherever I believe safety and efficacy are questionable. Evidence-based practice is the standard today, but studies of pregnancy and birth are frequently retroactive.

In most cases, evidence-based practice is driven by the pharmaceutical industry because of the ease of randomized controlled trials (RCTs) with a pill versus a placebo. However, RCTs are often difficult, practically and ethically, with pregnant women. For example, how could adequate nourishment be deliberately withheld in order to show that nutrition has important benefits for mothers and babies? (For that "data" one looks to pregnancy outcomes during famine.)

There is an impressive amount of clinical experience on nutrition from the work of Higgins, Brewer, and Luke, and it is on those grounds that I base my recommendations, risking criticism of "insufficient data" by those who accept only the stringent methodology of RCTs.

Another issue is quantitative versus qualitative obstetrics. The medical profession and insurance industry are increasingly invested in numbers — arduous paperwork documenting size, ratios, monitoring strips, and other test results — further driven by evidence-based practice. This preoccupation overlooks the effect of the "soft data" — psychosocial influences — which can be measured quite well. However, while *total* life stress score measures alone have been insufficient to differentiate increase in obstetrical complications, preterm birth, or growth retardation, prediction is possible using *perceived* life stress. Lewis Mehl-Madrona, M.D., published a study in the Fall 2002 issue of the *Journal of Prenatal and Perinatal Psychology and Health*. The research found that such factors do influence birth complications and that complications could be reduced if attention was paid to a woman's *fear of birth* and *lack of support from her partner*.

Scrimshaw at the United Nations University Food and Nutrition Program warns that psychological stressors cause metabolic responses that are qualitatively similar to those observed with infections. Infections, no matter how mild, increase catabolic nitrogen losses and divert protein for the synthesis of immune proteins. Loss of appetite is an early characteristic of acute infections, even before they are obvious. These issues are critical in the outcome of multiple pregnancy.

Regrettably, it is the rare clinician who has the time to help pregnant clients feel heard and respected as they describe their lives (which is where midwives and doulas can play a critical role). Women who were screened for psychological issues, once each trimester, were found to be 50 percent less likely to have a low-birth-weight or preterm baby.

A recent Japanese study found that one of the significant indicators of high maternal attachment to the unborn child was the statement by mothers who starting planning in pregnancy: "I plan the things I will do with my baby." For mothers of multiples, it is hard to imagine life with two or more babies, let alone plan for it, but this is a critical task discussed in this book. Almost half of pregnancies are "unintended."

My focus is on strategies for prevention. For this book, I read hundreds of studies and I quote from many of them, but I know that in a few years any or all of them could be contradicted by other studies. (Such was the case, for instance, with the controversial association between oral contraceptives and twinning.)

The emphasis upon family relationships and emotions differentiates family practice obstetrics from that practiced by conventional obstetricians. The days of ignoring women's feelings, stressors, social support, and her relationships by obstetrics are over.

— Lewis Mehl-Madrona, M.D.

God offers to every mind its choice
between truth and repose.
— Ralph Waldo Emerson

Alternative health strategies are rarely acknowledged or used by the medical establishment. Understandably, research into natural remedies and one-on-one consultation are more time consuming than simply prescribing one of the readily available products of the pharmaceutical industry, even if the evidence fails to justify their use. In modern society, the popular view is "better living through technology, drugs, chemicals" and usually the conception, pregnancy, and birth of multiples reinforce this position.

The Dangers of Drugs

A 1998 article in the *Journal of the American Medical Association* estimated that more than 2 million people require hospitalization per year because of the adverse side effects of drugs. Deaths due to prescribed pharmaceutical drugs total more than 100,000 annually. The number of patients killed in hospitals because of "medical errors" adds up to another 100,000 or so, according to the American Medical Association. Burton Goldberg points out that "the ordained guardians of our health kill as many people every week (in hospitals alone) as died in the September 11 terrorist attacks."

The Physicians' Desk Reference (PDR) — the "pharmaceutical bible" used by physicians — is compiled from information submitted by the drug manufacturers themselves! The FDA approves drugs by reviewing such studies, not by actual testing. Only two studies showing satisfactory results are required for FDA approval, despite the existence of other studies in greater numbers showing adverse reactions. Goldberg warns that many of the articles published in medical journals discuss the efficacy of a drug in studies paid for by the drug manufacturer. Physicians, academics, and scientists are often listed as lead authors to lend credibility to such papers. To read more about the many conflicts of interest between the FDA committees, their advisors, and the pharmaceutical and insurance industries, see http://www.alternativemedicine.com.

Old Traditions Linger Despite Research and Common Sense

Much medical care related to multiples is based more on assumptions than on valid research; for example, the often-prescribed routine Caesarean section and routine bed rest do not improve outcome. We must remember that multiples were all born at home and breast-fed in the old days! Today many women are confined to bed and pumped full of various drugs, only to deliver a few days later babies who will spend weeks or months in the neonatal intensive care unit (NICU). Some mothers eke out a few extra days, or occasionally weeks, of pregnancy under great duress.

So much more needs to be available to parents who are struggling every day to keep their babies alive before they are born and after. Unfortunately, the media glamorizes multiple births and that's the only side the general public sees or hears about until an unthinkable event happens to them. The devastation of losing one or both twins, for example, is long-lasting and affects every member of the family.

Most multiples are born to older couples whose expectations of themselves and their offspring have increased with the years they have waited to become parents. For these "premium pregnancies," Caesarean birth unfortunately is almost routine. High hopes are dashed if disability or death occurs among their multiples. In times of crisis, it is essential to have a comprehensive guide at hand. Twins may be healthy and bring double blessings, but they may also experience complications and developmental delays.

Walking the tightrope between providing comprehensive information and making common sense recommendations is a challenge. Mothers who have lost a multiple understandably advocate total surveillance and great caution. In contrast, those who enjoyed healthy pregnancies and naturally birthed their babies at term feel that describing complications, disability, or loss only makes parents fearful and sets them up to anticipate problems. However, letters from readers with unfortunate outcomes have made it clear how important it was for them to have the information and resources available when needed, even though they had skipped those chapters before.

I encourage mothers to trust their bodies and their intuition. We have all witnessed car accidents, but we retain enough confidence to keep driving. Likewise, the visibility of mothers with excellent outcomes must be high, as in the case of one who wrote, "Your advice to focus on hydration, nutrition, exercise and rest was key to my success in delivering 7 pound, 11 ounce and 8 pound, 9 ounce babies." Others have said that it was my commitment to natural birth that helped them stay committed. Such are an author's rewards.

My personal bias has always been toward respecting the body and Mother Nature, and against intervention unless medically necessary — which even then may lead to an ethical dilemma, such as when parents' wishes for their babies' well-being conflict with professional opinions. Circumcision is an example of this. No medical society in the world recommends it, but individual physicians still prosper from this mutilation and persuade parents to allow them to cut off a piece of their son's penis. (Two cases presently in litigation, brought by victims who are now adults, and the recent death in Vancouver, may soon end this practice in the United States and Canada.)

The Explosion of Multiple Pregnancies

Spontaneously conceived twins have actually been decreasing during the past couple of decades, but drugs that stimulate ovulation and techniques such as IVF (*in vitro fertilization*) have led to the current worldwide iatrogenic* increase of multiple births, often termed an epidemic in medical circles. In Sweden, for example, the incidence of twin deliveries has increased nearly 80 percent during the last twenty years in contrast with a decline in the 1930s to half the rate two centuries before.†

Assisted Reproductive Technology (ART) has become big business globally, and some women travel to countries like India to save thousands of dollars for these procedures. The medical questionnaire sent out by The Triplet Connection to its members listed fourteen types of ART in addition to spontaneous conception and adoption as ways to become parents of multiples! Since 1980, the rate of multiple pregnancies due to ART has been multiplied by 10. The prices paid are: increases in preterm birth (82 percent of deliveries); perinatal mortality (74 percent); and transfers to neonatal intensive care units (95 percent), which may not have room. In 1978, there were 68,000 twins born in the United States but by the year 2000 that number had jumped to more than 126,000! This does not take into account the rise in cost per child, which increased by a factor of 1.9 for twins and 3.7 for triplets.

The first surviving IVF twins were born in London in 1986. By 1998, in Australia, ART accounted for 1.5 percent of all births and the world's first IVF registry started there. Two-thirds of twins and triplets and almost all quadruplets and higher-order multiples are estimated to result from ART. A Swedish registry study showed a twentyfold increased risk

iatrogenic from the Greek word for physician, meaning "caused by medical intervention," for example, iatrogenic multiple pregnancy (IMP).

†Folic acid, now recommended for pregnant women to prevent neural tube birth defects, has also increased the twinning rate. In a 1994 study in Sweden, 2,569 women took folic acid supplements with a twin birth rate of 2.8 percent, compared with 1.5 percent in the general population. (However, the incidence of these defects began to drop before the enthusiasm for folic acid began, as explained in Chapter 8.)

of being born as a multiple from an IVF conception. The World Collaborative Report on IVF (1995) showed that about 45 percent of resulting births were multiples — 25 percent twins, 4.1 percent triplets, and 0.2 percent quadruplets. These rates are higher in North America.

In Canada during 1999, there were 8,864 sets of twins born, 384 sets of triplets, and 20 sets of quadruplets. In 1991, 28 sets of quads were born; that incidence has dropped. In contrast, the number of sets of triplets born in 1991 was 237.

Clinics specializing in ART publish statistics that indicate high success rates, such as pregnancy rate or number of babies born. However, the number of babies born is obtained at the expense of the problems associated with higher-order multiple pregnancies. Financial stress, increased potential for pregnancy and birth complications, and the challenges of caring for three or more babies can result from ART as it is currently practiced.

Clearly, the great increase in large sets of multiples stimulates further discussion about the rights, privileges, and responsibilities of such assisted conceptions. For example, in countries such as the United Kingdom that have a National Health Service, allocation of resources is an issue. In 1999, a singleton birth cost £167, twins cost £1,712, and triplets cost £7,185 — a staggering increase in cost per baby. The rate of triplets could be halved if only two embryos were transferred, resulting in, for example, ninefold fewer NICU costs in the United Kingdom (where 85 percent of litigation involves brain-damaged infants at a cost of over £500 million).

A policy of *birth per embryo transferred* would focus on achieving a healthy outcome from the transfer of a low number of embryos. However, other forms of ART are harder to control. For example, women respond very differently to ovulation induction (OI) — one mother conceived two singletons, triplets, and then quads, all on progressively *lower* doses of ovarian stimulants — and any physician can write the prescription. To further complicate matters, women often undergo both OI and IVF together, making outcomes even more unpredictable.

Consistent legal and professional standards in the administration of IVF have not yet emerged. For example, one survey found that twenty-two of thirty-seven countries permitted unlimited transfer of embryos. In the United States, usually three or four are transferred with a 40 percent multiple pregnancy rate. Between 1971 and 1998, the incidence of triplets increased more (by 500 percent) than that of quads (100 percent),

> Considerable medical and public attention is given to the higher-order pregnancies, as they represent the extreme achievements and, at the same time, failures of human reproductive physiology.
>
> — G.C. Renzo, R. Luzietti, S. Gerli, and G. Clerici

The very fact that there are two or more babies means that anything that can happen is already at least twice as likely to affect the pair.
— Jean Kollantai

twins (80 percent), and single births (10 percent). These numbers reveal the need for guidelines and greater prudence in the practice of ART. Moreover, each additional baby reduces the term of the pregnancy by about three weeks. Appendix 1 lists some differences between multiples conceived spontaneously and by ART.

The desire to maximize the chance of a successful pregnancy by creating or implanting several embryos is understandable, especially considering expense. Some couples undergoing fertility treatments may actually prefer to have twins and complete their family at the lowest cost rather than pay for future rounds of fertility treatments. Many women who delay childbearing and who are subfertile or single want to become mothers by any means possible. But when they request such assistance, they may be unaware of the possibility of conceiving and bearing (and later raising) twins, let alone more infants, and the risks associated with bearing them.

In the zeal to achieve a pregnancy, both doctor and patient frequently overlook the realities of life with multiples. Even the most well-prepared parents are challenged — thus it is important to recognize the stresses in advance. Scholz and team in 1999 assisted a birth of quintuplets who spent 714 days in the NICU, which cost $600,000. Even more sobering, their continuing care will cost more than $1 million. The father is a baker and the mother was described as overburdened and suicidal, often leaving the children alone. Although this case may seem extreme, it reveals the medical, financial, and care-related ordeals attending the arrival of higher-order multiples.

Since this book covers the many details involved in preparing for multiple birth and caring for the offspring, it will be helpful for *all those considering ART*.

More Babies = More Risks

ART has enabled the observation of early human development that has been described as "remarkably imprecise." With losses more frequent in humans than animals, up to 70 percent of embryos fail to implant and only 10 percent of transferred embryos produce full-term babies.

Although this book celebrates the special joys of bearing and raising multiples, it would be irresponsible to avoid discussing the additional risks involved. For example, the perinatal mortality is about five times higher among twins compared with singletons. Risks for multiples include preterm birth, smaller size, and a higher chance of disability or death occurring through the first year of life. One study found that 43 percent of pregnancies with quads produced one or more infants with cerebral palsy.

The risks associated with higher-order multiples is the price parents pay to enter the club where formerly "only God chose the members." Moreover, disabilities increase as birth weights decrease, leading to neonatal and pediatric costs up to fifty times higher than for singletons. Caesarean rates and prenatal and postpartum days in the hospital increase for both mother and babies. Not just the babies are at risk. A 2002 report from the Australian National Medical and Research Council and Australian Institute for Health and Welfare stated that pregnancy-related deaths (for all mothers) rose in the past three years by 70 percent! In the United States, the incidence between 1987 and 1997 almost doubled.

As well, there are often heavy educational and remedial costs in the early years. Indeed, the economic impact stretches beyond the health sector and over the infants' lifetime. Regrettably, two significant organizations that served this growth industry of multiples have met severe funding obstacles. Twin Services in California was forced to shut down, and the Multiple Births Foundation in the United Kingdom has downsized. They were flourishing models for the rest of the world to emulate. Many women, especially those with lower education, do not perceive the risks and do not have equal access to information. Furthermore, information alone does not translate into compliance with health guidelines and the financial means that can improve outcomes.

Changes in Medical Practice and in This Edition

The increase in the use of ultrasound since the last edition has made possible the early detection of a multiple pregnancy. Ultrasound can provide three-dimensional color images, and it is now a rare event to discover an extra baby at birth. However, today's machines are more powerful; and the bio-effects are downplayed by the institutions and individuals that profit from their use. Although the imaging of unborn babies has improved with ultrasound technology and fetal deaths have decreased, each edition of this book has reported an *increase in preterm births and low-birth-weight babies*.

Fetal reduction has become more prevalent as women expecting ART supertwins (triplets, quadruplets, and other higher-order multiples) "reduce down" to twins. Birthing fewer multiples in a set reduces the risks of preterm birth and low birth weight that are associated with cerebral palsy, which increases the burden of care. The decision, however, creates a wrenching dilemma for the parents. Furthermore, the parents, who are seeking to bear a child — not destroy a child — have to decide quickly. Clearly, couples who cannot grapple with this choice should never have more embryos implanted than they can willingly and safely bring into the world.

I have added a separate chapter on the feeding of multiple infants, specifically to encourage more breast-feeding — often the one mammalian function left for women whose multiples have been deposited and extracted by medical technology. The evidence continues to mount regarding the value of colostrum and breast milk for the future health and intelligence of offspring.

There are new chapters to guide you as your multiples grow, to help any siblings adjust, and to advise parents who have multiples with special needs or multiples who survive when one or more of the set dies.

In 1993, seventy-seven people from eleven countries co-founded The Cochrane Collaboration. An almost exhaustive list of reviews is now available on-line scrutinizing the evidence related to various medical practices. Medicine in general, and obstetrics in particular, engages in "information gathering" (many ultrasounds, for example) that may not improve outcome. Yet once a practice is entrenched as "standard of care," evidence showing it to be useless or even harmful is often ignored, such as routine bed rest in pregnancy or universal screening for gestational diabetes. In most of the Cochrane database reviews that I have searched, there is simply not enough evidence to make *any* recommendation!

Michel Odent, M.D., contrasts "circular epidemiology" (continuation of epidemiological studies "beyond the point of reasonable doubt") with "cul-de-sac epidemiology" — the publication of research on topical issues in authoritative journals that are shunned by the medical community and the media, and bypassed like a cul-de-sac. For example, a Swedish study published in 1990 by Bertil Jacobson led to the conclusion that certain obstetric drugs are risk factors for drug addiction in adult offspring. Despite drug addiction being one of modern society's main preoccupations, the results have never been confirmed or invalidated by further research. Likewise, Nobel Prize winner Niko Tinbergen studied autistic children and recognized risk factors for autism in the perinatal period, such as anesthesia during labor and induction of labor. It was found that the Kitasato University's method of delivery in Japan is a risk factor for autism. Their obstetric practices combine sedatives, analgesics, and anesthesia, together with an induced delivery a week before the due date. Further details can be found on www.birthpsychology.com/primalhealth, www.birthworks.org/primalhealth and www.michelodent.com.

The increase in availability of organic foods in regular supermarkets is another significant improvement in recent years. Good nutrition is easier to achieve today than it has been after decades of industrialization that progressively impaired our food supply.*

Finding the cause and prevention of SIDS (crib death) in New Zealand — wrapping mattresses to protect babies from the lethal gases — is some of the best news of the 1990s. Unfortunately, such a simple solution, like nutrition in pregnancy, does not readily find acceptance among those whose incomes are derived from research into the syndrome.

I myself have learned since the second edition to remove the words "don't" and "try" from my vocabulary — unless I wish to emphasize the negative! Recommendations are in positive language, which is important for communication skills and for effective parenting.

New terms have come into vogue, such as "multifetal" — which sounds as if the fetuses themselves are pregnant (like "multimillionaire")!

Telling It How It Is

Criticisms of my book have been posted on Amazon.com by readers who regard it as politically incorrect, for example, to question common medical practices, to present medical facts about the consumption of dairy products and the alleged adverse effects of ultrasound, and to discuss disability and death that strike multiples much more than single-born babies.

With ever-more multiples being generated these days and assisted conceptions resulting not just in twins, but in an explosion of vulnerable higher-order multiples, the need for the whole truth is even greater. My duty as an author is to inform, and to do so thoroughly. The reader has the choice of not reading any information that could be disturbing. But to gloss over the realities would be irresponsible. Indeed, the Multiple Births Foundation in the United Kingdom recommends that, at diagno-

*See Greg Critser, *Fat Land*; Michel Odent, *The Farmer and Obstetrician*; John Robbins, *Diet for a New America*; and Eric Schlosser, *Fast Food Nation*.

When I lost a twin in utero your book was the only resource I had at the time, since I did not expect a loss. It was through your book that I found CLIMB and a wealth of other resources. Second, I feel that including info on the loss of multiples will help parents of multiples who have not had a loss understand some of the issues that those of us with a loss have.

You might be puzzled as to why, even with the erupting sources of truth, the wall of silence remains standing. One explanation is that hard-held cultural beliefs are very difficult to change. It takes a "critical mass," that is, enough accumulated voices to be heard, in order for a societal shift in consciousness to occur. Each of our voices adds to this critical mass. . . Each time we tell the truth of our experience, we will be doing our part in exposing the emperor without his clothes.

— Susan Jeffers

If all prospective human mothers could be fed as expertly as prospective animal mothers in the laboratory, most sterility, spontaneous abortions, and premature births will disappear; the birth of deformed and mentally retarded babies would be largely a thing of the past.

— Roger Willliams, Ph.D., 1956

If we were all first time parents isolated on a deserted island without the advice of baby books, doctors, psychologists or in-laws — you would care for your baby instinctively — breastfeeding, holding and carrying your baby during the day and sleeping with your baby at night.

— William Sears, M.D.

sis of a multiple pregnancy, couples should be warned of the high risk of the loss of a twin in the early weeks.

Others question my discussion of natural, home, or water birth. Again, we must look at the most significant evidence — the outcome. The outcomes of such pregnancies usually reveal such methods to be far superior to the typical "medical brigade" of interventions. Every mother should know these facts and have a full array of choices.

Fewer women give birth vaginally to twins and triplets each year. With the perspective of thirty years in this field I know that women's bodies haven't changed, but obstetrical evaluations and interventions, as well as everyone's fears, have increased steadily. Unfortunately, such developments have *not* reduced two serious and persistent problems: preterm birth and low birth weight. In France, 80 percent of preterm labor results from iatrogenic multiple pregnancy — although the preterm birth incidence in that country is less than half what it is in the United States. (France also has a heterogenous population from many of its former colonies.)

Advances in *pediatric* care, rather than obstetrical screening and bureaucratic information-gathering, have allowed very tiny babies to survive. However, well-nourished mothers continue to deliver healthy multiples who do not need any obstetric or pediatric interventions.

People outside families of multiples often misunderstand the facts about twinning. It is up to parents, teachers, and others who live and work with multiples to provide education and help reduce "twinism" (the focus on the "cute unit" rather than the individuals). Society needs to support a sense of self-worth for each individual independent of the twinship or membership in a collective entity. Pregnancy is the ideal time to begin learning and sharing information — when everyone asks about your big belly!

I contend that if the money for expensive prenatal observation and intervention were proportioned to pregnant women for organic food, household help, regular exercise, rest, and personal care, most of their babies would be born healthy. When maternal lifestyle becomes the priority, outcomes will improve. The Web site BirthLove.com was founded in 1998 by Leilah McCracken, mother of eight, as a venue to share her birthing experiences, and to inform and inspire other women around the world about the beauty, safety, and power of childbirth. Since inception, this Web site has grown into a large and highly respected pregnancy, childbirth, and parenting portal.

The privilege of working in women's health has cemented my admiration for those who honor their power in childbearing — an activity that is what women *do*, like fish swim and birds fly. Every woman *knows how* — deep inside. Bearing more than one baby stretches one's limits, of course, and challenges the expansion of that power. The voices of successful outcomes on the pages that follow will guide you on your own path to parenting twins — and more.

Elizabeth Noble, 2003

HAVING TWINS — and More

1
The Fascination with Multiple Births

 Humankind has long sought explanations for the phenomenon of twins. Religious beliefs, cults, sanctions, rituals, hoaxes, and superstitions have developed around the idea of "instant siblings" in almost every culture. Myths and legends emphasized aspects, often bizarre, that set twins apart from the general population. Today, amazing coincidences, chance meetings of twins separated at birth, and large sets of multiples are newsworthy events that feed the public's curiosity. Horatio H. Newman, an early didymologist (twinologist), wrote that "everyone is interested in twins, or they should be." Twins can tell us more about ourselves — how identity is formed. They help reveal the borders between heredity and environment.

At least 12 percent of single-born individuals are surviving twins by the most conservative estimates. Even greater numbers — up to 80 percent — have been claimed. For three decades now, ultrasound has confirmed the "vanishing twin syndrome" (the medical term is *spontaneous fetal reduction*) in early pregnancy. Almost one-third of pregnancies screened with ultrasound during the first trimester are multiple.

Yet we still do not understand why a fertilized egg divides and why so many are lost. We are learning that the usually contrasted types of twinning have more in common than had been previously considered.

The Great Increase in Multiple Births and Survival Rates

More twins are conceived more commonly than higher-order multiples and experience fewer hazards sharing one uterus. Until the twentieth

> Through the ambiguity surrounding their identity, twins somehow challenge our own identities.
> — Ricardo Ainslie

century, multiples of more than three had little chance of the entire set surviving. The largest naturally occurring multiple pregnancy was nonuplets (all died). With advances in neonatal care, even septuplets survive now. The greatest mishap with fertility drugs concerned fifteen fetuses (quindecaplets) that were removed from an Italian woman during her fourth month of pregnancy in 1971.

Twinning and triplet rates in seventeen countries were studied by Yoko Imaizumi from 1972 to 1996. Twinning increased 1.2-fold in Austria to 2-fold in Denmark. The triplet rate showed a huge increase: the highest was found in Scandinavian countries — 3-fold in Denmark and 9-fold in Norway.

In 2000, there were 126,241 live multiple births in the United States, giving a rate of 29 per 1,000. Since 1980, the numbers of twins have increased by 74 percent and the rate of twinning by 55 percent. The increase in the twinning rate has been most pronounced among non-Hispanic white women — 41 percent since 1990. Twins accounted for 118,916 births, triplets for 6,742, and there were 506 sets of quadruplets. With 77 sets of quintuplets and other higher-order births, there was a total of 7,321 supertwins. Women forty-five years and older had the highest multiple birth rate (almost solely due to assisted reproductive technologies, or ART). Predominant among triplet mothers were university-educated women and women over thirty years. Among triplets, 43 percent were conceived with ART, 38 percent were conceived with stimulation of ovulation, and 20 percent were spontaneously conceived. The triplet rate was fifty times higher in 1998 than from 1971 to 1977. However, the birth rate of triplets of 181 per 100,000 in the year 2000 was down from 194 per 100,000 in 1995. Exactly the same number of triplets was born in 2000 as in 1999 in the United States — 7,325 — so the dramatic upsurge in the 1980s and 1990s appears to be leveling off.

Four Babies

The first known surviving set of quadruplets was reported in France in 1915. The St. Neot quadruplets, born in Britain in 1935, were the next to survive. The world's first set of surviving quads conceived through IVF was born in Australia in 1984. The heaviest set of quadruplets ever recorded was also Australian, born ninety-five years earlier. (The pregnancy went to term with each baby weighing about 7 pounds and delivered at home, three being in breech presentation. However, because of the poverty of the parents, all the babies died shortly after birth.)

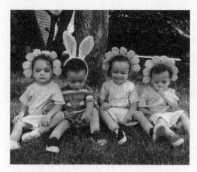

The Coppock quads in costume.

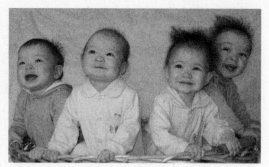

Four eager faces, four times the fun!

Until 1934, the word quintuplet was all but unknown. For the rest of the decade it was synonymous with the Dionnes.

It is not easy to recapture in words the public's infatuation with the Dionne quintuplets. They were international stars of the first magnitude — greater than Garbo or Barrymore or Harlow. Nobody, with the possible exception of Roosevelt, enjoyed a higher visibility.

— Pierre Berton, *The Dionne Years*

Five Babies

The Dionne quintuplets made headlines in Canada in 1934. They resulted from a single fertilized egg that split four times — this has never been duplicated. All five were born at home and survived despite a combined weight of barely more than 11 pounds. Their fame led to exploitation through the 1940s, when they were taken from their family and made wards of the government. Millions of spectators left their homes during the century's worst depression to drive into the backwoods of Ontario and wait in line to watch the five children playing together behind a mesh screen. Two cars per minute were clocked in July 1936! No photos were allowed, but the sale of souvenirs (including "fertility stones") generated income for the Dionne parents. In 1998, the last three survivors, Yvonne, Cécile, and Annette, were awarded $2.8 million in compensation by the Canadian government. Although they went their separate ways, two surviving sisters have now reunited and written a book about their experiences.

It took forty-six years after the Dionnes' birth before another set of quintuplets was born in Canada, and two more survived in the 1980s. In 1990, a record 78 sets of triplets and eight sets of quads were born in Canada; in 1999, those numbers had decreased to 13 sets of triplets and five sets of quads.

In the United States, there were at least 26 sets of quintuplets with all five living in 2002.

Six Babies

Worldwide, there are at least nine complete sets of sextuplets and an additional nine sets that have five survivors.

Seven Babies

In 2002, three sets of surviving septuplets were born. The Frustaci septuplets, born in 1985, were the first set with survivors in the United States. (The mother went on to have a set of twins in 1991.) In 1992, another set of four girls and three boys was born in Italy, with five surviving.

The McCaughey septuplets in Iowa, conceived on the fertility drug Metrodin, were born in 1997. The family has an agent to take care of payment for photos and other publicity to help with the astronomical costs of raising seven children, some of whom have disabilities.

A mother of six gave birth to septuplets in Saudi Arabia in 1998. (The father has two other wives and nine other children.) She was taking a drug only to regulate her menstrual cycle. Another Saudi Arabian woman gave birth to five boys and two girls in Washington, D.C., in 2001, making the third surviving set of septuplets in the world.

Eight Babies

In 1998, a set of Nigerian octuplets, seven surviving and healthy, was born in Texas. The mother took fertility drugs even though Nigerians have the highest natural twinning rate. An Italian woman also gave birth to octuplets, with four (three girls and a boy) currently alive in 2000. There have been nine other births of octuplets, but none where all eight survived.

The "Singular Phenomenon of Multiplicity" — Without the Help of the Medical Profession

A Texas mother bore quintuplets, quadruplets, three sets of triplets, and nine singletons. In North Carolina, a woman had delivered 20 children by the age of thirty-one. Only one was a singleton; the rest were quintuplets, quadruplets, two sets of triplets, and two sets of twins! Eight of these children were alive in 1960, when the last triplets were born.

Nebis Ramos in Chicago gave birth to four consecutive sets of twins.

A woman in South Africa bore two sets of triplets within ten months in 1960. A Chilean woman who in 1981 produced her fifty-fifth child gave birth to five sets of triplets (all boys!). Another woman conceived and lost a set of triplets but within two years had birthed another set. The world's most prolific mother, in Russia, reportedly gave birth to 69 children from 29 pregnancies. Between 1725 and 1765, she delivered a total of 16 pairs of twins, seven sets of triplets, four sets of quadruplets, and two singletons.

Reproductive feats like these are found not just in the *Guinness Book of World Records* but now on the nightly news, because of the increased use of ART.

Twin Experts

Long before the instant information of the Internet, such memorabilia was first collected by a "supertwinologist," Helen Kirk of Galveston, Texas. She has gathered "bits 'bout multiples" for more than sixty years, ever since the birth of the Badgett quadruplets inspired this hobby.

Nancy L. Segal, Ph.D., is a developmental psychologist with interest and expertise in twin research.* She is also a fraternal twin. Her recent book, *Entwined Lives: Twins and What They Tell Us About Human Behavior,* has many fascinating stories about multiples she has met and studied. She estimates that there are over 73 million twin pairs in the world, that is, 146 million "twindividuals." A professor at California State University, Fullerton, she has provided expert testimony in the courtroom for the significance of the loss of twinship in wrongful death, injury, and custody cases. Segal's experience with parent-child issues and the nature-nurture debate has enabled her to explain the unusually close relationship between "identical" twins.†

Debbie and Lisa Ganz are twin experts and media personalities in New York who are dedicated to helping multiples and their parents. They have launched the largest nonprofit organization in the world for twins, created a help-and-information line for multiples in the United States, and published a gift book of photographs about twins. They continue to develop programs furthering twin awareness and support. The Ganzes reunite twins separated at birth, hold twinless twin events, sponsor twins festivals, and cater to twin weddings, twin baby showers, and twin fundraisers. They organized a poignant gathering to raise funds for the families of the more than eighty parents of twins and adult co-twins who died in the twin towers of the World Trade Center.

*Dr. Segal is conducting a study of the relationships in families when the parents are identical or fraternal twins and one or both twins have children. This study is ongoing in the Psychology Department at California State University, Fullerton. To access the survey, which takes fifteen to twenty minutes to complete, go to http://psych.fullerton.edu/nsegal/twinparent/.

†See the Glossary for definitions of types of twinning and Chapter 2 for a complete discussion.

Adriana: I see two husbands or my eyes deceive me!

Duke: One of these two men is a genius to the other.

And so of these: which is the natural man,

And which the spirit? Who deciphers them?
— William Shakespeare,
The Comedy of Errors

One face, one voice, one habit and two persons . . .

An apple cleft in two is not more twin Than these two creatures
— William Shakespeare,
Twelfth Night

Their referral service, Twins Talent, is a unique agency exclusively for multiples around the world — casting for film, print, commercials, trade shows, TV, and corporate and other special events. Of course, the demand is mostly for look-alikes. However, sometimes "theme" twins are desired (e.g., red hair and freckles, or "biker" types). Debbie and Lisa founded Twins Restaurant in New York, staffed entirely by identical twins. More than 100,000 sets of multiples have dined with them, signed their twin guest book, been photographed, and received two-for-one drinks. Among their many "firsts" is TWINS and More, an annual calendar of baby twins, triplets, and quads.

T.W.I.N.S. — Twinsworld International Networking Society — is their nonprofit organization to promote and provide services for the support, education, enrichment, and well-being of multiples worldwide. For example, they aim to provide financial relief for the high cost of multiple births from pregnancy to early adulthood, particularly for parents of multiples with physical and mental challenges. They hope to persuade universities to offer discount packages to qualified multiples for tuition, housing, and school supplies. Another goal is to raise awareness of multiple births as a special needs sector, using educational brochures, support groups, on-line networks, twins festivals, outreach, and research programs.

Twins in History, Literature, Science, Film, and Art

Probably the most famous twins were Chang and Eng, conjoined twins born in Thailand (Siam) in 1811, who were the origin of the term *Siamese twins*. Despite being connected at the chest, they married two sisters and fathered a total of twenty-two children. One was an alcoholic and the other a teetotaler. As entertainers and curiosities, they traveled with Barnum's circus, becoming quite wealthy. They retired to a farm in North Carolina, where their deaths, as is often the case, were almost simultaneous.

William Shakespeare was the father of boy/girl twins; he used twins as a dramatic device in many of his plays, particularly in *A Comedy of Errors* and *Twelfth Night*. Playwright Peter Shaffer scored a Broadway hit with *Equus*, as did his identical twin, Anthony, with *Sleuth*. There is a French opera *Jumelles* (female twins). *Big Business*, a 1988 comedy film starring Bette Midler, deals with mistaken identities of two sets of twins mixed at birth. *The Man in the Iron Mask*, a film based on the novel by Dumas, describes the banishment of the twin brother of Louis XIV. *Blood Brothers* is a popular British musical about twins who were separated at birth and grew up as close friends without realizing their twinship. Thornton Wilder, whose twin died at birth, wrote a story of loss and pain around Estaban and Manuel in *The Bridge of San Luis Rey*. Prize-winning author John Barth (*The Sotweed Factor* and other titles) is a twin.

In Western literature, the popular notions of twinship revolve around those who are physically indistinguishable, with common themes of mistaken identity, falling in love with the same person, spouses tricked by the twin-in-law, and so on. Twin likeness and intimacy lend themselves to exaggeration in modern fiction, with themes of narcissism, homosexuality, and even murder. In *Brave New World*, Aldous Huxley created the image of ninety-six identical twins working ninety-six identical machines — a "major instrument of social stability!"

Twins Ross and Norris McWhirter founded and compiled *The Guinness Book of World Records*, which, of course, has many amazing entries on the subject of multiple births.

Elvis Presley was a twin; his brother Jesse died at birth. Other famous twins include Maurice and Robin Gibb of the Bee Gees rock group, Ann Davis of *The Brady Bunch*, Anita Bryant, Heloise, Muhammad Ali, and the late Shah of Iran. Ann Landers and Dear Abby were twins who chose the same career of giving personal advice as newspaper columnists. Australians Steve and Mark Waugh are test cricketers. Derek and Keith Brewer are identical twins and fashion models from California. David Suzuki, a Canadian scientist and TV personality, is a twin.

Famous parents of twins include actors Al Pacino, Ingrid Bergman, Cybill Shepherd, Debby Boone, former *Today* host Jane Pauley and her cartoonist husband, Gary Trudeau, former congressman from Massachusetts Joe Kennedy, former governor of Massachusetts Jane Swift, and U.S. President George W. Bush. Margaret Thatcher, the former British prime minister, delivered her twins between the two parts of her bar examination.

The Detmold twins, who were born in England in 1883, shared an equal talent for art. Their superb collaborations have been exhibited at London institutes and galleries. Today, also in England, Indian twin sisters Amrit and Rabindra Singh also work together on the same paintings and have published their collection *Twin Perspectives: Paintings by the*

Two nations are in thy womb, and two manner of people shall be separated from thy bowels; and the one people shall be stronger than the other people; and the elder shall serve the younger.

— Genesis 25:23

And the first came out red, all over like an hairy garment; and they called his name Esau. And after that came his brother out, and his hand took hold on Esau's heel and his name was called Jacob.

— Genesis 25:25–26

And Isaac loved Esau, because he did eat of his venison, but Rebekah loved Jacob.

— Genesis 25:28

And it came to pass, when she travailed, that the one put out his hand; and the midwife took and bound upon his hand a scarlet thread, saying, This came out first. And it came to pass, as he drew back his hand, that, behold, his brother came out: and she said, How hast thou broken forth? this breach be upon thee: therefore his name was called Pharez.

— Genesis 38:28–29

Authors. Chicago plastic surgeon and photographer David Teplica has created a magnificent collection of twins in unusual poses.

Biblical Twins

Jacob and Esau are the best-known twins in the Bible — a family story of hostility and division. The dispute over who would be first-born began in the uterus.* Esau was actually born first, but Jacob sought his revenge at the deathbed of their blind father. Dressed as Esau, Jacob received his father's special blessing for the first-born, an important rank in such societies. Jacob was helped in this deception by his mother because he was her favorite twin.

Pharez and Zarah are another pair of biblical twins, whose struggle began in the uterus. Pharez was born first, although the midwife had already seen and identified the hand of Zarah. Considered the second-born, nevertheless, Pharez became the father of King David, while his twin brother did not distinguish himself.

Greek and Roman Mythology

In contrast to the differentiation and competition between twins in the Old Testament, harmonious bonds were stressed in Greek mythology.

Castor and Pollux were the most famous twins in Greek myths, which also included Apollo, the sun god, and his sister Artemis, the moon goddess, as well as Hercules and his twin brother Iphicles. Castor and Pollux are the two main stars in the constellation Gemini (which means "twins"), the third sign of the zodiac. Leonardo da Vinci depicted this myth in his painting *Leda and the Swan*, which hangs in the Louvre. Actually, Castor and Pollux were members of two different sets of twins conceived and carried within one pregnancy. Pollux and Helen were fathered by the god Zeus, who disguised himself as a swan to seduce Leda. That same night another pair of twins, Castor and Clytemnestra, were also begotten by a mortal father, Leda's husband. Four children resulted from these two separate matings. This myth plays down the human levels of twinning to explore fantasies of divine paternity and dual conception.

*Identifying the first-born is still an item of interest, if not an issue of primogeniture (inheritance) — a tiresome nuisance for multiples, who are often asked about their birth order. The order of birth depends not on superiority or strength but on convenience of position. (This is altered during Caesarean section, which is often routine for multiples today.) The Mischnagoth and Talmud prohibited primogeniture when twins were born by Caesarean section and waived the purification rituals for women delivered by surgery.

Another Greek twin legend concerns Narcissus — the word *narcissistic* means "self-love" and "self-absorption." The most common account is that Narcissus was so vain that he fell in love with his own reflection. However, another interpretation explains that Narcissus had an identical twin who died, and it was his brother's image that he constantly sought.

The Greek myth of Amphion and Zethus is similar to the better-known Roman legend of Romulus and Remus — twins who were abandoned at birth and raised by a female wolf. Zeus was the father of the twins Amphion and Zethus, who took the form of a satyr to impregnate their mother, Antiope. Romulus and Remus owed their divine heritage to their father, the god Mars. In both tales the twins survived a hazardous beginning, abandoned in the countryside until rescued by a shepherd. In later life both sets of twins founded a famous city, Thebes and Rome. The Forum in Rome contains a temple built in honor of Romulus and Remus, which housed the standards of weights and balances — symbolizing the balancing forces of twinship. In 1989, the Sixth International Society for Twin Studies Congress was held in Rome, and after a reception by the

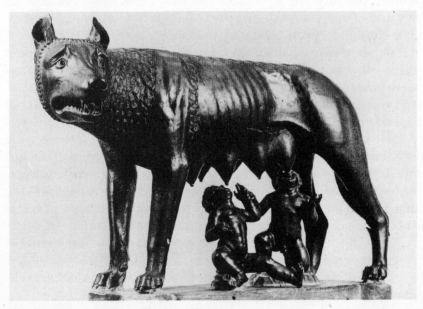

Romulus and Remus, twin founders of Rome.

mayor, we toured the Capitol and saw the original sculpture of Romulus and Remus being nursed by the wolf.

Twins are a recurring theme in Mayan mythology of the Quiche Indians who lived in Guatemala. The exploits of several sets are mentioned in the Popol Vuh, the most important text in the native languages of the Americas.

Cultural Attitudes and Customs

Multiple births have always evoked surprise and curiosity about the laws of nature. Historically, if the conception and paternity of a single child were beyond comprehension, then all the more so was the arrival of two or more individuals. Anthropologists have documented various attitudes and customs that arose in response to this phenomenon. Where the birth of two infants was thought to indicate two fathers, the tradition of the particular society established whether the extra father was evil or divine. Some social groups viewed twins as punishment and the work of the Devil, but others welcomed twins as a gift from God, rewarding the parents. If a society believed that twins were reincarnated ancestors, special privileges were extended to the twins and their parents.

"Double paternity" in some societies was considered evidence of adultery and of intercourse during pregnancy. Where a taboo against intercourse during pregnancy existed, twins were sacrificed in the belief that the father was an evil sorcerer. In other situations, despite being viewed as offspring of divine paternity, they were sacrificed because they were held to be beyond the claim of earthly parents. Sometimes just one twin was sacrificed; whether the first-born or second-born was chosen depended on the culture. The sex of the twins sometimes determined their fate. In the Pacific island of New Britain, both twins were permitted to live if they were the same sex — if they were not, the girl was killed. In New Guinea, however, it was the boy who was unacceptable. In parts of Africa, less drastic measures were taken to diminish the twinship. One of the twins was sent away to live with relatives, or sometimes both were confined together and excluded from certain tribal activities. Yet in other parts of Africa twins were and are still celebrated in the *Ibeji* cult (see next section).

The former dictator of Uganda, Idi Amin, included in his lengthy self-appointed list of titles "Father of All Twins."

A mother with twins was held in very low esteem in some cultures because of the association with animal litters. Sanctions would operate against the parents, the twins, or even the whole family. For Australian tribal aborigines, some of whom still live within a complex structure of myths (*dreamtime*) regulating every aspect of their daily living, twins posed a threat to their secret and sacred traditions and invoked fear of the supernatural. Although against the law today, one twin was frequently killed where resources were scarce.

The Inuit (Eskimos) formerly killed one twin of a pair for the same reason that they disposed of members of the older generation who became a burden. Sometimes one of the twins was given away, but child rearing necessarily had to be kept to the bare minimum for the group to survive.

According to Elizabeth and Neil Carman, authors of *Cosmic Cradle*, the Chippewas and the Ojibwas believed twins were related to superior beings, the Thunderers or the Thunders. The Mojave insisted that souls of twins always existed in heaven with no earthly parents, unlike ordinary souls that spring from the state of "aliveness" after conception. Twins never return because the one life is all they desire. The Cocopa women of the Southwest dreamed of their twins during pregnancy. Twins who chose to leave their pleasant Twinland, one of the cosmological realms of the four-storied sky world, named themselves around age three with the names they had recalled from heaven. They further distinguished themselves by piercing their noses and ears and making tattoos on their chins. The Akwa'ala Indians in southern California believed twins "are always going back and forth and being born to different mothers." The unborn twins' spirits leave their earthly mother and "return to their own country." The parents requested help from the shaman Jackrabbit to communicate with them.

In Asia, where the fewest multiples are born, they have not always been welcome. The Tunguses of Manchuria apparently held twins in such distaste that they felt that ill luck would result if anything were bought or borrowed from the mother.

In Indonesia the father of twins could request an amulet from the priest to guard against a subsequent birth of twins.

Until recently in Japan and other Asian countries, the birth of twins could bring shame on a family. A set of quadruplets was born in South Korea in 1959, but their father refused to take them home. Perceiving them as freaks, he blamed them for his wife's death from eclampsia. Sadly, the babies were placed in an orphanage until adopted by an American couple.

The pastor in the birthplace of the Dionne quintuplets announced that they were God's reaction to those who advocated birth control!

On the other hand, the luck of twins in France, especially a boy-girl pair, is considered *le choix du roi* — the "choice of the king"!

The Ibeji

In Africa, where twinning rates are the highest in the world, especially among the Yoruba in Nigeria, elaborate customs developed around the high number of twin births and, in the past, deaths. Before the arrival of Christianity in the nineteenth century, twinning was considered a bad omen in much of Nigeria, especially among the Igbo and Efik ethnic groups in the southeast. In these cultures, twins were either drowned at birth or cast into the so-called "evil forest" to die. Apprehension was expressed in some areas by the ominous curse "May you be the mother of twins," gestured by two outstretched fingers.

In other parts of Nigeria, such as among the ethnic Yoruba in the southwest, twins are traditionally regarded as special gifts from God and harbingers of good luck; outside Lagos a temple is dedicated to the twin deity for twin pilgrims and their parents.

Ibeji means "to beget two" and is also the Yoruba linguistic term for twins. As good omens, twins are believed to have considerable powers and to bring prosperity to their parents. They play an important role in the polygamous family because their mother is promoted to favorite wife.

If one or more Ibeji should die, carved effigies are created. An Ibeji is never said to be dead, but in transition, traveling or "gone to the market." The wooden statues are carved in the likeness of the dead twin and are suitably clothed. They are cared for, offered food, adorned during parties and certain rituals, and sleep next to the survivor. The mother cares for the statue as if it were human until the surviving twin is able to take over. These fascinating customs are based on the belief that twins share one soul and thus the living twin could not be expected to live with only half a soul. The statuette serves as companionship for the surviving twin or the family, provides safe refuge for the spirit of the deceased, and protects the living against torment.

When members of the community come across an Ibeji, they recite the eulogy called *ijuba*, which recognizes that twins are set apart for their assumed royal lineage.

The custom of fixed names has been found in at least seventy-five African tribes. The first- and second-born twins and the elder and younger siblings have a name that describes their family position. These names are the same in every family with twins. Among the Yoruba, the first-born is considered the younger — sent ahead by the elder twin to check out the world. Pediatrician Elizabeth Bryan in her book *Twins in the Family* describes a Nigerian mother who brought her twin daughters to a clinic. They were called Taiwo ("The One Who Has First Taste of the World") and Kainde ("Who Lags Behind"). They had several pairs of twin cousins also called Taiwo and Kainde. Taiwo is considered to be the risk-taker, impatient but with a quick wit. The second-born shows his or her greater wisdom in a slower pace.

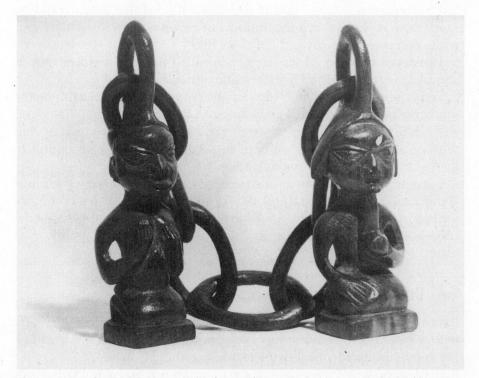

Ibeji carvings of twins. These are used in West African rituals to ensure the health of twins.

Superstitions

In Africa, India, and among the Native American West Coast tribes of North America, twins were believed to have power over the elements. In cultures where such power was considered threatening, twins were killed to prevent natural disasters or else elaborate purification rituals were required, as in Bali, to restore the balance of natural forces. Twins were highly regarded where their power over nature was considered beneficial. The Mohave Indians considered twins the incarnation of immortals or an older person returned to earth in a double form. Believing that twins could cause thunder, lightning, and rain, in a drought they would pour water over the graves of twins.

Kwakiutl Indians in British Columbia regarded twins as a sign of plenty, and their birth heralded a good year of hunting and fishing. These Indians believed that the wind is the "breath of twins" and that disease could be cured by twins using the wooden rattles from their birth ceremonies. Some Hindus in India believed that crops could be saved from hail and rain if the buttocks of a twin were painted black and white and then faced toward the elements.

Parents of twins in Africa have been called upon to perform rites to stimulate reproduction in livestock and agriculture.

Sometimes bearing twins helps emancipation. In one African tribe the mother of twins is identified by having half her face and legs painted red and white and half her hair shaved. Held to be the incarnation of clan fertility, she is obeyed by all and allowed the privilege of joining in men's conversations and making jokes.

Superstitions around twins also existed in Western Europe. Warnings about eating a double grain of rice or double nuts and fruits are described in French literature. A well in Scotland was believed to cause the conception of twins if a woman drank more than half a cupful of its water.

Double Paradoxes

French twinologist René Zazzo suggested long ago that genetic effects tend to be erased by environmental influences when twins live together. For certain traits, identical twins reared together are actually *less* similar than identical twins reared apart. Zazzo points out that many twin studies do not take into account that twins are also a "couple." Like any cou-

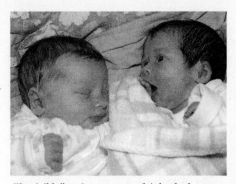

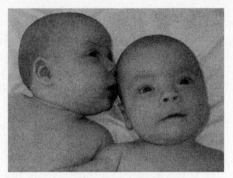

*"Invisible" twins; most multiples look un-
alike, even at birth.*

But a boy and girl can look identical.

ple, individuals settle into roles, divisions, or separate tasks, such as "Minister for the Interior and Minister for the Exterior." These relationships (whether the twins get along or fight) begin in the womb, as revealed by the ultrasound studies of psychoanalyst Alessandra Piontelli in Italy, and continue in the same vein in later life. The environment is doubly complex for twins because they interact with each other and with society as part of a unique bond. They can be a "gang of two" and behave in ways that a single child would never dare to do. When identical twins pair up with other identical twins, sometimes in marriage, they provide the spectacle of duplicate couples!

Whether or not multiples are physically identical, they are not psychologically identical, and they experience their multiplicity differently. Zazzo considers that the chief value of twins lies in their demonstrating, despite their identical heredity and shared environment, the principle of singularity.

Twin studies make a valuable contribution to research on health, disease, and social and psychological development, especially anatomical and genetic questions. Research with twins reared apart has shown that heredity is much more significant than formerly realized. As Segal points out, "it is counter-intuitive, but true, that sharing a womb *reduces*, rather than enhances, identical twin resemblance." Experiences differ depending on the positions of the babies and their birth order, "lateral versions" or "physical reversals" such as mirror imaging of hair whorls, handedness, and shared blood circulation. Identical twins, raised apart or together, are *equally similar*, showing the greater influence of common genes over common rearing.

Some readers . . . may say . . . that it was a fainting fit . . . or be inclined to give it some other names. But what will such people divine when I inform that my brother-twin during the same afternoon when we were 15 miles asunder was afflicted in exactly the same manner?

— John Dixon,
The Twin Brothers, 1826

Extrasensory Perception

Twins frequently experience parallel clairvoyance, when they feel each other's illnesses and traumas. Louis Keith (who wrote the foreword to this book) and his brother Donald were featured on the TV program *Unsolved Mysteries* because Louis in Chicago was astounded that a pain he felt in his groin was experienced at the same time by Donald, miles away in Washington, D.C.

The Time Factor

The horoscopes of individuals born close together are of interest to astrologers, who determine the differences and the similarities between such individuals through interpretation of the stars and planets. Astrologers explain that the (changing) ascendant star influences the individual characteristics, causing "identical" twins to be different.

Sets of twins within the same family may also have common birthdays. Nancy Sutherland, one of the founders of the New Zealand Federation of Parents Centres, conceived three sets of twins in the month of May. While the appropriate sign of the zodiac (Gemini) operates from May 21 to June 21, twins are not born in greater numbers at this time.

Twins may also be born in different years if there is an interval of hours or days at the end of a year. This has been an obstacle to multiples separated at birth when they later sought their co-twin or co-triplets but searched birth certificates in the wrong year.

Sometimes twins die of the same cause at the same time, thousands of miles apart.

Accounts of amazing series of coincidences between total strangers born at the same hour and latitude may be found in the astrological as well as the twin literature. Such people are considered "twins by fate" and are sometimes included in anthologies about twins.

"Virtual twins" are unrelated siblings of the same age who are adopted into the same family at nearly the same time. They offer another opportunity to research the effect of shared environment. Sometimes a woman will conceive while waiting to adopt; my assistant has such a combination — two boys with a six-month age difference.

Organizations for Twins and Twin Studies

Physicians, psychologists, geneticists — indeed much of society — like to distinguish multiples. Therefore they classify and contrast, for example, by size, birth order, personality, and appearance. To be human is to be unique, and we naturally look for the defining differences when individuals arrive in pairs or sets.

Proper scientific investigation is important for multiples themselves and society. Twin studies are used in the perennial debate of "nature versus nurture" first proposed by Charles Darwin's cousin Sir Francis Galton in 1875. As well, they provide a vital control group — a "living laboratory" — for research into the heritability of biomedical and personality variables in all kinds of human experience, including diseases.

Today there are dozens of social and research organizations around the world as well as periodicals. Some groups focus on gemellology (the study of twins), other groups are formed for multiples themselves, and others are organized by parents of multiples. Medical research focuses on improving the outcome for babies who are mostly preterm and of low birth weight (although the incidence has not been reduced in the three decades since I began research for this book; in fact, it has steadily worsened).

Research Organizations

The Gregor Mendel Institute of Medical Genetics and Twin Studies in Rome was named after the founder of genetics, who made his early discoveries with botanical twin pairs of sweet peas. For several decades, this institute, under the leadership of the late Luigi Gedda, provided free medical and dental care for more than 15,000 twin pairs and in 1952 began the international quarterly *Acta Geneticae Medicae et Gemellologia*, adding the subtitle *Twin Research* in 1979. This pioneer founded the International Society for Twin Studies, and in 1980 he was honored by the establishment of the Luigi Gedda Institute in Jerusalem.

The International Society for Twin Studies (ISTS) is a nonpolitical, nonprofit, multidisciplinary scientific organization that fosters research and social action in all fields related to multiples. Members include scientific researchers, clinicians, multiples, and parents of multiples. Collective membership is granted to official groups such as Twins Clubs and Mothers of Twins Clubs. In addition to sponsoring an international congress every three years, the society conducts interim working groups on obstetrics, the standardization of twin data collection and analysis, and also behavioral research.

The Center for the Study of Multiple Birth in Chicago was organized in 1977 by Donald and Louis Keith. Louis is an obstetrician-gynecologist and Donald works in private industry. The purpose of the center is to stimulate and foster medical and social research into multiple birth and to help mothers with the special problems they and their offspring will encounter. The center also sponsors scientific conferences on the care of twins and other multiples and encourages funding for the support of medical and social research. Major concerns of the center include improvement of clinical standards, early diagnosis of multiple pregnancy, better care through the childbearing year, and a reduction of maternal and fetal complications. The first institution of its kind in the United States, the center has become a leader in the field of multiples, and its Web site has links to major organizations throughout the world.

The Louisville Twin Study at the Child Development Unit, University of Louisville School of Medicine, Kentucky, was organized in 1957 by Frank Falkner, M.D., a pediatrician interested in twins. Topics of research have included psychological development of personality, temperament, intelligence, language and reading ability, and physical growth. The study draws from all segments of society to ensure a sample that is representative of the general population. Both "identical" and "fraternal" twin pairs are studied to identify features of behavior and development that are most sensitive to genetic control. In recent years the focus has been on temperament development from the newborn period through adolescence. Twins have been assessed in the newborn nursery for spontaneous and reactive behaviors during sleep and while awake. The evaluations of newborns have looked at constitutional and genetic influences on behavior and the relation of newborn behavior to later development. Testing has been done in the laboratory several times a year for the first few years of life, and yearly thereafter. Researchers posit that the progressive development of intelligence and personality may be intimately related to the structure and lifestyle of each family, and information is gathered from parents and from the home environment. Details also are obtained from teachers about the twins' behavior in school. Follow-up studies have been made of the twins as young adults, and second-generation twins are recruited when the original participants have twins of their own.

Perinatal influences on development, such as preterm birth and low birth weight, also have been investigated. A current study is evaluating the interaction of characteristics of twin infants and their mothers, together with assessments of the environment, to determine how information about the match between infant and mother in areas of temperament/personality, family/environment stress, and cognitive abilities leads to better outcomes for both twins and mothers. The study is focusing on twins from birth through eighteen months of age. The birth of twins creates physical and psychological stressors on mothers. In addition, twins have more perinatal complications and are at risk for developmental problems that include speech and language delays, as well as behavioral problems. There also is a behavioral gene-mapping study to locate the genes that influence the development of individual differences in behavior. The study includes twins, their siblings, and their parents, and the twins' and siblings' children. The research is designed to help clarify the developmental timing of genetic effects and the interactions among genetic and environmental influences.

The East Flanders Prospective Twin Survey (EFPTS) registers all multiple maternities in one of the ten provinces of Belgium. It has quarters at the Universities of Leuven and Gent, and at the University of Maastricht, the Netherlands. It focuses on obstetric and neonatal management. The EFPTS encourages accurate determination of type of twinning (discussed in detail in Chapter 2) so that twin studies can be used by researchers in related fields such as genetics. The EFPTS also maintains a databank with detailed information about several thousand twin pairs.

The La Trobe Twin Study, started in 1976 by psychologist David Hay, explored all facets of speech, reading, and behavioral development at home and at school of 2,000 children (twins, their siblings, and cousins). Hay investigated how twins differ from single-born children, and methods for predicting long-term behavioral problems.

Hay's systematic study of the needs of multiples in school began in 1985 with a survey of 85 percent of all primary school teachers in South Australia. This was followed by a nationwide survey of twins in primary school and resulted in the booklet *Twins in School* that is widely used in Australia, the United Kingdom, and other countries.

Since 1991, Hay and Florence Levy have run the Australian Twin Attention Deficit Hyperactivity Disorder Project (ATAP), which now involves some 18,000 family members. The results of their genetic studies can be found in their 2001 text, *Attention, Genes and ADHD*. In Western Australia, Hay and colleagues have developed the WA Twin Child Health Study (WATCH), which uses the unique record linkage in that state to identify and follow all multiples in terms of progress, disability, and death. The Web site www.twinsandmultiplebirths.org offers many resources for teachers and families.

The Minnesota Center for Twin and Adoption Research received much publicity in 1979 when a pair of identical male twins was brought together for study by Professor Thomas Bouchard of the University of Minnesota Department of Psychology. The men had been separated at three weeks of age and met again for the first time thirty-nine years later. The similarities in their separate existences were remarkable. Each man had been named James by his foster parents, each worked in law enforcement, and each married a woman named Linda for his first marriage and a woman named Betty for his second. Each twin had a son named James Alan, and the twins drove the same make of car. After they met, they were able to switch roles and speak to the other's wife on the telephone without arousing suspicion about their identity.

Among more than 200 individual twins reared apart, only one set was afraid to enter the soundproof chamber in his lab, and they were identical twins reared apart. Each one also entered the ocean backward! In the decade since this unique study began, the Minnesota Center for Twin and Adoption Research, appropriately located in the "Twin Cities," has interviewed more than 130 twin pairs reared apart. (New twins are no longer being recruited into the project, which has shifted into a data analysis phase.) Bouchard's work goes beyond the actual searching for and uniting of twins reared apart — his research is germane to all of us about how we become who we are, what paths we choose in life, and our fundamental sense of identity.

The International Twins Association (ITA) is a nonprofit, family-oriented organization that promotes the spiritual, intellectual, and social welfare of twins and multiples throughout the world. Its first reunion of twins was hosted in 1930 by Rev. Edward M. Clink and his twin sister, Elsie, with 13 sets of twins present from his congregation in Indiana. Since 1939, the convention sites have moved throughout the United States and Canada.

The annual Twins Day Festival is always held in Twinsburg, Ohio, between Cleveland and Akron. Begun in 1978, it was named in honor of a pair of twins, Moses and Ariel Wilcox, who donated land and funds toward the town's first school. Several thousand multiples, enjoying their "twinness" to the hilt, attend the yearly festival that includes a parade, games, contests, exhibitions, entertainment, and fireworks. Most valuable, however, is the opportunity for research, and many twins stop by booths in the scientists' pavilion to complete questionnaires and undergo various examinations.

Resources for Expectant Mothers and Families of Multiples

A century ago, the mothers were at greater risk, whereas today the babies are. Emphasis is now shifting from postpartum rescue to prenatal prevention — my longtime focus. Indeed, preterm birth and low birth weight are obstetric challenges. The importance of the prenatal environment, including the mother's health and nutrition even before conception, is slowly gaining recognition. The Multiples Clinic in Ann Arbor, Michigan, founded by Barbara Luke, D.Sc., M.P.H., R.D., was an example of practical solutions that achieved impressive results through enhanced nutrition. The Antenatal Care of Multiple Pregnancy Centre in Toronto serves the obstetrical and psychosocial needs of multiple birth parents, providing specific prenatal classes for multiples and links with Multiple Births Canada and other appropriate organizations.

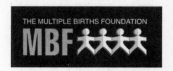

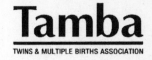

The Multiple Births Foundation in the United Kingdom was founded by British pediatrician and author Elizabeth Bryan. Together with the Twins and Multiple Births Association (TAMBA), she established several twin clinics in the United Kingdom at Queen Charlotte's and Chelsea Hospital in London, and in Birmingham and York (these last two are now part of the National Health Service and as such are the only multiple birth clinics in the United Kingdom). Parents may bring their twins to a children's clinic for routine assessments of language, behavior, growth, development, emotional and behavioral problems, disabilities, and testing for type of twinning. Monthly prenatal talks are given to expectant parents. The clinics also serve as a teaching forum for professionals, and volunteer research opportunities are available. In a support room, volunteers from TAMBA provide practical help, information, advice, and refreshments as well as look after other children so parents can talk with a pediatrician. Special clinics are held every three months for supertwins, twins with special needs, and families suffering the loss of a twin. Parents can call a hotline about such issues as sleeping, feeding, biting, and toilet training.

There are many clubs around the world and one of their most important services is a hotline for instant advice. The Internet has made chat rooms possible that link housebound and isolated parents of multiples.

National Organization of Mothers of Twins Clubs

The National Organization of Mothers of Twins Clubs, Inc. (NOMOTC), formed in the United States in 1960, is a support group for parents of twins and higher-order multiples. It is a network of local clubs nation-

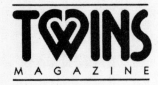

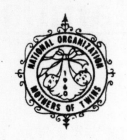

wide whose basic purposes are research and education. As such, NOMOTC's focus is to assist parents as they face the challenges of raising multiple birth children.

NOMOTC distributes a bimonthly newsmagazine, *MOTC's Notebook*, and a pamphlet *Your Multiples and You* for expectant parents and parents of newborn multiples. They publish numerous booklets on topics including placement of multiple birth children in school, higher-order multiples, and bereavement, and they have compiled the book *Twins to Quints* that covers all stages of parenting multiples.

NOMOTC provides a four-part Support Services program geared to individual concerns. This program particularly benefits those needing support that is unavailable locally. A Special Needs "pen pal" program aids mothers of multiples who have children with disabilities or illnesses and also assists parents who may themselves have disabilities that affect their parenting skills. A Bereavement support program reaches out to those parents who have experienced the loss of one or more of their multiple birth children. The Single Parent support program offers widowed, divorced, and never married parents opportunities to share information. The Higher-Order Multiples support program offers information to parents of triplets, quadruplets, and more.

NOMOTC also completes its own organizational research on selected issues, and maintains a Multiple Birth Data Base with details on the birth and parenting of multiples. Plus, NOMOTC liaisons with researchers who wish to recruit participants for their studies.

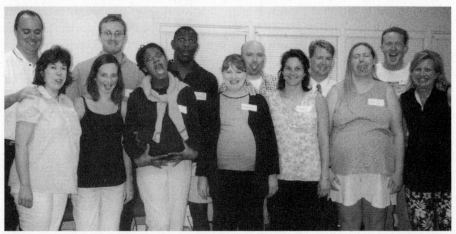

A childbirth class for expectant P.O.M.s (Parents of Multiples).

The annual convention is held each July in varying locations. Numerous workshops cover topics such as research, parenting multiples, and family issues. One of the lighthearted activities of the convention is the "Show, Tell, and Sell" night, when member clubs can display and sell T-shirts, buttons, bumper stickers, booklets, and other creations.

Parents of multiples can check the on-line referral database on the organization's Web site www.nomotc.org to find the nearest local club. A booklet is available that explains the process of starting a local Parents of Multiples chapter, if none exists in your area. Individual affiliate memberships are also available if a local club cannot be located or formed. Professional affiliate memberships are available for researchers who have a specific interest in the area of multiple birth children.

Member clubs often have their own newsletters, with such titles as *Reflections, Twinette Gazette, Twinsville, Double Dilemma, Double Delight, Twincerely Yours, Doubly Blessed, Double Exposure, News of Twos,* and *Twofolders,* which offer child care tips, recipes, and birth announcements for mothers and their "twinfants."

The Triplet Connection

The Triplet Connection in California was founded by Janet Bleyl, a mother of ten including triplets. Since its establishment in 1983, this organization has helped guide more than 20,000 families of multiples worldwide. The network has more than 200 expectant mothers and families at any time. There is a quarterly newsletter with extensive listings of expectant and new parents that is sent to 8,000 locations and 2,000 expectant parents each year. An information packet is sent to expectant parents that explains how to minimize the risks of supertwins. A telephone hotline and an annual convention are offered to members. If you are a parent of multiples, please complete the group's medical questionnaire to add to their pool of more than 15,000 questionnaires; this is a crucial source of information for you and other parents of multiples. There is a list of names and phone numbers of MOMs (mothers of multiples) who are available to provide personal support for every issue you can imagine — truly networking at its best. Visit www.thetripletconnection.com.

Mothers of Supertwins (MOST)

Mothers of Supertwins is an international nonprofit charity support network for families who have or are expecting triplets, quadruplets, or more. Founded in 1987 by a small group of mothers on Long Island,

Unless you have had triplets, you just can't really know what it is like. My local club has helped me keep my sanity.

It is so reassuring to meet others in the same situation. You think you are the only one who feels that you can never give your twins as much love as one child. But then you realize others have those same feelings.

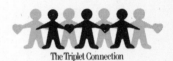

The Triplet Connection

New York, it has trained volunteers who are spread out over the globe (with the vast majority residing in the United States). MOST supports families from the early pregnancy decisions a couple may face all the way through school-age experiences to help parents become informed consumers of health care and education for their families.

MOST has a research database of pregnancy, birth, and neonatal experiences of thousands of families of higher-order multiple birth children to assist medical professionals in research and analysis. *Supertwins* magazine is their quarterly publication, which focuses on the unique issues faced by higher-order multiple birth families and their extended support systems. There are articles on pregnancy, infancy, toddlerhood, school age, special needs, siblings, issues facing mothers and fathers, grandparents, larger families, breast-feeding, loss and bereavement, crafts, cooking, and resources and networking in your community.

Visit their award-winning Web site www.MOSTon-line.org, which has over 400 pages of resources for member families. Through their Member Only on-line networks and forums, families gain pregnancy and parenting support and information. MOST also coordinates special on-line networks such as a grandparent network, quadruplet, quintuplet, and sextuplet family network, the larger family network (families with five or more children), and special needs network (for families who have one or more surviving higher-order multiple with ongoing medical or developmental challenges). Annually MOST sponsors (through its daughter organization, PreemieCare) an RSV (respiratory syncytial virus) awareness program. Different parenting packages are available to member families on a range of issues including toilet learning, cerebral palsy, and loss of a multiple.

Multiples Clubs Abroad

In other countries, similar organizations concerned with "twindom" include the Australian Multiple Birth Association (AMBA), Multiple Births Canada (formerly Parents of Multiple Births Association — POMBA), the South African Multiple Birth Association (SAMBA), TAMBA in Great Britain, and the ABC Club for higher-order multiples in Germany. TAMBA has created a Multiple Birth Excellence Award to raise the standards of maternity units in the National Health Service. A global umbrella organization for them all, Combined Multiple Birth Organizations (COMBO), is headquartered in London. See Appendix 2 for the Declaration of Rights and Statement of Needs of Twins and Higher-

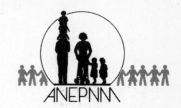

Order Multiples. These volunteer organizations arose because most government services and professional care providers do not recognize or assess the needs of families with multiples which include: physical and emotional health, financial burdens, lack of home help, and social isolation, all of which are intensified by single parenthood, disability, or bereavement.

Twin Registries

Twin registries are important for collecting data not just about multiple pregnancy and birth, and multiples themselves, but also for what they contribute to our understanding of heredity, environmental influences, and family diseases. Registries provide critical follow-up, although the lack of distinction between Twin A and Twin B in some registries limits the research. There are registries in Australia, Belgium, Canada, China, Denmark, Finland, Germany, Italy, Japan, Korea, Netherlands, Norway, Poland, Sri Lanka, Sweden, United Kingdom and several in the United States (including the U.S. National Academy of Sciences-National Research Council (NAS-NRC) Twin Registry, the Vietnam Era Twin Registry, the Mid-Atlantic Twin Registry, and the Southern California Twin Registry).

The Swedish Twin Registry at the Karolinska Institute is the largest in the world with more than 140,000 twins. It was started in the early 1960s and its first landmark study showed that smokers developed lung cancer more often than non-smokers. In 2000, after scrutinizing 90,000 twins, a Swedish team reported in the New England Journal of Medicine that diet and smoking are more likely to cause cancer than inherited genetic defects.

The Minnesota Twin Registry is a birth-record based twin registry begun in 1983. It includes data for 4,307 surviving intact pairs born in Minnesota between 1936 and 1955, as well as data on more than 1,300 other pairs born since 1904. In addition to studying events like divorce, and personality variables like authoritarianism, the researchers are interested in "emergenic" traits determined by the interaction of genetic influences rather than their sum. Thus, genetically identical twins will tend to show the same traits, while for unlike twins the combination of genes may be rare enough so that the traits do not "run in families," even though they are highly genetic.

There is a discussion group at: www.twinregisters-subscribe @yahoogroups.com.

2
How Are Multiples Formed?

Multiple births are rare in large, long-lived animals with pregnancies lasting more than 150 days. Mammals such as humans, horses, and elephants typically produce only one offspring, whereas the Texas armadillo consistently bears four identical quadruplets, all arising from one egg. Twins from two eggs are the usual offspring for the marmoset and occur quite often in sheep.

It is common knowledge that there are two kinds of multiples: those with identical genes and those whose genes are different.* Triplets and higher-order multiples are commonly a combination of both types. The incidence of *identical* twins (*monozygotic, monovular,* MZ, or "true" twins), who have identical genes and look alike, has been fairly uniform throughout the world, about 1 in 250 births. With the use of ART, the incidence is rising, especially in Holland and Sweden. Twins whose genes are not identical and who look no more alike than brothers and sisters are commonly called *fraternal* (*dizygotic, binovular,* DZ, or "false" twins). This more usual type results from double ovulation, which varies with race, maternal age, and number of children a woman has previously borne.

The incidence of mixed-sex or opposite-sex (OS) twins, who are dizy-

My husband and I were making a purchase and the clerk asked us if our twins were identical; and when we said they were, she then asked if they were a boy and a girl. Some people have no idea what identical and fraternal mean.

*The terms *identical* and *fraternal* are familiar labels, but they describe only the external appearance of twins and not their genetic origin, or *zygosity*. Furthermore, the labels encourage stereotyping of the individuals. *Identical* favors the prejudice of duplication — that twinship is a bond of two equal halves. *Fraternal*, meaning "brotherly," is equally imprecise; it would make more sense to describe unlike twin sisters as "sororal." In this book, I will use the more precise labels of zygosity in their abbreviated forms *MZ* and *DZ*, which are discussed in detail in this chapter.

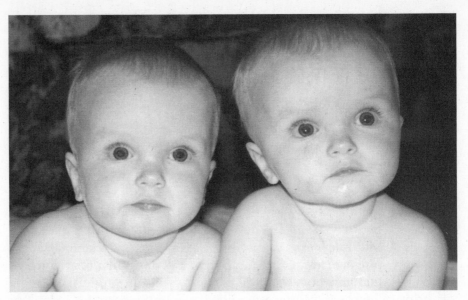

MZ girls may not look identical.

gotic, accounts for about one-third of all twin births. Clearly, if twins are of opposite sex, they cannot be identical, although many people don't understand this fact (parents of twins are often asked if their boy-girl twins are identical!). In the case of same-sex (SS) twins, the type of twinning may be obvious at birth, but microscopic examination of the placenta, blood groups, or even DNA testing is necessary when it is not.

Geneticist Charles Boklage of East Carolina University (also the father of very similar DZ twins) believes that both types of twins arise from variations of the cellular events that occur when a normal single embryo develops. Rather than contrasting the two types of twins, he believes that they have much in common that we do not yet understand, and I will return to his theories later.

Boklage *conservatively* estimates that twinning occurs in about 12 percent of all natural conceptions but statistics show that only 3 percent of all births involve twins (not all twin pairs survive to term, however; see *spontaneous fetal reduction* in Chapter 22).

Fertilization

Around the middle of a normal menstrual cycle, the ovary releases an egg (*ovulation*), which travels through the fallopian tube to the uterus. If

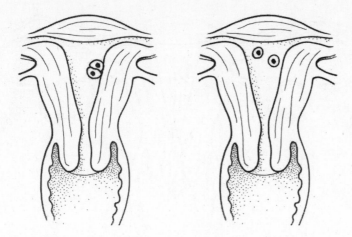

One or more eggs may be fertilized to produce a multiple pregnancy.

unprotected intercourse takes place around the time of ovulation, millions of microscopic sperm make their way through the female reproductive tract. When one sperm successfully penetrates the egg, fertilization — the union of male and female cells — is achieved. Timing is important, as fertilization must occur when the egg is viable — in the outer third of the tube and within about twenty-four hours of ovulation. A fertilized egg divides and expands as it travels down the tube to implant in the uterus. If the egg is not fertilized, it is shed with the preparatory lining of the uterus during menstruation, and the cycle is repeated the following month.

Although unusual, it is possible for conception dates of twins to differ. As long ago as the second Talmud, the phenomenon of *superfecundation* was acknowledged. Two eggs may be released during the same reproductive cycle and fertilized on two different occasions. As the conceptions will be only a week or so apart, such a slight difference in age and growth may pass unobserved at birth. It is also possible for each twin to have a different father (as in the myth of Leda and the swan described in Chapter 1). A case of double ovulation and superfecundation was reported in Germany in 1978, where the resulting twins were clearly of different parentage — one was black and the other white. The mother had intercourse with two different men a short time apart but within one menstrual cycle. Another report concerned a mother who claimed that her twins were fathered by two different men, which blood typing indeed confirmed. *Parade* magazine reported a case in 1983 of a

My dates were vague and even after the pregnancy test I had a sort of period. All through the pregnancy I just felt that one twin was very different. I know the second one wasn't ready to be born — he squirmed like a squirrel and didn't want to come out.

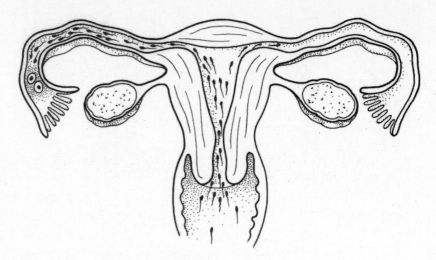

Fertilization occurs in the outer third of the fallopian tube.

Nigerian mother and a Caucasian father who had dizygotic boys, one black and one white; however, this was not a case of superfecundation but simply genetic potluck.

Superfetation occurs when a second egg is fertilized in a subsequent reproductive cycle. Marked difference in the weight of the twins at birth may indicate such an occurrence. Superfetation is theoretically possible anytime in the first three months of an established pregnancy, but it is unlikely because once a pregnancy becomes established the resulting hormones usually prevent ovulation. In these rare cases, low hormone levels at the beginning of such a pregnancy do not adequately suppress ovulation. This may be due to a gene that acts to reverse the normal suppression of ovulation. I have a friend who married into a family with triplets. At birth, one weighed 8 pounds and the twins weighed around 4 pounds each. The attending doctor explained to the parents that two separate conceptions were involved.

"Identical" Twins: Monozygotic

The events of fertilization determine the type of twins that develop. Monozygotic (MZ) twins result from the union of one egg and one sperm. The cause of monozygotic twinning remains a mystery — there is a delay in the division process of the fertilized single egg or a delay in implantation. As a result, the 46 chromosomes that carry the genes dou-

Monozygotic Twins Result from the Union of One Egg and One Sperm

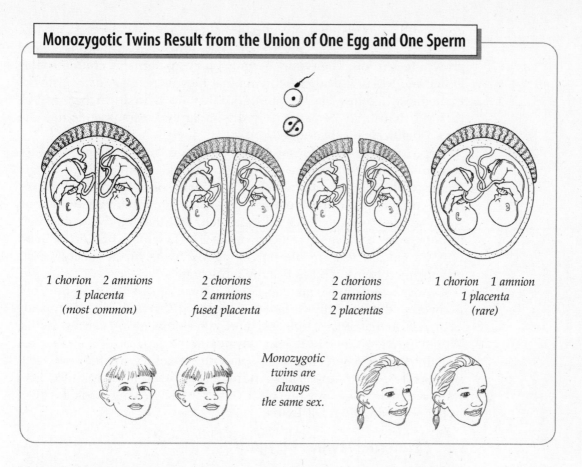

1 chorion   2 amnions
1 placenta
(most common)

2 chorions
2 amnions
fused placenta

2 chorions
2 amnions
2 placentas

1 chorion   1 amnion
1 placenta
(rare)

Monozygotic twins are always the same sex.

ble and the fertilized egg splits into equal halves. Each twin develops from an identical half of this original fertilized egg. The term *monozygotic* means "one-cell union" (the term *monovular*, "arising from one egg," is occasionally used). An interesting question to ponder is whether there is a single or a dual influence.

About one-third of all twins are MZ, with an equal distribution of male-male and female-female pairs, although among higher numbers of MZ twins resulting from assisted conceptions, there is an unexplained increase in female pairs. Monozygotic twins are always the same sex and have identical features — hair and eye color, blood groups, body scent, dental impressions, and so on. They also have very similar electro-encephalograms and cardiovascular measurements and may even make the same errors on tests. However, lyonisation can be asymmetrical (random) with a different balance of paternal and maternal genes.* One MZ twin may arise from far fewer stem cells, for example, which leads to growth restriction. There may be more active paternal X chromosomes in one and less in the other, showing that they were not equally cleaved. Pathologist Geoffrey Machin points out that few twin researchers realize that MZ twins may be genetically dissimilar and recommends that the term "identical" be abandoned.

Approximately one-quarter of MZ twins are "mirror twins" because certain identical features are on the opposite side as in a mirror image. For example, a whorl or cowlick, a birthmark, or even internal organs (most commonly the heart) may be on reverse sides. In mirror twins, one is left-handed and the other right-handed, and they tend to cross their thumbs, arms, and legs in opposite ways. The first tooth may come in on opposite sides. These are late-separating MZ twins; further delay would be conjoined twins, who also show mirroring.

Genetic endowments are laid down at the moment of conception, but prenatal and postpartum influences lead to differences in size, appearance, emotional characteristics, and development of certain skills. Within the uterus, one twin may develop at the expense of the other, especially if they share the same placenta resulting in different birth weights (feto-fetal transfusion syndrome, explained in Chapter 7). Birth trauma may involve only one twin. In fact, MZ twins may look *less* alike in the beginning than DZ twins.

"Fraternal" Twins: Dizygotic

The more common type of twinning is dizygotic (DZ). Two eggs, which may be from one or both ovaries, are fertilized by two different sperm, just as one egg is joined by one sperm in a singleton pregnancy. Two separate unions, or zygotes, result; hence the term *dizygotic* (also called *binovular*, "arising from two eggs").

Approximately half of dizygotic (DZ) twins are same-sex (SS) pairs and half are male-female (OS). However, in Holland and Sweden, because of the use of ART, same-sex dizygotic (SSDZ) twins now occur 10 to 15 percent more often than OS pairs.

---

*Lyonisation is the random inactivation of one of the two X chromosomes of the cells of female mammals. In consequence, females are chimeric — may share cells from each other — for the products of the X chromosome.

Twin Types

MALE-MALE		MALE-FEMALE	FEMALE-FEMALE	
Monozygotic	Dizygotic	Dizygotic	Monozygotic	Dizygotic
1/6	1/6	1/3	1/6	1/6

Dizygotic Twins Result from the Fertilization of Two Eggs by Two Sperm

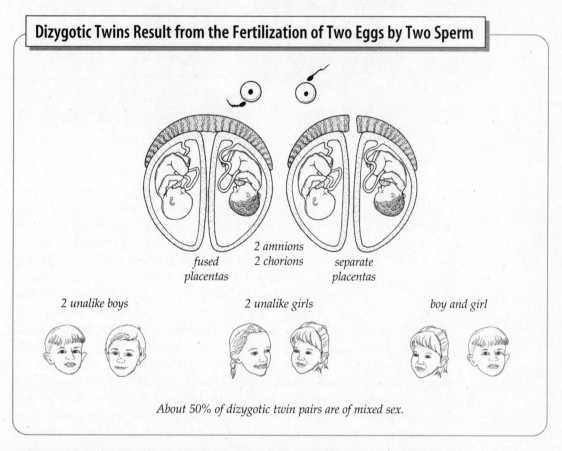

fused placentas · *2 amnions 2 chorions* · *separate placentas*

2 unalike boys · *2 unalike girls* · *boy and girl*

About 50% of dizygotic twin pairs are of mixed sex.

Dizygotic twins may or may not look alike. This type of twinning is simply a double birth, as commonly happens in other species. Dizygotic twins are siblings with the same birth date who shared the same uterine environment and they have between 25 to 75 percent of their genes in common.

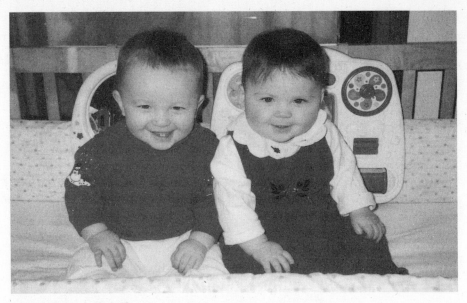

Most twins look dissimilar.

Having differentiated the two types of twinning according to conventional understanding and terminology, I now return to the questions raised by Boklage. He claims that there is "no sound evidence of a two-egg origin for *natural* DZ twins." He suggests that the cellular events of MZ and DZ twinning can be part of the same process, with DZ twinning occurring before fertilization and MZ after. Boklage's research shows that DZ twins are not developmentally the same as singletons, and that single-born siblings of twins also differ from singletons in families with no twins. Observed developmental differences between MZ twins and singletons are at least equally present in DZ twins.

These differences include asymmetry in the development of the brain, face, heart, and handedness. Monozygotic and DZ twins equally are more often non-right-handed* than singletons, a tendency they — and their singleton siblings — inherit from their parents, which has nothing to do with any aspect of twin gestation. The teeth of MZ and DZ twins also show less of the normal asymmetry found among singletons. Both DZ and MZ twins — and their siblings — share greater-than-normal incidences of the most common major fusion/midline malformations (particularly neural tube defects, congenital heart defects, and clefts of the

*includes left-handed and ambidextrous

lip and/or palate). These occur more frequently in twins and siblings of twins than among singletons in families without twins. These malformations in twins are not seen just in MZs as previously believed. Also, the incidence of fetal and neonatal deaths in SSDZs is at least as great as among MZs. Boklage explains that

> the failure to see this before is one of many fundamental mistakes that have been made in the past by taking results from OSDZ twins to represent the development of all DZs — a convenient assumption which has apparently simplified a great deal of research but certainly made it at once hopelessly wrong.

Furthermore, explains Boklage, DZ twins are often chimeric, with one or both carrying some cells that originated in the other twin's body. The actual frequency observed to date may be greatly underestimated. (Other tissues of the body need to be examined for mixed cells.) Blood is the easiest tissue to sample in order to examine large numbers of genetic markers simultaneously, and, if DZ twins indeed come from double ovulation, an exchange of blood via placental vessels is about the only way the observed sharing could happen. The examination of many hundreds of DZ twin placentas makes it clear that signs of DZ blood cell exchange via placental vessels is *far less common* than chimerism appears to be. If, however, DZ twin embryos often arise from single egg cells, as Boklage believes, they would be expected to begin embryonic development inside a single egg membrane, and it would seem likely that complete or partial fusion of two such embryos would be much easier than completely separate development. As well, it would be quite likely that mixing of cells in tissues other than blood would be *much more common* than mixing in blood alone.

A Third Type of Twin:
A Third Phase of Egg — Sesquizygotic* (SZ) Twins

A "third type" of twinning has been mentioned from time to time — the concept of a single ovum dividing and each half being fertilized by different sperm. The common term "splitting" is an outdated metaphor for the replication and segregation of chromosomes.

Boklage has found that it is possible for two sperm to fertilize two egg

Sesqui is Latin for "one and a half."

Sesquizygotic Twins Result from One Egg and Two Sperm

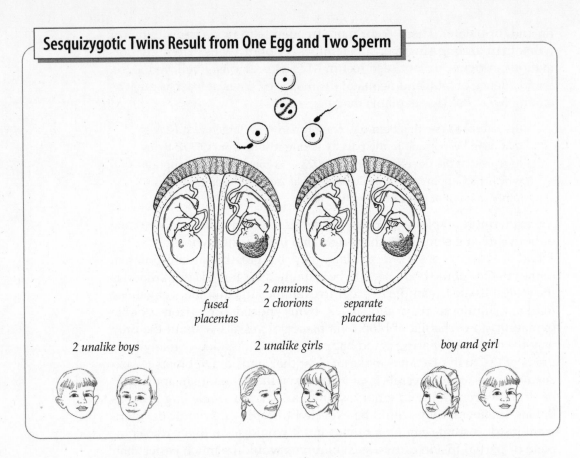

2 amnions
2 chorions

fused placentas   *separate placentas*

2 unalike boys   *2 unalike girls*   *boy and girl*

cells derived from a single secondary oocyte (the egg cell that is usually fertilized). The secondary oocyte has two half-sets of chromosomes — one more than is necessary. The extra set usually goes into a small accessory cell called the second polar body immediately after fertilization. For several reasons, including delayed fertilization, the secondary oocyte may divide before fertilization. In that case, a roughly equal division occurs instead of the usual asymmetrical division, and this produces the zygote and the much smaller second polar body. The two daughter cells from such a division can now be fertilized by different sperm.

It has been thought that multiples derived from single egg cells by such a process must have all the same genes from the mother. Were that correct, such sets would be easy to identify. Unfortunately, the normal reassortment of the grandparents' genes (by the process of recombination when the sperm and egg are formed) makes that supposition incorrect and the identification very difficult.

Fertilization by two sperm is called *dispermy* (and this occurs in about 20 percent of hydatiform moles). Feng and Gordon in 1996 estimated that 7 percent of eggs are penetrated by more than one sperm.

Twins that occur along the entire spectrum between MZ and DZ are termed sesquizygotic twins (SZ). Resulting from two different sperm, they may be SS or OS. They resemble DZ twins but have more similarities in their maternal gene makeup because these components remain the same during the second division. (DZ twins are assumed to begin as two separate eggs.)

In rare cases, before and during fertilization, differences in the timing may result in mixing of genes from both parents. Timing is critical in twinning; heterochronic (of different times) SZ twins will have identical paternal genes but different recombinations of maternal genes. Asymmetries result from some kind of "instructions" in the embryo prior to cleavage. In certain families, paternal influence has been shown in both MZ and DZ twins.

Families with twinning in the paternal line provide an opportunity to research chimeric twins. Dispermic chimeric twins, according to Lichtenstein et al., are always the same sex. This explains difficulties in research where a small percentage of twins cannot be defined as MZ or DZ according to appearance (phenotype). Chimeric heterochronic twins will be SS but have a different appearance despite being MZ. These differences can have important medical and social implications. In difficult cases, apparently, it will take two generations of molecular analysis.

Boklage is studying this third type of twinning, occurring perhaps in the majority of DZ twin conceptions, by way of the *tertiary oocyte*, an egg in a third phase of pre-fertilization division. Although this has been mistermed "polar body twinning," Boklage points out that the name "polar body" belongs to a very particular cell that cannot be fertilized nor is it capable of further development.

According to Boklage, the few studies seeking this kind of twinning in humans have been limited by one of two factors. First, the researchers were looking for twins identical for all maternal genes, which is impossible after the mixing of genes produced by recombination. Second, some researchers acknowledged this but lacked the technology for investigation. With the specific exception of DNA sequences in or very near each chromosome's centromere (the part of the chromosome involved in sorting during cell division), such twins do not differ in resemblance from any pair of nonidentical siblings.*

Boklage believes that events of both types might occur in daughter cells of the same single egg cell, to yield DZ triplets — MZ twins plus one — the most common natural type of triplet set. To further his research of this type of twinning, Boklage is seeking biological samples from such triplets and their parents, and pays the costs incurred. (There is an on-line questionnaire at http://members.tripod.com/klowed/twinhome.htm.)

Supertwins

Triplets, quadruplets, and other multiples may be a combination of MZ and DZ twinning (PZ or polyzygotic) or just one of these types. The phenomenon of MZ quadruplets — the Morlok quads born in Poland in 1930 — is rare in humans. The Dionne quintuplets also were MZ, the result of one egg splitting into four divisions after fertilization. Likewise, MZ triplets are the least frequent type. More commonly, triplets arise from three separate eggs or a combination of monozygotic twins and one singleton. (It is also possible that the pregnancy began as two pairs and that one embryo of one of the pairs was reabsorbed; see Chapter 22.)

The percentage of females increases with the number of multiples in a set. For example, females are 48 percent of singleton births, 49 percent of twins, and 51 percent of triplets. Chorionicity (see "Zygosity and Chorionicity" later in this chapter) plays a role in the sex ratio, too. For every male set that has only one inner and one outer membrane, there are two female ones.

The use of hormones in cases of infertility inflates the number of supertwins well beyond the normal incidence. Multiple births that result from such hormone therapy are commonly DZ, but with two particular types of therapy (IVF and GIFT — gamete intrafallopian transfer) there is an unexplained increase in MZ twins.

Prior to the use of fertility drugs, calculations for the ratio of multiples were based on Hellin's rule: Twin deliveries averaged 1 in 90 of all live births (about 2 percent of all live babies) and 97 to 98 percent of all plural deliveries. Triplets occurred once in n^2 (90 x 90) or 8,100 pregnancies, and quadruplets once in n^3 (90 x 90 x 90) or 729,000 pregnancies. How-

---

*Only within the past few years has it become possible to study centromeric sequences directly.

Supertwins Can Develop in a Multitude of Ways

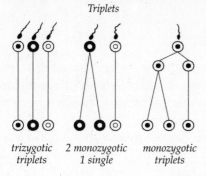
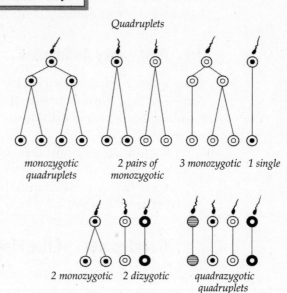

Triplets

trizygotic
triplets

2 monozygotic
1 single

monozygotic
triplets

Quadruplets

monozygotic
quadruplets

2 pairs of
monozygotic

3 monozygotic

1 single

2 monozygotic

2 dizygotic

quadrazygotic
quadruplets

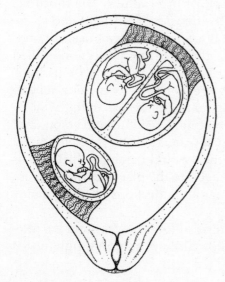

Triplets may be a combination of monozygotic twins and one single.

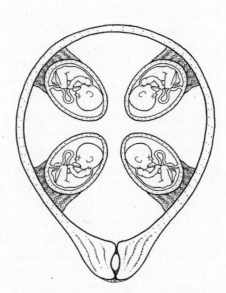

Quadruplets are commonly formed from four separate eggs (quadrazygotic).

ever, in the year 2000, the ratio of multiple births per 1,000 total live births reached 29; almost 3 percent of plural births were triplets or higher-order multiples.

 ## Pregnancy Anomalies

On very rare occasions an *ectopic* twin pregnancy occurs. In such cases, a fertilized egg grows outside the uterus, usually in the fallopian tube. Combinations of one ectopic and one uterine pregnancy have been observed.

Women have also miscarried a twin, sometimes without realizing it, but delivered the remaining baby at term. Rarely, evidence of an undeveloped twin compressed into the placenta is observed at birth or can be found later in a tumor.†

 ## Development of the Placenta

During the first week after conception, the fertilized egg reaches the uterus and the *placenta* begins to develop in the wall of the uterus. The placenta, composed mostly of maternal and some fetal tissue, grows to be at least six inches across and a couple of inches thick. The functions of this important organ are more than the transfer of nutrients and waste products between mother and baby. It is a source of hormones, antibodies, and electrolytes. Exchange occurs through tiny projections called villi, which are bathed by the mother's blood, and this "villous tree" grows during the first four months of pregnancy by branching repeatedly, and the fetal capillaries increase in number and size. In this way, an initial terminal villus can become an intermediate villus and so on until a surface area is formed of more than 150 square feet! The fetal blood vessels within the villi, if linked together, would be about thirty miles long. The umbilical cord connects the baby to the placenta and thus indirectly to its mother's circulation. Drugs and infectious organisms may also cross the placenta.

The mature placenta (from the Latin word for "cake" — and we celebrate with birthday cakes) is shaped like a disc and at term weighs about

---

†*Fetus papyraceous* or *compressus* occurs once in 200 births and results from a death in the second trimester. Incomplete development appears as a hydatiform mole in 1 in 1,500 pregnancies in the United States; see Glossary.

500 grams. The fetal surface is smooth with the umbilical cord attached near the center. In contrast, the maternal surface is rough and raised into 10 to 38 cotyledons (see diagram). You can understand how important your nutrition and hydration is during the early months so that your placenta attains full development and function, with a high number of cotyledons.

There is an International Federation of Placenta Associations (Japan, Australia and New Zealand, Europe, and the Americas) and a specialized journal, *Placenta*.

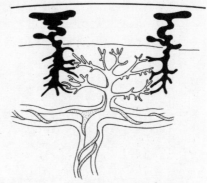

The babies' development depends on the growth and development of the placenta. Although the maternal and fetal circulations never mix, nutrients and waste products are exchanged through the villi.

During ultrasound scans, babies have been observed stroking the placenta and burrowing into it like a pillow. They hear the continuous whooshing song as the blood perfuses it and they touch and feel their pulsating cord. After birth, children may cling to a soft toy or old blanket at night — these represent transitional objects for the placenta.

Write in your birth plan that you want to examine the placenta. Certainly your doctor should be checking it carefully for the reasons explained below. You may, as I did, want to plant this miraculous organ in the garden under a special tree. A tree is symbolic of a placenta, and this custom can be found in many societies. In fact, many cultures outside the industrialized world treat the placenta with appreciation and sometimes even awe.

Sometimes women in developing countries stay away from modern maternity services for fear of losing control over their placenta. Mammals generally eat the whole placenta, and some humans have eaten a tiny piece to prevent a postpartum hemorrhage. In hospitals the placenta is either tossed in the trash or it is used for the extraction of hormones. The umbilical cord is used for grafts, as are the amputated foreskins of baby penises. (Make sure you protect any sons you may have against circumcision — take the *whole* baby home.)

As well as being the biological center for the regulation of food and oxygen, the placenta can be considered as the first instrument of the unconscious — where we literally have "blood ties." This concept becomes even

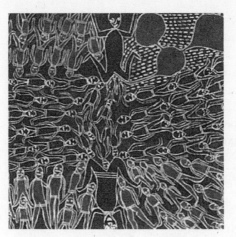

An Australian aboriginal bark painting showing the Earth Mother, symbolized as the Placenta giving birth to two spirits.

more interesting in the case of those twins who share the same placenta.

Welsh homeopaths Kathy Briggs and Linda Gwillim have made available a remedy called Placenta (stocked only in the United Kingdom; see http://www.helios.co.uk.com). The benefits of this remedy can also be found (in German) at the following Web site: http://www.homo eopathieforschung.de/placenta. htm. Although I have no clinical experience at all with this remedy, I have always been impressed by homeopathy, which brings great benefits with few side effects. It will be interesting to see how expectant mothers in preterm labor and preterm babies in a neonatal intensive care nursery (NICU) and surviving multiples might fare with this remedy.

Universal Symbols of the Placenta

For singletons, the placenta is their "twin"; it is genetically identical! Anthropologically, the placenta has been called the "double," "soul," "secret helper," or "brother." It was either buried or placed in a tree or on the top of a pole. Placental fetishes that have continued into modern life include the crown, scepter, robe, banner, or flag, representing the source of all blood power. In Egypt, the pharaoh led processions preceded by his actual placenta, affixed to the top of a long pole with a dangling umbilical cord. Placental symbols since antiquity have been seen on temples, seals, shields, and cave paintings. The treelike, snakelike, or mazelike qualities of this organ may be emphasized. All mythical stories about trees represent this "tree of life" — the placenta.

Adequate development and function of each placenta are essential to the growth and well-being of each multiple.

Each baby develops in a membranous sac filled with fluid that provides freedom for growth and movement, acts as a shock absorber, and

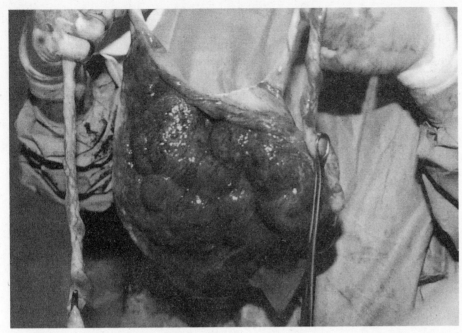

The maternal surface of a single MZ placenta.

maintains an even temperature. The sac consists of two *membranes* that arise from the edge of the placenta. The outer membrane is the *chorion* and the inner layer is the *amnion*.

Placentas and Membranes Differ Among Multiples

The chorion is more opaque than the amnion, it contains blood vessels, and it is fused to the underneath surface of the placenta. A ridge felt on that surface of the placenta indicates the attachment of the chorion. When two chorions attach to the placenta, there is an obvious line where they join.

The amnion is a clear shiny membrane with no blood vessels. It can be easily pulled away from the placental surface of adjacent membranes. The dividing septum on the fetal surface of fused placentas can be examined for two or four layers. Careful attention in such cases reveals that there are two amnions and two chorions without any connecting blood vessels.

Thus, twins of the same sex — with what appears to be a single placenta — can be DZ, and separate placentas can occur with MZ twins. If, on closer examination, the inner layers can be eased apart with no evidence of the outer chorionic tissue between them, one outer sac and one original egg — MZ twins — are likely. However, sometimes microscopic analysis reveals chorionic tissue sandwiched between two amniontic layers.

Membranes Affect Outcome

Placentas are described in terms of both amniotic and chorionic membranes — *mono-* for a single membrane, *di-* for two. Ultrasound can assess chorionicity as early as the fourth to fifth postmenstrual week using transvaginal sonography (TVS). Amnionicity can be determined between the seventh and eighth week or in late second and third trimesters (more difficult). In the first trimester, the chorionic sacs can be seen and counted. Also, the number of embryos can be measured by the sixth week. The number of yolk sacs can be counted at least two weeks before the number of amnions can be determined and their number correlates with the number of amnions.

There are three types of membrane structure for twins — DC (dichorionic), MC (monochorionic), and MCMA (monochorionic and monoamniotic, also known as MoMo). This increases to six possible combinations in triplets, as many as ten types for quadruplets, and fifteen for quintuplets! The ultrasound diagnosis of chorionicity and amnionicity in the second and third trimesters can provide information on:

1. Fetal gender (different gender indicates DZ twins, same gender may be MZ in 25 percent of cases).

2. The number of placental sites: two separate placental sites indicate DC placentas. A single or fused placenta is more difficult to evaluate and occurs in about 40 percent of all DC placentas.

3. The membranes: origin, thickness, and the number of layers. In DC twins, the area of fusion between the placentas forms a wedge-shaped zone termed the *Lamda* or *twin-peak* sign. In MC twins, this structure is absent and the junction between the two amniotic sacs and the uterine wall creates a T-shaped appearance. Counting the number of layers and measurement of their thickness is important: in MZ twins there are only two membranes which are thin as opposed to four layers of thick membranes in DZ twins.

MZ twins can have separate placentas!

An MC placenta proves MZ twins but the converse is not true. Two separate placentas occur (rarely) in MZ twins when the division begins on the fourth day after fertilization. Dizygotic twins usually have two entirely separate placentas, but they are sometimes fused. This is a racial characteristic. Among Africans, fused placentas are the least common type, whereas among the Japanese, separated DZ placentas are the least frequent. In the United States, the incidence falls in the middle.

The cell division that results in MZ twins usually occurs within the first week following fertilization, before the amnion develops (about day nine); therefore, each MZ twin almost always grows in his or her own separate inner sac. The chorion is formed around day four; MZ twins who split in the first couple of days will each have their own "safety net." With such twins there is less difference in growth (discordance), fewer complications, and the best outcome. One-third of MZ twins are DC (as are all DZ twins).

DZ twins are always DC. MZ twins may be DC or MC. Most MZs are MC.

Zygosity and Chorionicity

Zygosity (genetic determination of the type of twinning) differs from chorionicity (number of membranes). Chorionicity refers to the identification of the number of chorionic sacs (MC, DC, TC, QC), and amnionicity refers to the number of amniotic sacs (MA, DA, TA, QA).

The combination of placentas and membranes can reveal much, but not all, about zygosity. For about half of all twins, who are SSDC, their zygosity can be determined prenatally only by genetic tests like amniocentesis or chorionic villus sampling. Thus, the placenta should always be carefully examined at birth and samples sent for testing if the zygosity is not clear. Parents are often told that the babies cannot be identical because there are two placentas, which is wrong and makes no sense to them either in the presence of their babies' carbon-copy resemblance!

The fewer the dividing membranes, the greater the risk for complications. Disruption of the supply of nutrients occurs if connections between the blood vessels favor one baby. The circulations between DC twins are never shared; therefore, the demise of one does not cause the pathology that can happen to an MC co-twin if one twin succumbs. The chart shows why chorionicity is so important obstetrically. It can be established only during pregnancy — as early as the first trimester — or at

Differences in Genetic Make-up and Structure of Placenta and Membranes

Monozygotic, monovular, "identical"	MZ	Arising from one fertilized egg
Dizygotic, binovular, "fraternal"	DZ	Arising from two fertilized eggs
Trizygotic, triovular, "fraternal triplets"	TZ	Arising from three fertilized eggs
Quadrazygotic "fraternal quadruplets"	QZ	Arising from four fertilized eggs
Monochorionic	MC	One chorion (outer membrane)
Dichorionic	DC	Two chorions
Monoamniotic	MO	One amnion (inner membrane)
Diamniotic	DI	Two amnions
Dichorionic diamniotic	DCDA	Two amnions and two chorions (< 4 days)
Monochorionic diamniotic	MCDA	One chorion, two amnions (4–7 days)
Monochorionic monoamniotic	MCMA/MOMO	One chorion, one amnion (8–13 days)

birth. Once the membranes and placenta have been disposed of, the evidence is lost. (Placental tissue, rich in DNA material, can be frozen for later analysis to determine zygosity.)

Zygosity can be established from ultrasound only if the twins are monochorionic (= MZ) or OS (= DZ). If the babies are SS or unknown, and there are two chorions, zygosity will be determined after birth. Indeed, zygosity testing can be done at any future time. There are poignant stories of twins who found out in later life that, contrary to what they had been told, they were indeed MZ.

Dichorionic Twins

When division occurs within the first four days, each twin will have both an inner and outer sac. This is always the case with DZ twins and occurs in about one-third of MZ twins. Twins with separate chorions and amnions (DCDA) always have separate placentas, although in some cases the placentas become fused. With these early-division MZ twins, there will be minimal birth weight difference because with separate placentas there is better growth.

Monochorionic Twins

An MC placenta is proof of MZ and enables about 20 percent of twins to be so identified immediately. About 60 percent of monozygotic twins have their own separate inner membranes and share one chorion. Monozygotic twins with one chorion always share and compete for the one placenta; they are more likely to suffer malformation and to develop transfusion problems. Twins with one chorion and two amnions (MCDA) have divided a little later, and there is a greater difference in birth weight among female pairs than males.

Monoamnionic Twins

Twins formed after the first week of fertilization will be contained within one common inner and outer sac (MCMA) and can be diagnosed around eight weeks. Only 1 to 2 percent of MZ twins arise from this most delayed type of duplication (another day or so of delay and conjoined twins result). They can be diagnosed prenatally by ultrasound and amniocentesis (see Chapter 9).

Intermediate and later division means more connections between blood vessels, which lead to circulatory imbalance. For unknown reasons, late division means a greater proportion of female twins, up to 75 percent, according to Robert Derom in Belgium. Anomalies may be present such as a single artery in the umbilical cord instead of two, or insertion of the cord into the membranes instead of into the placenta. With no dividing membrane, cord entanglement is possible. Therefore, it is very important to determine chorionicity as soon as possible.

Zygosity Testing

Some people regard zygosity as unimportant unless an organ transplant is needed or if there is a risk of genetic disease. However, multiples and their parents do not know when such information might be needed and then it may not be available. (Mothers who have lost multiples usually wished they had known their zygosity.) For multiples and their parents, as well as for medical research, zygosity should be determined routinely and paid for by health insurance. With same-sex twins, the placenta and membranes may reveal the zygosity if carefully examined by an experienced doctor. Testing is necessary in only 25 percent of twin deliveries because different sex of the twins is evidence of DZ.

Parents and twins themselves are not always correct in their assessment of zygosity, especially MZ. Physical appearance and skin color provide important evidence as the twins grow older. (At birth, even MZ twins may look very different, even less alike than DZ if they have been

At 14 weeks, I had an ultrasound and they told me our twins were monoamniotic. At 17 weeks, they told us they found a separating membrane. I had monthly ultrasounds following that but it was never brought up again. At 34 weeks, I delivered vaginally to find that our twins' cords were completely entangled and our second baby came out not breathing. Luckily, they were able to revive her immediately and both babies were fine. However, my doctor was really upset about the misdiagnosis. The hospital said they didn't make an error though, but that the membrane had disintegrated (they had supposedly heard of one other case like that). I feel cheated by the hospital because I feel as though they're not really being honest with me, but just trying to cover up for a mistake. Also, even though my twins look completely alike, there are subtle differences so in the back of my mind (because of what the hospital did) there is always a worry that they may not be identical after all.*

*It is precisely for such parents that I explore the formation of twins in great detail.

As triplets, we always thought we were one fraternal and two identical twins. Only when we were in our forties and all had blood tests because of a special illness that one of us developed did we find out that we were three DZs.

Everyone had always thought we were fraternal twins. After four pregnancies, I developed severe kidney disease and my sister and I underwent tests to see about a transplant. After three decades, we learned that we were identical after all. Now I have one of my twin's kidneys.

From the ultrasounds, they looked like fraternal girls (two placentas, amnions, and chorions). But after the girls were born, they were so identical we literally kept them labeled with pen for four months. Eventually, feeling like such a failure as a mother because I was so unable to tell them apart, I paid to have a genetic test. And they are identical.

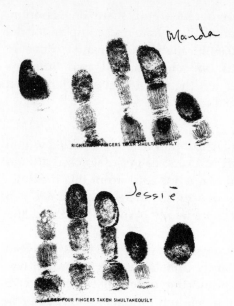

Not even monozygotic twins have the same fingerprints.

subject to an unequal blood supply in the uterus, discussed in Chapter 7.) If nonfamily members cannot tell the multiples apart in childhood, and they have the same eye color, weight and height, and hair color and texture by about the age of two, they are probably MZ. A parent report questionnaire devised in the United Kingdom found that for 95 percent of a sample of eighteen-month-old twins, zygosity was correctly determined (and it was 96 percent at three years of age). This questionnaire is available on-line at http://statgen.iop.klc.ac.uk/twinzyg.html.

The blood groups ABO-Rh-MNS from each multiple's umbilical vein can be compared (although DZ twins can show great similarity). Alkaline phosphatase, an enzyme test, can be done, as well.

Dental characteristics are also identical for monozygotic twins. While handprints and footprints of monozygotic twins are similar, each one's fingerprints are unique.

The ultimate zygosity test is DNA "fingerprinting," which has nothing to do with hands but distinguishes microscopic features called polymorphisms. Samples of DNA are typically collected from blood or a swab of cells from inside the cheek (buccal sample) but any tissue will do. Results are reported as a likelihood ratio of being MZ versus DZ if both parents are tested. If only the twins are tested and no DNA difference is detected, it is probable that the twins are MZ. There is only one chance in 16,000 that all the markers in a set of chromosomes will match another person's DNA. This test, which is required only for same-sex DC multiples whose zygosity cannot be established by other methods, can be done for under $100 by sending for a kit from Australia (see Resources for ordering information).

The Importance of Zygosity

- To understand why only one twin may have a problem (discordant congenital anomalies)

- To research the heritability of conceiving multiples

- To estimate the chance of having a subsequent multiple birth (increased after DZ twins)

- To reduce the high mortality of multiples

- For each multiple's sense of identity

- To answer the common question: Are you identical?

- For accuracy if parents and multiples participate in research studies

- For understanding rates of growth and development. Dissimilarities between MZs are a warning. However, for DZs, differences are to be expected as with any siblings.

- For teachers and parents to know if the twins are MZ in order to treat them as individually as they would treat DZs

- Learning correct zygosity in the future may be a difficult adjustment for twins and their family.

3
Who Has Multiples?

Births of twins and other multiples are recorded by statisticians and analyzed in population studies. Many of the statistics are difficult to decipher and compare because of differences in the populations and discrepancies or uncertainties in reporting, collecting, classifying, and analyzing the data. Generally, studies rely on volunteers and self-administered questionnaires. The picture is further confused by undetermined zygosity and type of conceptions (artificial versus spontaneous). Today, with the use of fertility drugs and reproductive technology, it is no longer possible to discern the true characteristics of the population that has "multiple luck." White women over age forty-five had the highest number of multiples in 2000, compared to 1987 when both blacks and whites aged thirty-five to thirty-nine had the most twins.

My own research has been thwarted because much data concerning multiples has not been analyzed. I have contacted various government departments and parents of multiples clubs, but either the questions have not been asked, or the numbers are unavailable, or the trends have not been computed. Even the National Center for Health Statistics (NCHS) publishes only an occasional report on multiple pregnancy and claims it does not have the resources to provide the analyses that would answer many questions. I have had the raw NCHS data analyzed for this book.

In estimating the incidence of multiples, statistics deal with the births, but we now realize that many more twins are lost than was formerly known — from induced abortions, miscarriage, and spontaneous fetal reduction (discussed in Chapter 22). Similarly, stillbirths are often excluded from the twin tally, and it is not always clear if twins are counted when there is only one survivor or triplets are noted when two survive.

Twinning peaks have varied with different times in the same population and in different populations. They depend on the mother's age of menarche (onset of menstruation) or the age at which the mother had her first child or even socio-legal circumstances such as the availability of abortion. The content of the diet as well as adequacy of nutrition may play a role in predisposition to twinning and thus explain geographical and ethnic differences.

As we saw in Chapter 2, the types of twinning are not well understood. The strongest trends have been observed with DZ twins and are associated with race, age, family size, seasons, geography, hormones, and heredity. Some of these factors may coexist. For example, if an increase in twin births is related to both maternal age and the use of oral contraceptives, societies in which women postpone childbearing by taking the pill may show a higher number of twins in the older age group. In addition, it is not uncommon for women to ovulate twice a month, as can be learned from basal temperature charts.

Variations by Race

Twinning rates, zygosity, and types of placentas vary considerably with race. The greatest number of twin births occurs among the Nigerians, particularly the Yoruba — about 45 per 1,000 births. A Nigerian town called Igbo-Ora proudly welcomes visitors to "The Land of Twins." Among this farming community of about 60,000 "the town lacks electricity, drinking water, and a doctor at its run-down general hospital, but not progeny." There are no reliable population figures and no census has been conducted for a decade. However, of the 25 homes visited by a journalist, 19 had twins or triplets!

The fewest numbers of twins are born to Asians. Twins occur among Japanese and Chinese at the rate of about 4 per 1,000 births. However, while DZ twins are more common than MZ twins in general, among the Japanese there are two sets of MZ twins for every set of DZ. For a mixed group of Asians, such as Malays and Indians, the rate is about 8 per 1,000 births. The incidence in Europeans and white Americans falls between these two extremes. We know very little about multiple births among the Hispanic peoples of Central and South America.

The racial factor is thought to have a hormonal basis, because higher

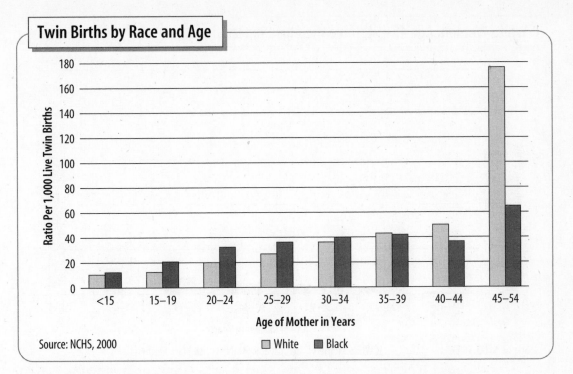

Twin Births by Race and Age

Age of Mother in Years

Ratio Per 1,000 Live Twin Births

Source: NCHS, 2000 ☐ White ■ Black

levels of circulating hormones that stimulate egg production in the ovary are found in mothers of twins generally, and blacks in particular. The rate for multiple non-white births in 1960 was 36 percent higher than that for white multiple births, but in 1985 the difference between the races decreased to 24 percent. In 2000, by contrast, MZ twins occurred with almost uniform frequency in all racial groups — between 4 and 5 per 1,000 births. The rate is less than that of DZ twins except in Asia, where they are about the same.

The Effect of Age

It has long been observed that the older the mother, the more likely she is to have twins. Although fecundity generally declines with age, the paradox of an increased risk of twinning in certain women is due to apparently deficient feedback mechanisms between the ovary and hormones.

With aging, higher levels of hormones are produced, which encourages more eggs to be released from the ovaries (see "The Influence of Hormones" later in this chapter). The incidence of twinning peaks between

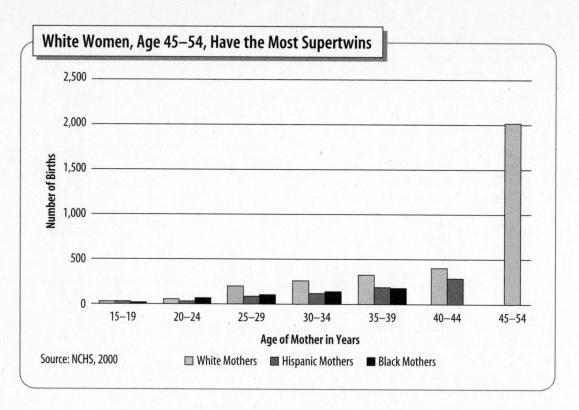

White Women, Age 45–54, Have the Most Supertwins

Number of Births

2,500
2,000
1,500
1,000
500
0

15–19   20–24   25–29   30–34   35–39   40–44   45–54

Age of Mother in Years

Source: NCHS, 2000   ☐ White Mothers   ■ Hispanic Mothers   ■ Black Mothers

the ages of thirty-five and thirty-nine for white Americans (27 per 1,000) and black Americans (31 per 1,000). The rate after age forty diminishes except for black women, for whom the incidence of twins increases through age forty-nine. Although there is a general decrease in twin births for mothers aged 40–44, this age group had twice as many supertwins in 2000 as in 1980. In 1971, there were 18 twins per 1,000 births; the figures rose to nearly 22 per 1,000 by 1987 and by 2000 was 29 per 1,000. One hundred and three of the 255 births by women aged 50–54 were multiple from ART.

According to the National Center for Health Statistics, over the last 20 years multiple pregnancies in the United States have increased 400 percent among women in their thirties and 1,000 percent in women in their forties. This trend is due in part to the fact that more older women are requesting infertility treatment. As a woman grows older, she has less chance of higher-order multiples; however, 4 percent of women over age forty who use ART will have triplets.

The National Institute of Child Health and Human Development

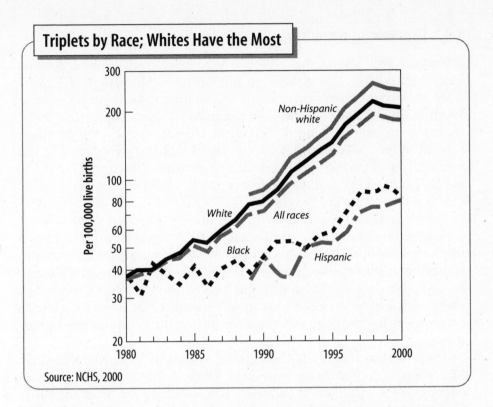

Triplets by Race; Whites Have the Most

Per 100,000 live births

Non-Hispanic white

White · All races

Black · Hispanic

Source: NCHS, 2000

(NICHD) found in a September 2002 study that triplets born to older mothers actually fare better than triplets born to younger mothers. Many older mothers of multiples conceive through ART and the offspring are more likely to be non-MZ. Additionally, mothers who conceive multiples via ART tend to be monitored more closely.

The Relationship to Family Size (Parity)

Twin-bearing families are more fertile, and statistics show that the more children a woman has, the greater her chance of conceiving twins. However, because an increase in family size also parallels an increase in maternal age, the two factors are associated.

The ratio of MZ twins to DZ is considered a marker for human fertility because double ovulation (if that is the mechanism of DZ twinning — see Boklage's comments in Chapter 2) increases the likelihood of a conception in a given cycle.

The Role of Heredity

It has been well known that a mother who has already borne DZ twins has a higher chance of conceiving another pair. Mothers of DZ twins often show more than one egg ripening in a reproductive cycle. Grace Wyshak, Ph.D., has done extensive research on the inheritance of genetic factors in twinning, using the excellent records kept by the Mormon Church in Salt Lake City, Utah. She found that the gene favoring DZ twins passes along the female line. If a woman has a history of DZ twins in her family on her mother's side or if she is a twin herself, her chances of conceiving twins are increased.

However, not all women who are genetically disposed to have twins actually do so. The genetic component in twinning is modified by environmental factors. These factors include psychological stress, nutrition, climate, and intercourse after sexual abstinence, which may stimulate hormone production. Environmental influences may affect the egg, the uterine environment, or both. We must remember that an egg links three generations, having begun its existence during the grandmother's pregnancy.

The influence of heredity through the paternal line in general, and on MZ twinning in particular, is unclear. While it was formerly acknowledged that the incidence of MZ twins has been constant, since the 1970s the MZ rate has increased by more than 50 percent in Sweden and northwestern Europe (but with no paternal effect on MZ twinning, according to the Swedish twin registry in 1998). In some families the same heritable traits may contribute to both MZ and DZ twinning. Machin and Bamforth studied fifteen sets of spontaneously conceived triplets: six were MZ, seven were DZ, and only two were TZ.

Women who are MZ twins have an increased chance of conceiving MZ twins; some intriguing cases of MZ twinning have been reported. Four sets of MZ twins were discovered in one extended family, and there are cases in which a mother had MZ twins by two different husbands. Similarly, a man had MZ twins with two different wives. A 1985 case in Italy of three ART eggs resulted in all MZs, making sextuplets.

Mrs. Gehri in Switzerland, mother of the first set of quadruplets where all survived past sixty years, showed a strong genetic influence in her family line. Twins occurred seven times in her maternal line and five times in her paternal line. Her maternal grandmother produced twins twice. Mr. Gehri was the son of a twin, but that was the only pair in his family tree.

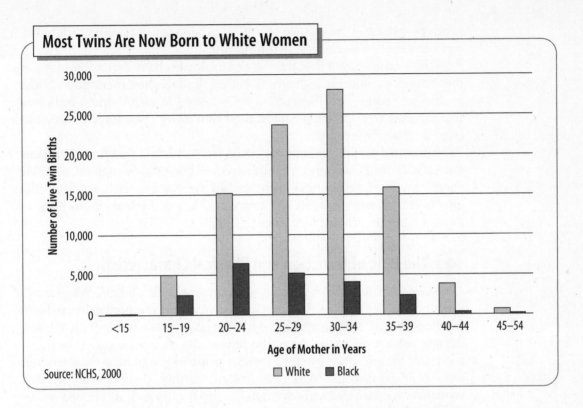

Most Twins Are Now Born to White Women

Number of Live Twin Births (y-axis)

Age of Mother in Years (x-axis)

Source: NCHS, 2000

☐ White ■ Black

Quadruplets were born (with three surviving) in Australia in 1905 to a woman who had previously given birth to two sets of twins, as well as triplets.

The Influence of Hormones

Mothers of DZ twins, especially Nigerians, show high levels of gonadotropin hormones (that cause the egg to ripen and burst from the ovary). The normal ovary has about half a million eggs, but only about 400 actually mature in the 30-to-40-year span of a woman's reproductive life. Gonadotropins such as follicle-stimulating hormone (FSH), human chorionic gonadotropin (HCG), and the drug Pergonal stimulate ovulation, as does clomiphene citrate (Clomid, Serophene). All have been used successfully to treat human female infertility and in animal husbandry to increase litter size.

Studies attempting to link oral contraceptives and twinning have been largely inconclusive: they have shown that the use of oral contraceptives increases the chance of a twin pregnancy, makes no difference, or even causes a decline in twinning rates!

Wyshak has shown that mothers of multiples have an earlier onset of menstruation, shorter menstrual cycles, and earlier menopause than mothers of singletons. Research on Orthodox Jewish women indicates that women who conceive late in their ovulatory cycle have a threefold chance of bearing twins.

Hormones in the food supply come from animals that have been fattened with estrogen and pollutants that become estrogenic as their chemical structure changes. Plant-based substances with estrogen-like effects (phytoestrogens) in soy products do not increase twinning, as Asians have the lowest incidence.

The Role of Nutrition and Physical Characteristics

Older, heavier, and taller women with several children have the greatest tendency to bear twins. Denmark, Norway, and the Netherlands have the most twins among whites. Africans have more twins than whites. Asians, who are smaller, have the fewest. Women who conceive twins naturally weigh more for their height prior to pregnancy than women who bear singletons. With the use of fertility drugs, small-framed women can conceive twins or higher-order multiples but often have difficulty gaining and comfortably carrying adequate weight.

Since twinning rates fall during wartime, the influence of nutrition is considered significant. Evidence of this fact has been shown in animal husbandry: if sheep are fed a better diet, more twins are born.

African women who were themselves twins or children of twins were not found to be more likely to bear twins than women with no family history of twinning. As this is contrary to what occurs in white populations, environmental causes have been sought. The incidence of twinning is higher — 62 per 1,000 — in the classes of African society where a native diet is consumed and lower — 15 per 1,000 — in the upper strata, whose members eat a more Western diet. The reputed high estrogen content of agida, a local yam root tuber used as a staple in Nigeria, is often given as a reason. However, Robert Asiedu, a yam specialist at the International Institute of Tropical Agriculture in Ibadan, argues against this: "Nobody has provided any scientific explanation or evidence that could prove that yam consumption can cause multiple births." In fact, there are even species of yams cultivated, especially in Asia, for contraceptive purposes!

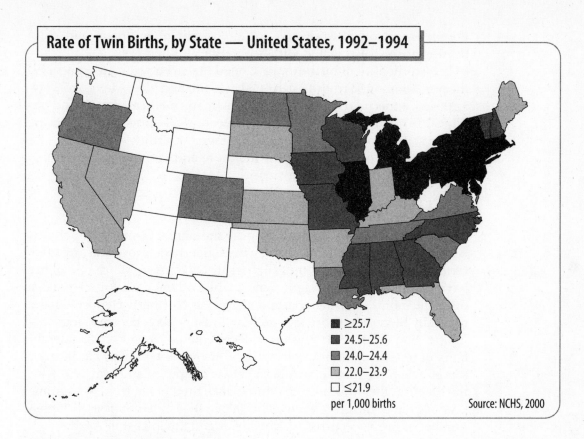

Rate of Twin Births, by State — United States, 1992–1994

- ≥25.7
- 24.5–25.6
- 24.0–24.4
- 22.0–23.9
- ≤21.9

per 1,000 births   Source: NCHS, 2000

Geographic Differences

Although Scandinavians show twinning rates similar to those of Europeans and Caucasian Americans, a very high incidence has been observed among some Finnish island communities. The rate was 15–20 per 1,000 until the 1960s, when it began to decline, compared with 7–11 per 1,000 for Europe in general. A possible explanation is that the exposure to light of certain glands, such as the pineal and pituitary, following the long northern winters stimulates double ovulation. The decline in multiple births in these formerly isolated communities over the past 30 years is attributed to population increase, urbanization, and changes in marriage and migration patterns.

Twinning has always been more common in rural than in urban areas. Explanations include the larger stature and superior physical fitness of rural women as well as better diet and less environmental pollution.

Population characteristics and social customs of marriage and childbearing are also associated with geographical differences.

In a study of twin births in the United States between 1992 and 1994, the number ranged from 19 per 1,000 in Idaho and New Mexico to 28 per 1,000 in Connecticut and Massachusetts (many medical schools and hospitals!). Six of the ten mountain states accounted for the lowest rates, and eleven states mandated insurance coverage for fertility treatment.

Like studies of seasonality, the literature on twinning and geography reveals a mixed bag of conclusions.

 ## Seasonal Effects

Twin births do not usually occur under the sign of Gemini. Actually, the reverse was found in a 1976 survey in England: the probability of a twin birth was lowest in May and highest in November. Many researchers have found no seasonal significance, while others have found peaks in different months. Twins conceptions in the Northern Hemisphere are generally highest in February and March, as the days become longer and lighter. Some interesting random facts emerge out of a considerable body of research. For example, in Italy, increased twinning has been observed when the mother was born between January and May and when the grandmother was born in winter; also, mothers born in the summer produce fewer mixed-sex twins. In 2000 in the United States, the highest number of births occurred in November and the lowest in April.

 ## Sexual Activity

Despite the common correlation between maternal age and the incidence of twins, other research has found that twins are most frequently conceived within the first three months of marriage, presumably because of higher levels of sexual activity. There is an increase of DZ twins conceived outside marriage and after a period of abstinence, apparently with intercourse stimulating ovulation. Likewise, a post-World War II study found that twins were conceived more promptly than singletons after veterans returned home.

In contrast, the observation has also been made and strengthened by recent evidence that twins occur more often in single mothers (who are usually younger); and the explanation may involve the irregularity of sexual intercourse. (I know of several cases in which a single woman conceived twins with one sexual encounter.) The twinning rate in one Swedish study was 40 percent higher for single than for married mothers. In the year 2000, 45 percent of the births in the United States were to single mothers, but it is not reported how many of those births were plural.

Yet increased twinning has been associated with an increased number of marriages — again presenting more opportunities for intercourse.

Another Swedish study reported that OSDZ twins were more common in younger mothers, who engaged in intercourse more frequently than older women. The investigation assumed that the sex of the offspring is related to the phase of the menstrual cycle when fertilization occurs. Human ovulation, as in the rabbit, can be triggered by sexual activity, particularly by orgasm, as well as influenced by higher centers in the brain.

It is clear that the causes of twinning are many and complex and there is much that we do not understand. The chances of having twins are not increased just because twins "run in the family." Even if DZ twins have occurred in the mother's family, she may never conceive DZ twins or, by a stroke of fate, may actually have MZ twins! Today twins can be easily arranged with ART even after menopause. A woman's age, hormone levels, nutrition, emotional state, sexual activity, and environmental conditions (including season and latitude) all play a role along with her genes in the natural conception of multiples.

4
Awaiting Multiples: Parents' Feelings and Practical Considerations

 Pregnancy is a transition with special psychological states for expectant mothers and fathers. You will experience mood swings, emotional changes, and dreams that are normal and necessary. Both of you are moving into a new phase in your lives with its attendant choices, anxieties, and expectations. Fathers-to-be report more headaches and stomach upsets and are absent from work more often than at other times. Couples who make the best adjustment are those who are aware and accepting of the fluctuating feelings in pregnancy and explore them with each other. Despite your multiplicity of blessings, you are facing more of the unknown and unexpected than ever before, beginning with the big news.

If I, myself upon a looser creed
Have loosely strung the Jewel of Good Deed,
Let this one thing for my atonement plead:
That one for two I never did misread.
— Omar Khayam, *Rubaiyat*, 12th century

Detection* of Multiple Pregnancy

Few multiples pregnancies are a surprise now that the use of ultrasound is practically routine. Contrast this with the situation in 1962, when the Mothers of Twins Club in Illinois surveyed its 2,631 members and found that only 510 knew of their twins in advance! Statistically, however, obstetric outcome has *not* improved with timely detection, probably because "early diagnosis" is the start of a powerful nocebo effect.

Almost every pregnant woman, at some time during her nine-month pregnancy, wonders if she is carrying twins as she contemplates the astonishing growth of her abdomen. If there is a history of twins in the

*I am using the term *detection* instead of *diagnosis* because it is important to avoid the nocebo effect that results from the medicalization of natural events especially through choice of words.

With this third pregnancy, my clothes stopped fitting by about 2¹/₂ months. I had horrible morning (and afternoon and evening) sickness—when I had none with my first two pregnancies. I was exhausted. I had an ultrasound two days later. I went alone because my husband was visiting his identical twin brother for the weekend. Sure enough, twins. I just laughed and laughed. What else could I do?

At my 10-week ultrasound, I got the shock of my life when two babies popped up on the screen. I was shaking with the uncertainty at the prospect of having twins, but after the initial shock, I was elated.

My sister and I got pregnant around the same time, and she was due three weeks ahead of me. I started getting bigger than she was and kept thinking we were having twins. I also had dreams about twins. When I went to my doctor at 12 weeks, she thought my uterus was larger than it should be but heard only one heartbeat and never mentioned anything about having multiples — she thought maybe I was further along. I had an ultrasound at 14 weeks that confirmed our twin pregnancy. It was surreal finding out because I felt like I had known about it all along.

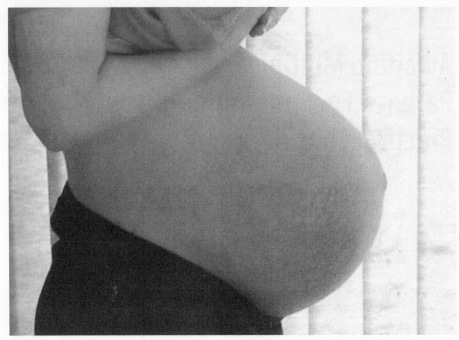

An amazing s-t-r-e-t-c-h of muscle occurs when mothers eat well.

family, relatives are usually the first to suggest this possibility. Children, siblings, or even complete strangers have intuited a multiple pregnancy!

The earlier you know you are pregnant with two or more, the more time you will have to adjust and make adequate preparations. It is best to learn the sex of your babies when seen on the scans to enhance bonding before birth, and to resolve any "gender disappointment."

The confirmation of a pregnancy will be welcome if it was planned. Not all unplanned pregnancies are unwanted, by any means, and those that have been anxiously awaited arouse ambivalence at times. Even women who have been taking fertility drugs or undergoing ART may have very mixed emotions about their "sudden abundance." With multiple births, the extra baby or babies are usually unplanned, but with so much ART today, not always unexpected. Nevertheless, most families are poorly prepared for news of a multiple pregnancy, let alone some of the prenatal restrictions and monitoring that invariably follow. Some couples take a tape recorder to appointments because taking notes of what is being said can be distracting.

Mode of Disclosure

As with all major life events, your reaction depends to a large extent on the manner in which the news is given. Joking during an ultrasound scan is an undesirable form of disclosure and so is the question "Have you been taking drugs?" Sometimes the woman may wonder what is wrong while the technician goes off to find the physician (who is the one supposed to relay any findings to the "patient"). Disbelief is usually the immediate response when twins are announced. "Get me a chair," "It must be a mistake," "Are you *sure*?" and "Why *me*?" are typical comments. Some women miscarry or go into preterm labor following an unexpected detection of a multiple pregnancy; therefore, the news should be conveyed with great sensitivity and support. The woman should sit down when told the news! The doctor should take time right then to answer her questions; at the same time she should be given literature and contact information for local organizations for multiples, especially if she does not have access to the Internet. Ideally an experienced mother of twins (or whatever size of the detected set) should call the expectant mother *that same day*, at the doctor's request.

The Internet offers unlimited information from the science of twinning to chat rooms for parents of multiples. A wide range of equipment for multiples can now be viewed and bought on-line. The World Wide Web is especially helpful for expectant mothers who may be on bed rest (and later for housebound new mothers of multiples).

The initial shock may pass quickly as first-time parents realize the advantage of having two children for the time and effort of one pregnancy. If there are already other children at home, the news may bring dismay. Unexpected extra children can present a major burden on space, time, income, careers, and lifestyle. On the other hand, if twins complete the number of children planned, the parents are thrilled. In cases where a fourth child was wanted but the twins make five, acceptance can be difficult, as when the parents are hoping for a girl and two boys are on the way. It is very important to allow and validate whatever feelings emerge without reassurance or judgment. This helps parents to move on to greater acceptance and an easier adjustment. Sharing emotions with other parents of multiples is the most helpful of all.

The feeling of being different, or treated as being different, starts as soon as the twins are detected and continues, with people saying things like "Oh twins, we have never had them in the group before" or "I don't

I usually wear size 12 maternity clothes but found that I needed a size 16 or 18 to go around my huge abdomen. I ate six small meals a day and paid special attention to my diet. One week, my doctor kindly announced that I had the biggest uterus in town!

When my husband heard I'd had twins, he forgot where he had parked the car. He even forgot where the elevator was.

My husband and I were overjoyed. We think it is the most exciting thing that ever happened to us.

My parents kept saying, "Oh, you're going to have twins." Then when I told them I really was going to have twins, the joke was on them — they didn't believe me!

We both felt that planning to have a child is a serious life decision. People today make that choice responsibly. It is a shock, then, when you find that you are having twins. Suddenly you realize you had no control over this unplanned event. I'm getting used to the idea, but I need to have those babies in my arms. Then they'll be more personal and less amorphous.

We had the perfect American family — a boy and a girl. I was so upset when I knew I was pregnant. I was one of a threesome and I hated it. Learning they were twins saved the day. I would have had to balance the numbers and now we are all square.

I wasn't worried about paying for the birth. My thoughts raced ahead to two tennis rackets, two cars, and two kids in college together.

I nearly fainted when I heard the news. But what could I do? I can't send one of them back.

Twins run in my family, so I kind of expected it. I don't know why people make such a fuss about twins.

Because I was infertile, when my best friend had twins I really felt that one of those babies should have been mine. So when we went to the adoption agency, I put in my order for two. After waiting 18 months, we suddenly had 36 hours' notice that "something" was coming. We didn't know we would really get our twins until we went to the hospital. "Baby A" and "Baby B" were embroidered in a heart on each twin's jacket.

know how this would apply in your case because you have triplets."

Confirmation of triplets or quadruplets can be very frightening. In addition to the enormous amount of care needed by higher-order multiples, there are the challenges of a supertwin pregnancy and birth. Parents are understandably anxious as they grapple with the ramifications of such a large and sudden increase in family size. At the same time, the possibility of fetal reduction (see Chapter 19) may be proposed, an issue they may have never heard of and are certainly unprepared to explore when multiples are first detected.

Fathers, after the drama of discovery passes, usually become very excited. Two babies obviously involve the father more than just one, and participating partners look forward to being needed. Even when dads have to take on an extra job to make ends meet, they may do so with great pride. Congratulations on their fertility and jokes about aphrodisiacs and sexual positions can be expected. Finances usually come immediately to the father's mind — not just the expense of the doctor and hospital fees but long-term projections for the children's education.

The attitudes of family members also influence the couple's response. One of the mothers I interviewed was separated from her husband, in school full time, and on welfare. With time marching on, she decided she wanted a child whom she would raise on her own. She selected a genetically satisfactory "temporary partner" for the conception — but little did she expect that twins would result! However, the predicament of twins helped her family swallow their disapproval and come to her assistance — they had ostracized her earlier in the pregnancy.

Another woman was considering an abortion for the unplanned pregnancy, but when she found out there were twins, they were "too special" so she kept them.

Time eases all adjustments. With early detection today, parents have months to prepare for the birth of multiples, gather supplies, and make necessary shifts in their self-image to prepare for their new roles. Extra hunger, fatigue, weight gain, and swelling make sense when you know from the outset that you are carrying more than one.

When twins used to be discovered at birth, it was a shock for everyone — doctor and staff as well as parents. The couple often would be so preoccupied with the arrival of the first baby that they hardly heard the nurse remarking, "I think there is something else inside" or "Whoops, here comes another one!" In former times, a second twin might be named by the nurse or doctor, during the parents' bewilderment!

Psychological Adaptation to a Multiple Pregnancy

Your adjustment to a multiple pregnancy depends on such factors as partner and family support, marital status, age, economic situation, other children, fertility history, general health, acquaintance with multiples, and you and your partner's own births and upbringing.

The following chart describes two opposite poles of reaction. Most women will fluctuate along the continuum — ambivalence in pregnancy is common. It is important to recognize if you lean strongly toward the negative side so that you can seek timely counseling.

Reactions to Pregnancy

NEGATIVE	POSITIVE
Insensitive disclosure of twin pregnancy by technician or doctor	Suspected twin pregnancy, confirmed with sensitivity and support
News experienced as a shock	News received as a wonderful surprise or dream come true
Unplanned pregnancy; unwilling to bear multiples	Planned pregnancy/conscious conception, optimistic about outcome of fertility treatments
Perceives large abdomen as "too fat"	Enjoys blossoming of her body
Feels like a sow having a litter	Grateful for abundance — "two babies for the price of one"
Resents size, appearance, social comments	Welcomes questions about large belly, due date
Anxious about high-risk pregnancy and going to term	Strongly motivated to learn about achieving a healthy term pregnancy and parenting skills
Irritated by bodily changes and discomforts of pregnancy	Views adaptation of body with sense of wonder and appreciation
Unaware of differences between babies; just feels kicks	Begins prenatal bonding with babies as a unit and individually
Fears labor, sees Caesarean as an easy way out	Looks forward to labor, finds providers to support natural birth
Rejects idea of breast-feeding	Joyfully anticipates breast-feeding
Feels overwhelmed by the thought of having and caring for two or more babies	Understands the need for assistance and sets up support systems for birth and postpartum in advance

Some mothers are intensely angry about being pregnant with multiples. They don't want the physical, emotional, and financial burdens of the extra child or children. Parents often are congratulated on their luck, and any ambivalence they feel about two babies or more may be met with little sympathy, especially if ART was used.

On the other hand are women who desired and consciously conceived twins. They feel proud and empowered to have exercised that choice. Such mothers are thrilled to have the bonus of an "instant family." In families with a history of multiples, the couple may have secretly hoped for twins.

If this is your first pregnancy, you will also be adjusting to the idea that you will never be just a couple again. You can be an ex-spouse but never an ex-parent! A common concern of couples is the change in their relationship that the "group arrival" will bring. The notion of "double trouble" or three or more of the same age understandably may raise doubts about the parents' ability to rise to the challenge of their care.

Rare events attract attention and publicity and multiples are special — particularly the larger sets. Your success depends on how supportive your extended family is and the help you can arrange, beginning in pregnancy.

Choosing Your Team

You will soon be warned about the potential hazards of a multiple birth, discussed in Chapter 7. Twins in recent decades have been classified as high-risk rather than a bonus, although a better term is "special needs." If a home birth had been planned, the midwife or doctor may insist on a hospital delivery, although some twins continue to be born at home, in birth centers, and at communities like The Farm in Tennessee. There may be the option of staying with your midwife and doctor with additional consultations from a perinatologist, if indicated. Ask your doctor how many sets of multiples he or she has assisted with, the length of the pregnancies, the birth weights, and the Caesarean rate.

Progressive doctors will counsel you about nutrition, sensible exercise, and rest and thus encourage the placebo effect. Midwives spend more time discussing your concerns and helping you feel that this special pregnancy is normal. For the same reason, I recommend that you find a doula, a trained woman who will support you *before* the birth and during labor and visit postpartum (see www.dona.org). Mothers of quadruplets and more can expect to be referred to a perinatologist at a Level III medical center; indeed, twins and triplets are often "layered up" too. You should ask how many observers might be in the room when you give birth (you have the right to refuse) and whether zygosity determination is available at the hospital.

The Path of Pregnancy

Your adjustment to pregnancy follows certain phases. Prenatal bonding is more of a challenge with multiples because you have to integrate the "extra" baby or more since you probably expected just one.

Feeling Your Babies Move

Although you may have seen your babies move during an ultrasound scan, feeling them move is a more powerful form of connection. Multiples create more movement than singletons and you feel the movement earlier. As with palpation, it is not just two moving parts, but several, that suggest twins.

An in-tune mother may notice different activity levels between her babies. Toward the end of pregnancy, there is little room for them to change position and it is easier to identify each infant. Mothers themselves can record fetal movements. Share any new observations in your pregnancy with your midwife or obstetrician. Trust your intuition and demand medical assistance if you feel something has changed for the worse. (This point was emphasized to me by mothers who had lost one or more babies during pregnancy.)

Usually the same traits and patterns of interaction displayed by babies in the uterus are seen after birth. The parents' observations of their babies' characteristics during pregnancy likewise affect how they view them in infancy and thereafter. A child who is considered to have a certain behavior from pre-birth days tends to have it reinforced later. On the other hand, the child who did not have as much room to move around in the uterus may become the active crawler, making up for lost time. In such cases, parents can encourage movement for the baby who was less active before birth.

Experiencing Physical Changes

A multiple pregnancy is associated with exaggerated and earlier onset of the customary signs and normal discomforts. Before the routine use of ultrasound, 37 percent of respondents to a 1987 survey by *Twins* magazine suspected they were carrying multiples because of their increased weight and abdominal size. Physical changes are always more pro-

When our twins are born, we will have four children under four. The difficulties of parenting are obvious; the nice aspects are not so easy to put into words. It is taking us a little while to get used to this pregnancy, although we know we'll love the babies when they arrive.

I am 5'2" and my pre-pregnancy weight was 115 pounds so by the time I got to 35 weeks I was very uncomfortable to say the least. I had gained 50 pounds and measured 46 inches around my belly.

One baby did somersaults to the left and the other one to the right. I was glad when things quieted down in the last two weeks.

What I remember is pressure. Everywhere, from my bladder to my ribs. It was impossible to find a comfortable position.

People often said to me, "You're huge — you must be having twins," which only made me feel even more large and dependent.

I got so sick of strangers saying to me, "You shouldn't be out shopping when it's so close, dear." My husband told me to just lie about the due date when those busybodies asked.

nounced in subsequent pregnancies than the first, but growth with twins is much faster in the early weeks than with a singleton. From weeks 13 to 20 much of your weight gain is water and fat that build necessary reserves.

By the sixth month you may be so large that you tire of friends and strangers asking if delivery is imminent. At 32 weeks the size of a uterus with twins is the same as for a singleton at term (40 weeks). During the last trimester you may be overwhelmed by your huge body, aching legs, swollen ankles, heartburn, and constipation! Itching of the abdominal wall, a common irritation in pregnancy, is often worse with multiples. The greatest itching, burning, and sometimes numbness or even pain is localized around the upper ribs and breastbone. (Friction massage from a physical therapist and stretching exercises can help.) Other discomforts include exhaustion, nausea, awkwardness, and difficulty breathing, sleeping, and walking. Increased hormone levels also encourage fluid retention and relaxation of the walls of the blood vessels, perhaps leading to varicose veins. For others, body size and lethargy become issues only at the end. Some women are "born to carry twins" and feel wonderful through the entire pregnancy with few of these annoyances.

The work of the lungs, kidneys, heart, and circulatory system is doubled and fatigue sets in easily. Family and friends may treat you like a queen or an invalid, forcing you to feel that your condition is abnormal rather than a doubling of a physiological state. However, in many countries, including the United States, pregnant women work too hard and too long, and this duress is worse for those expecting two or more. Pregnancy lasts only nine months, often less with multiples, and the welfare of your babies must be your top priority. It should be society's, too.

Getting Enough Rest

The heaviest demand on your heart and circulation is when standing. As you now service two or more extra hearts and circulations, you need to get off your feet at regular intervals. However, lying flat on your back when your uterus is large enough to compress major blood vessels is also undesirable. Instead, recline or lie on your side or even on your front with a Bodycushion® or use some of the giant pillows available today.

Regular rest is not only essential for your body during this challenging time of growing two babies or more, it is also an opportunity for interaction. You can play games with your babies: if you pat a moving part and say a certain word (name of baby, pat, kick), you can encourage your babies to respond. This is the time to state your goals of healthy outcome, reassure them that all is well, they are safe, and there is enough room and nourishment. (See Chapter 5 on bonding.)

If you do heavy lifting or have other physical stress at your job, you must reduce these liabilities. Ask your doctor to prescribe "disability" for you to compensate for the inadequate maternity leave in the United States.

Leave from Work

Ideally, mothers of multiples quit work by 24 weeks. However, unlike France and Scandinavia, in the United States the Family and Medical Leave Act provides only twelve unpaid weeks a year on 30 days notice (except emergencies) *if* you and your employer qualify. The Pregnancy Discrimination Act may be of use, if other employees get benefits for medical conditions. You can check your local Department of Labor to see if your state has temporary disability insurance. Since 1985 in Sweden, mothers of multiples may leave work from the twenty-fourth week at 90 percent of their pay.

Mothers in Finland have maternity leave for 105 days (Sundays and other holidays excluded). It starts no later than 30 days before the due date. In the case of a multiple birth, maternity leave is lengthened by 60 workdays for each additional child that is born. In the case of a preterm birth, maternity leave is extended by as many workdays as the birth occurred before the due date, minus 30 workdays. During this maternity leave mothers are entitled to an allowance. Compensation for the costs arising from pregnancy, childbirth, and medical care is also available, excluding hospital charges. Mothers are entitled to a special maternity allowance if in performing their work or at their workplace they are exposed to a chemical substance, radiation, or an infectious disease that is considered a danger to fetal development or to the course of the pregnancy, and if suitable alternative work cannot be found. Entitlement to parenthood allowance begins immediately after payment of the maternity allowance ends. The mother and the father can take turns receiving

My doctor asked me how my days were going and I told him I was no longer able to meet the goals I had set for hydration, nutrition, exercise, and rest while I was working. Without hesitation, he authorized short-term disability (at 29 weeks). I'm convinced that my ability to focus on those basic needs allowed me to avoid bed rest and carry my babies to $38^1/_2$ weeks. I was able to swim every day for 30 minutes, nap 2 hours every day, and focus on a high protein diet with lots and lots of water.

the parenthood allowance. This benefit is voluntary; if it is not used, the parent returns to work.

Fathers residing in Finland who live with the mother and participate in childcare are entitled to up to 18 days of paternity allowance (and leave from work, of course), divided between two periods: 6 to 12 days while the maternity allowance is being paid to the mother, and six days during the maternity or parental allowance period. In both of the cases, the allowance is paid retroactively in one installment. Fathers who are on paternity or other leave from national military or alternative service may receive the minimum allowance. Similar support for childbearing families can be found in the other Scandinavian countries and parts of Europe. In contrast, the United States is negligent with its dismal maternity leave.

Seeking Assistance

Husbands/partners provide the most important help. They should have a chance to discuss their concerns in private, ideally with other fathers of multiples. Relatives and friends may give welcome encouragement during the pregnancy or they may actually cause added stress. Well-meant advice may focus heavily on the potential problems of multiple births or raise doubts about your ability to care for two or more offspring together. You may feel alone and isolated. There may be no history of twinning in your family and no multiples among your friends and neighbors. Yet some first-time mothers of twins feel that the situation is easier for them than for women who have had other pregnancies — they know nothing else! Experienced mothers, who remember the time it took to meet the needs of one baby, may be more nervous at the thought of nurturing two or more. The various clubs for parents of multiples and the Internet provide major sources of support (see Resources).

Friends and neighbors who share your excitement and enthusiasm typically gained their experience with single children. I strongly recommend that you seek out and visit at least two or three families of multiples to plan your postpartum life. Compare a mother who works with one who stays at home, perhaps with no help, part-time help, or even live-in help. Visit families who have other children if you already have children. Observing mothers of multiples who nurse and those who bottle-feed should convince you that breast-feeding saves time, money, and energy as well as being an intimate, fulfilling experience that offers your babies the best health. Breast-feeding is more efficient because you can nurse twins for the same amount of time as a mother of a single baby. Breast-fed babies have an average IQ ten points higher than that of babies who are fed formula.

It is also a good idea to visit a mother of multiples on bed rest in a hospital. This could be the time to check out the maternity unit and the neonatal intensive care nursery (NICU). You could offer to help daily after she returns home and learn in advance about life with multiples. This is a free networking service that all mothers can provide for each other, since unlike in the Netherlands where a "baby-caregiver" is provided for the first eight days, mothers in the United States have to find such people themselves.

Learn from the Experts

Multiple birth organizations like the Mothers of Twins and Supertwins Clubs are your lifeline; they provide information that a family with multiples — as well as their health care providers — needs to receive before, during, and after birth. Join one right away for guidance from those who have been there. Attend meetings and establish a relationship with members of your club *before* the birth so that advice will be easy to get when you need it. Through these clubs you can also find used clothes and equipment, thus saving money for items like a diaper service, an extra freezer, or home help. Many of these mothers still have young multiples and mutual baby-sitting exchanges can be set up.

The La Leche League (*leche* means "milk" in Spanish) is an organization of volunteer mothers who promote breast-feeding. As with Mothers of Twins Clubs, I strongly advise that you contact a member *prior* to the birth. It is easier to call on someone you have already met when you are in the hospital or during the first weeks at home. Mothers of twins and supertwins who have successfully nursed are happy to provide free counseling and moral support. Such encouragement is essential because busy hospital staff and doctors tend to push bottle-feeding in general, and with multiples in particular. Some expectant mothers get the very wrong idea that breast-feeding is a chore and nursing twins or other multiples is just about impossible. On the contrary, breast is best, and nursing is a joy. A double supply of formula costs from $5,000 to $8,000 a year for twins — money that could be better spent considering you can make breast milk for just the cost of your meals. Some people recommend bottle-feeding because it offers the advantage of the father's par-

At the La Leche League meeting, I got tips on how to prepare my breasts — checking the nipples and exposing them to sunlight to toughen the skin.

... the unalterability by time of the repressed ... seems to offer an approach to the most profound discoveries.
— Freud, 1932

ticipation, but he can help by changing diapers and taking care of plenty of other tasks. (See Chapter 13 for specific advice about feeding.)

Exploring Your Personal and Family Agendas

Family Time Bombs

Having one baby (or more) is a momentous event; you need to be clear about hidden agendas. Research by Australian psychiatrist Averil Earnshaw has demonstrated that for four out of five people, their life events have eerie parallels to those of their parents. She explains:

> When we reach the age of a parent (usually a same-sex parent), the age the parent was when the next child after us was born, our lives change in some way which is often clearly observable . . . in the cases of youngest and/or only children, the eventful year is the one in which we reach our parents' age, when we ourselves were born.

Figure out these events and dates in your own case. Then draw your family tree and add to the usual chronology of births, deaths, and marriages the really interesting material such as illnesses, divorces and affairs, miscarriages and abortions, adoptions, episodes of sexual abuse, major life events (travel, immigration, graduation, job and career changes) *with their dates*. (This is called a geneagram.)

In my personal experience and professional work, I have found Earnshaw's concepts to be most helpful in resolving some intergenerational patterns, especially regarding reproduction and reproductive loss. As Freud observed, "the remembering is repeated in the action."

Get as much information as you can from your mother and medical records about your own gestation, birth, and infancy. How were you born? Were you early or late? Did you spend time in a neonatal nursery? Were you breast-fed? For how long? What sibling if any was born after you? You can ask these same questions about your mother's prenatal and perinatal experiences. Did she have a stillbirth or miscarriage?

Are you the same age now as your mother was when the next sibling was born (a red flag)? These are *your* realities, more powerful than any text on these subjects. Talk to your parents about your beginnings and let any demons out to clear the way for the next generation to begin afresh. The questionnaire in Appendix 3 can be done by both parents and is a memorable record of valuable information for your babies.

Setting Your Own Goals

Break down your challenges into a list. When tasks are divided and written on paper, they are more manageable. Put each topic on a separate index card in a box divided into trimesters.

Write down your goals, and read them aloud every day, preferably on arising and retiring. Stating your goals will affirm to your unconscious mind what you want to achieve. There are many books written about the power of such autosuggestion (a classic being *Think and Grow Rich* by Napoleon Hill, who in 1960 wrote using only the masculine pronoun!). Patients after heart surgery also did better when their cardiologists prayed for them.* The power of positive thinking is ours to harness if we believe it: I recommend the 2001 book *Excuse Me, Your Life Is Waiting* by Lynne Grabhorn or *The Dynamic Laws of Prosperity* by Catherine Ponder, originally published in l962, to introduce these principles.

Use the present tense when writing goals because it is more concrete than future and future conditional tenses. For the same reason, choose actual dates and numbers. These can be modified at any time. In fact, goals should be constantly reviewed and rewritten to program your direction in life.

Turn every worry into a goal. You could spend time becoming anxious over something such as your doctor's order for a repeat ultrasound scan. Stop the mental chatter by picking up a pen and writing down the outcome you desire — "The ultrasound shows the placentas of all three babies functioning perfectly." When the worry-monkey starts chattering again . . . take a breath and repeat your goal to yourself as often as needed. Talk to your babies the same way. Other examples of goals are listed on the following page. However, it is more powerful to create them yourself using your own words.

---

*One of the first and most striking findings of the nocebo effect concerned women who believed that they were prone to heart disease, thereby increasing their risk of death by a factor of four. Their fatalistic attitudes were self-fulfilling. Another group lost their hair, believing that they were receiving chemotherapy! In fact, the IVs contained only saline.

Everyone told me that twins come early, so I packed one month ahead of time. All that happened was that dust collected on my bags. My twins were two weeks overdue.

Examples of Goals

- My babies are born vaginally at term the last week of July (or whenever your due date is). Paste some photos of full-term twins, triplets, or quadruplets on your bathroom mirror or refrigerator. Watch videos of vaginal births of multiples.

- I am in excellent health and successfully nourish my babies who are born weighing xx pounds (the weight you desire).

- My babies are healthy and growing well.

- My boss doubles/triples my maternity leave. (Include your wishes, for you never know what may come true!)

- Three days after their normal birth, my healthy babies are home with me.

- My breast milk nourishes them for xx months and our bonds of love strengthen each day. Nursing gives me time to rest and my satisfied babies sleep well (attach photos of sleeping multiples).

- I am grateful to the Universe for this experience of abundance. I receive all the assistance I need, financial and emotional.

- A compatible live-in helper answers my ad.

- [Your partner]'s bonus pays for xx (whatever you need and can't afford).

Planning Ahead for the Babies

Multiples often arrive early; therefore, it is a good idea to have everything ready and organized by the seventh month (while setting a positive goal for birth at the ninth month!).

A diaper service cuts down on laundry but multiples use plenty of clothes, sheets, and towels; therefore, a washer and dryer are essential. Apartment dwellers can find portable washers to save them trips to the Laundromat. Parents of multiples can often afford such items with savings they gain by purchasing used items. It's an excellent idea to discuss all equipment you plan to buy with an experienced parent of multiples.

Assess your living arrangements with the view to your mobile equipment. Note the width of doors, accessibility, and whether you have indoor or covered parking for inclement weather. Lack of elevators may oblige you to move. Infant car seats should be obtained beforehand. In most states and countries today the law requires that the babies be secured for their first drive home from the hospital. Most car seats can be used indoors as infant seats, and it is easier to pick up two handles than two babies (although that is an important skill to learn as well). However, dual-purpose car seats have to be detached and repositioned each time. Their advantage is that the babies are happily seated in familiar surroundings in strange new places (a stroller for multiples offers the same benefit). Mothers who do not buy a stroller for two, three, or more may end up pushing two, which really requires a second person. (More details are given in Chapters 14 and 16.)

Battery-operated swings with lift-up trays give you some quiet time, and the babies love the movement. A four-door car is a priority to spare your back. If you are expecting a large set of multiples, you will need a van that makes loading of the strollers much easier.

Friends and family want to bring useful gifts. Disposable diapers for travel or a few weeks (or months!) of diaper service are obvious suggestions. Parents of twins can expect 4,500 diaper changes the first year. Warn everyone ahead of time that visitors should bring a casserole or be prepared to help! You will appreciate practical baby clothes more than fancy matching outfits. There will be no time to iron anything and easy-care fabrics such as stretch terry cloth are essential. Extra clothing is needed so you don't have to do the laundry daily. Large tote bags for outings with the twins are another gift idea. Best of all is the card that says "Gift certificate for 100 hours of house cleaning"!

Layette and Supplies for Twins

- Diapers: You will need about 100 a week for twins and 150 for triplets if you use a diaper service (highly recommended, and the incremental costs are reasonable because there is just one delivery charge). If you buy and launder cloth diapers you will need fewer, especially if you wash a load each day. Disposable diapers, handy for outings and travel, are expensive and the problem is *their* disposal!

- 8–10 wool diaper covers: These covers are expensive but allow air circulation and are preferable to plastic pants.

- 6–10 fitted crib sheets (unless the babies join you in the "family bed")

- 4–6 blankets or baby afghans

- 8–10 terry cloth one-piece stretch suits with snaps at the crotch

A survey of the mothers in our club showed that a dryer was the most appreciated piece of household equipment.

When I was six months pregnant, I started to make extra soups, sauce, lasagna, pies, muffins, cookies, etc., and froze them. We had enough food to get us through the last month of my pregnancy and first few weeks after birth.

- 8–10 cotton undershirts

- 8–10 cotton nightgowns with ties or elastic at the bottoms to keep them down

- 4–6 machine-washable sweaters, if the climate warrants

- 2 one-piece snowsuits, if applicable

Bassinets are optional. Sleeping with your twins in the family bed (see Chapter 15) is the easiest solution, or the babies can be put down in padded drawers, laundry baskets, a mattress on the floor, or even a large box. Twins shared the uterus for nine months and prefer to stay together — indeed, separation may upset them. Keeping a larger set of multiples together poses more of a challenge but they can be grouped — for example, quads are often paired. There are lots of chat rooms on the Internet where such topics are discussed, but every family makes these decisions by trial and error.

Although the idea of a pair or a unit is foremost in your minds before birth, select different clothes for your multiples (just a few because you will receive more gifts than you expect and most will be matching).

It is easier to shop in bulk if you have storage space. Products are cheaper by the case, and several months' supplies of nonperishables can be bought, allowing more time between shopping. Make as many meals as possible and freeze them ahead of time. Consider buying an extra freezer.

Consolidate all the baby clothing and equipment in one room, particularly if your house has a second floor. Place a spare bed, chaise longue, or a large comfortable chair with a footrest in the room so that you can rest and nap with the infants in the early weeks when they are fed so often. A gymnastic ball makes a very suitable footrest and can be rolled up under your knees. By itself, it is a comfortable seat as well and an effective way to bounce and soothe a baby.

A changing table of the right height is essential because mothers of twins bend over twice as often. Foot controls on diaper pails leave your hands free but the containers are usually too small. A large trash can works better and it is a good idea to set up a second "changing station" if your house is large.

For your clothes and for the babies, the greater the quantity you can afford, the less often you will have to launder. You can buy attractive maternity and nursing outfits these days at stores like Pickles and Ice-cream or on the Internet at www.motherwear.com. Remember that two-piece outfits work best for nursing twins. Nursing nightgowns, for example, are usually designed for nursing one baby at a time and are difficult to use with twins nursing together. During winter, clothes or nightshirts worn over an old T-shirt with two big holes cut out will keep your upper body warm.

Household Help

Very few parents are prepared for the realities of raising multiples. Some will have greater practical difficulties, especially if there are financial problems. Others may have plenty of assistance and living space but are challenged emotionally by the simultaneous demands of their children.

In the beginning you need the most help at night so you can sleep and the babies can be fed with the minimum of stress. Later you need help to give you a respite from the constant caring for so many babies. While you will get support from mothers of multiples clubs, friends, and families, you still need regular help, and this often means a paid professional worker.

The foundation of your postpartum recovery is your timely organization of others: to bring you meals, to assist with baby care, to ensure you get regular rest and sleep — especially if you have other children at home. Arrange household assistance *now* for when you return from the hospital. This basic need of all new mothers is more pronounced with twins or triplets, especially after the very likely Caesarean section. I repeat: Night help is needed as well as help during the day.

Many couples no longer live near their family and have to rely on friends, neighbors, or hired help to clean, cook, and baby-sit. Sometimes your expectations of grandparents and other relatives are not met and it is hard for them to rise to the occasion, which mostly requires the services of a full-time worker. Unless their help is organized and systematic, it may actually contribute to your stress. They, like friends, rally around in the beginning, but after a month or so their visits may taper off because they figure you have everything well under control — but this is usually when the babies are more active and you need it even more! Ideally, you need someone to coordinate the assistance you require, as you will be much too busy with your babies.

My neighbors banded together to help me. I had a different neighbor come over every Monday through Friday for approximately 2 hours. This gave me a much needed break each day. I was able to shower, nap, and get out of the house. My neighbors did this from the time my boys came home from the hospital until they were 3 months old. It quite literally saved my life and my marriage!

My neighbors set up a schedule and wrote it down for me so I knew who was coming on each day and what time they would arrive. I so looked forward to that time each day. It was a huge help and now my twins are very comfortable with a variety of different people and our going out, because they know we will return, as we always have.

Twins are really a strain. You wonder if you'll ever get enough sleep or even have any time for yourself again.

My pediatrician's advice to us when we left the hospital was, "Cancel all engagements for the next eighteen months."

I had no experience in childcare at all, and there I was at home with my twins — outnumbered. I could have used an extra pair of arms.

You have to set priorities every day. I often used to take the telephone off the hook, especially when the babies were asleep and I took a rest.

We had a live-in graduate student to help with the twins. We did not have to pay her anything, as we took care of her room and board. I don't know how we would have managed without her cooking and baby-sitting.

People you haven't heard from for years suddenly come to visit you now that you have had twins.

Twins are simple to take care of — if you are prepared to give up sleep!

I really missed having time for myself. Even getting a shower and brushing my teeth required planning far ahead. I spent a lot of time crying in those early months, mostly because I was physically exhausted. If I had to do it over again, I would cry out for more help. I would tell others how desperate I was instead of saying I was doing fine.

I gave up the idea of being a superwoman long ago and enjoy being a single mother of twins.

Perhaps your local middle school, high school, or senior citizen center can help you find someone who can assist you for a few hours. Some preteens are quite mature and helpful. Many schools require their students to volunteer for community service.

It is the ongoing daily maintenance that helps keep the house clean and tempers calm. Encourage visitors to cook meals or do laundry. Make a list, or place a calendar or box of index cards at the front door, so visitors choose a task as soon as they arrive and sign up again before they leave.

By preparing your support system well ahead, you will avoid feelings of low self-esteem when the reality of caring for two or more hits home. Couples who imagine they will cope alone then feel guilty when they can't and are reluctant to request help at that point.

If you already have someone who cleans for you, perhaps she could increase her hours. You need this type of work from someone you know and trust rather than a "baby nurse" (discussed in Chapter 13) because such an "expert" may sabotage your success at breast-feeding, albeit with the best of intentions.

Make sure that you have someone lined up who can help on short notice in the event of an emergency.

Shopping will be a challenge with two or more babies — just getting out with them as well as selecting and carrying the groceries. One woman solved the problem ahead of time. Before the babies were born, she drew a detailed map of her local supermarket and made photocopies. Each week she had only to visually review the product aisles and check off the items she needed. This made it easy for her to remember everything while making the shopping easier for visitors or neighbors who offered to help. You may be able to find a store that delivers or use an on-line service.

Costs

Families of the first surviving sets of higher-order multiples (the Dionnes, Morloks, Dilegentis) had zero hospitalization costs because the babies were born at home. Today the cost of maternity care is astronomical, as described below.

An understandable concern is the reduction of family income to one salary when expenses are doubling or tripling, although giving up work earlier than you had planned may be very good for your health. In

France, the preterm birth rate for multiples was drastically reduced by allowing mothers to stop work. It makes a huge difference, of course, when the government provides financial benefits to compensate.

The costs of having your children arrive all together are multiplied. Many couples need a larger house or a larger car and often both. Hand-me-downs don't work with babies all the same age. Special equipment, such as strollers for multiples, is expensive because it is not mass-produced. Whereas a mother usually has her hands full looking after a single baby, extra help needs to be employed to take care of multiples — another expense. Perhaps there is something you can do during pregnancy to "earn credit" for help when the babies arrive or maybe you can find someone to live in, like a student.

Some parents of multiples organizations, particularly in the United Kingdom, have arranged discounts with various chains. Always ask about discounts for multiples — store managers may never have considered it and may be happy to oblige. If you save all the receipts for baby clothing and equipment, the store may duplicate each item at no cost or at half price or offer some other deal. Multiples draw much attention from shoppers as well as from store clerks, and businesses like to encourage good will.

Because of the prevalence of multiples today, commercial enterprises are less enchanted with the publicity opportunity and unlikely to donate items. In addition, publicity may come with a heavy price if it disturbs your home life and invades your privacy.

Health insurance in the United States rarely pays more for twin births than for single births, although some physicians charge double. Check with your obstetrician, pediatrician, and hospital for their fees as well as with your insurance company for its reimbursement. Hospital nurseries charge for both twin occupants, but the cost can be reduced if you keep your babies with you in your room (rooming-in). The expense of hospitalization for mother and child can be staggering: Hospital admissions during pregnancy cost at least $1,000 a day (and each day in NICU costs about $3,000 *per baby*). The doctor may prescribe a Home Uterine Activity Monitor Device (see Chapter 19) at a cost of up to $10,000, and it may not be covered by health insurance.

Almost half of all births in the United States were to single women in 2000. Single mothers and others below a certain income level in the United States may be eligible for state assistance such as Medicaid and food stamps. These programs and their criteria for eligibility vary from

I had to learn to accept help! Having always been independent, it was a change to let strangers open doors and help carry groceries to the car. Then I realized they enjoyed helping or they wouldn't have offered. We should all help each other more.

The nuclear family is a bad idea anyway, and with multiples you really miss the extended family. It is foolish to think two parents can raise multiples without help. Don't even try to do it all by yourselves!

I felt certain that I could manage my babies by myself, because I knew that other people did, so I struggled on until their first birthday, by which time we were all miserable. In retrospect, I bitterly regret not having acknowledged that I needed some kind of help so that we all might have enjoyed that time more.
— Sally Salveson

My parents were unable to visit from Hawaii, but they sent money instead, which we used for household help.

I found it difficult to respond when people asked me, "What can I do?" or "Let me know when you need help." So, a friend helped me create a postcard simply listing the things I needed help with (Food, Care for My Older Children, Household Help), including very specific examples of what people could do. On the card, I requested that people call me with what specifically they wanted to do and when. This way I didn't feel inhibited by asking someone to do something they didn't want to do or couldn't do.

state to state, so check with your state Department of Health. Women, Infants and Children (WIC), a federally administered program, provides vouchers for food and formula as well as counseling and medical review of recipients who are at risk. State welfare benefits vary also but they increase for an extra child. Parents of higher-order multiples, with persistence, may discover some state support. Each state's Department of Health should provide loans of infant equipment; education on nutrition, birth, breast-feeding, and parenting; counseling for prematurity and disabilities; and childcare or homemaker services for single parents, teen parents, and parents of multiples.

Barbara Luke during 1991–92 investigated whether it was prematurity, being a multiple, or being a premature multiple that determined the length of hospitalization and total cost of neonatal care. The most significant factor was preterm birth. For *each infant* born between 25 and 27 weeks, the cost was more than $195,000 for an average stay of 71 days. It decreased to $91,343 if the birth took place between 28 and 30 weeks with a hospital stay of 39 days. Between 31 and 34 weeks, the stay was reduced to 12 days at a cost of $18,367. Only four days were needed for babies born between 35 and 38 weeks at a cost of $4,308 and this cost was reduced further for babies born between 39 and 42 weeks — only three days costing $2,230 per infant. Data from a 2001 multicenter study headed again by Luke reinforced the anticipated conclusion that the best outcomes had the lowest costs. Twins born between 38 and 39 weeks and their mothers spent five days or fewer in the hospital for a cost of $8,065 for the mother and $5,005 for the twins. The average weight per baby was 2,842 gm. On the other end of the spectrum, twins born before 28 weeks (averaging only 829 gms) spent *an average of 61 days in the hospital for a tab of over $190,000.* The mother's average stay of ten days cost more than $14,000.

Social Services

In different locations, help may be available through community nursing services, special twin agencies, day-care grants, and allowances for families with multiples. An organization called The Care Team Network (www.CareTeam.org) trains teams to provide such services. Maybe there are some people in your community who would be interested to learn such skills if there is no existing local resource affiliated with this organization. There is also a volunteer pilot association, *Angels of Mercy*, that will fly people to their destinations in times of need.

In Australia, a grant from the Department of Maternal and Child Welfare provided a free postpartum service of household help from women who are themselves mothers of twins or triplets and have completed a training course in hygiene management and baby care. These helpers share their experience and give advice as well as help with housework and feeding sessions. Twin and triplet baby carriages are lent free to members of the association and sales or rental of other equipment is also offered.

In some countries like Australia, France, and Canada, a bonus is paid to the mother for bearing a child, but it is not always increased for multiples. A friend of mine in Paris who has triplets was able to stay home to raise them because of the generous French allowance for her four children plus the additional income from a live-in student. Recently, in my home state of South Australia, a wonderful system of postpartum assistance was set in motion. Young unemployed women were trained for six months and provided with a car to help with baby care, cooking, cleaning, and so on. Unfortunately, some of the local obstetricians reacted with scorn and derision that such a service could replace a couple of days of professional care in the hospital! I hope that their nocebo effect will not sabotage this excellent solution to two problems.

The need for assistance is especially critical for poor, black, single, and teenage mothers. These are the ones who are often too busy, too tired, or too uninformed to reach out for support, but they need it the most. Housing assistance, welfare, food supplements, extended leave from work (which is often used up before the birth with bed rest), home care covered by insurance, and home visits for help with breast-feeding will be necessary.

Most multiple births clubs, such as Multiple Births Canada (www.multiplebirthscanada.org), provide literature for single parents who have multiples. The National Organization of Mothers of Twins Clubs in the United States has similar information as do MOST and The Triplet Connection. Information is provided for parents, grandparents, counselors, and others who may be working with single parents of twins, triplets, or more. Single parenting situations can arise for a number of reasons: divorce, widow/widower, military postings, job demands, or choice.

Having triplets qualified me for aid in my county. Ask your local social service agencies if help is available.

When my children reach tax-paying age, the Government will benefit from two taxes at the same time at the same rate. Children's Benefit should follow the same principle.
— Parent in England

Naming

Infant names are usually finalized before you leave the hospital. Each state has its own requirement for completion of the birth certificate and if you change the names later, a fee is involved.

These days you have time to choose names well in advance, unlike parents of multiples a couple of decades ago who often let hospital staff name their unexpected babies! The Morlok MZ quads, born in 1930, were named by an x-ray technician at the hospital who won a competition organized by the local newspaper to name the four identical babies. The girls were named Edna A., Wilma B., Sarah C., and Helen D. The first initials of their names correlated with the initials of the Edward W. Sparrow Hospital, and their birth order was denoted by their alphabetical middle initials!

Knowing the gender of each baby before birth makes naming easier. An individual's name is key to his or her identity, so choose names carefully. Although twins are part of a pair, and thus share one social unit, their names should be clearly their own. Favoritism in one name, such as that of a special relative or illustrious person, is unfair to the other twin. "Tweedledee and Tweedledum" names emphasize twinship over individuality, and parents as well as children often regret them later. One set of quadruplets was called Annette, Suzette, Bernadette, and Yvette. The famous Badgett quads were called Joan, Jeanette, Jeraldine, and Joyce.

Confusion abounds with names like Rigby and Digby, Marlene and Darlene, Elaine and Germaine, Helen and Ellen, and Dale and Gale. Research at the Twinsburg Festival turned up the fact that 27 percent of identical twins have first names that rhyme, and the names Ronald and Donald show up among twins at nearly five times the rate in the general population!

Other names may not rhyme but are clearly couplets: George and Georgia, Kristen and Kirsten, Wendy and Wanda, Jack and Jake, Robert and Roberta, Francis and Francine, Taylor and Tyler. Occasionally, parents favor fancy paired names such as Samson and Delilah or Mary and Joseph.

Triplets born on Christmas Day have been named Noel, Carol, and Merrie. A set of twins born on December 7, 1941, was called Pearl and Harbor. Birth order is sometimes indicated in the names, as in Anthony and Barrie or Oliver and Timothy. More obvious are the triplet names

Awaiting Multiples · **85**

Prime, Secondo, and Terzo (first, second, and third in Italian). Triplets have been named Franklin, Delano, and Roosevelt; Faith, Hope, and Charity; and Tom, Dick, and Harry. These names emphasize the collective entity, as do names of seasons, April, May, June, or flowers — Daphne, Violet, and Daisy. Frequently, multiples share names with the same first letter: Jenny and Joanne; Richard and Roland; Timmy, Tommy, and Tammy. All such combinations can be confusing. It is important to have different initials for each multiple, not only for individuality but for future convenience — school, correspondence, the phone directory, and the government departments.

Repeat each infant's name as often as possible to confirm his or her identity and to enhance one-on-one bonding. Another benefit of repeating the name at every opportunity is that multiples themselves are often slower than singletons to refer to themselves by name.

Sibling Preparation

The advent of multiples has an enormous impact on the entire family, and their needs push siblings very much into the background. Parents, of course, are usually sensitive to these issues, but other people often are not. The single sibling has the hardest time with twins: they are a pair, the parents are a pair, but she or he is solo. It is natural for children to feel displaced and jealous of any new arrival, although the many distractions that accompany higher-order multiples may help diffuse jealousy. Siblings need to be well-prepared for a multiple birth and Chapter 17 focuses on the older sibling's adjustment after the birth. Books for children listed under "Children's Books" in the Further Reading explain twinning and provide an opportunity for feelings to be explored.

Be ready with a greeting gift from each multiple to the older child after the birth and vice versa. It is a good idea to arrange in advance some special treats or activities such as a playgroup for the other children when the babies come home.

Use the time before the birth to become acquainted with the special features of twinship while you still have time to read! Also explore with your partner the views you each have about parenting in general and parenting multiples in particular. Discuss ways in which you can honor the special bonds of multiples while affirming each one's individuality. Start educating grandparents and friends, too, on the importance of identifying each member of the set and relating to them individually.

I was worried about the impact of four babies on a two-year-old. I mentioned my concern to my doctor, who said that if the adults don't stress how unusual it is to have four babies, it won't occur to a two-year-old.

During our baby shower, my husband and I opened one gift after another for the expected babies, and I realized our older child was watching, and feeling very left out. If you do have other children, make sure there is something for them, too.

We bought twin dolls for our daughter, and she was very happy playing mother with her own pair.

5
Bonding with Multiples

 The importance of early attachment between parents and infants gained attention in the 1970s. The pioneering work of pediatricians Marshall Klaus and John Kennell and obstetrician Frederick Leboyer revealed that babies are much smarter than we ever thought.

The term *bonding* implies a seal, a kind of "glue" that binds individuals together emotionally, but this is a process that can take time. The flourishing of attachment after birth depends also on how profoundly your emotional connections were established during pregnancy.

Detection of Multiple Pregnancy

The parents' adjustment to the news of an extra baby or babies is affected by the timing of its disclosure and the manner in which it is conveyed. The public is aware of the great impact of such news because the most common question mothers are asked is "When did you find out?"

I strongly recommend that you collect all available information from ultrasound scans and any prenatal tests. Knowing your babies' genders enables you to name them and get acquainted with them individually, thus enhancing the bonds between you and your multiples.

Prenatal Bonding

The natural time for bonding to begin is while you are all connected before birth. The prenatal phase of bonding is the foundation of the subsequent relationship; therefore, this chapter comes early in the book. I have led many sessions with guided imagery, touch, art, and music to help pregnant women relate to their babies. I was impressed with their value and I learned that many mothers need guidance like this to feel more connected with their babies.

During the months of pregnancy, a personality forms just as a body develops. Research presented in books such as my own *Primal Connections: How Our Experiences from Conception to Birth Influence Our Emotions, Behavior, and Health,* and *Tomorrow's Baby* by psychiatrist Thomas Verny, and *The Mind of Your Newborn Baby* by psychologist David Chamberlain shows us that unborn babies are very sentient beings. They are always awash in their mother's emotions and their biochemical effects.

Today with ultrasound, some parents start observing their babies from as early as six weeks. Mothers may develop a clear perception of each baby, its individual position, level of activity, and confirmation of sex from ultrasound. The doctor and ultrasound technicians will name your babies A, B, and C, depending on their proximity to your cervix. (See Chapter 9 for a discussion of the safety of ultrasound.)

Attachment is experienced on intuitive and hormonal levels as well as consciously. The more you can identify with each baby while he or she is within your body, the more expanded is your sense of self. This is crucial for your confidence and optimism.

Parents interact with their babies before birth through stroking, tapping and talking games, singing, meditation, prayer, visualization — whatever means you choose to connect to them emotionally and spiritually. Involve any other children you may have, too. The more connected an older child feels with the babies, the better their acceptance when they are born.

The mother usually bonds with the baby she envisages when she learns she is pregnant. However, when she finds out there are more than one, she will need to bond twice or three times, which can be compared to falling in love with two or three people simultaneously! Do this in your own way and in your own time. Parents learn to love more than one child, but it is much easier when they arrive years apart.

Your best source of inspiration is other mothers of multiples, whom you can find by contacting one of the multiples clubs *before* the birth. With preparation, encouragement, and time, mothers of multiples are able to receive and love two babies or more.

It is often easier to focus on the unit, especially when you are still coming to terms with the fact that you are having multiples. You can take turns making contact with one of the babies as well as both together. This process will change and evolve as you notice their differences.

Ideally, bonding starts with a conscious conception, which is explained in a book of that name by Jeannine Parvati Baker. You can start a journal for your babies at their absolute beginning if you know it!

Guidelines for Optimal Prenatal Conditions

Integrate these guidelines with your goals (see Chapter 4).

1. **In a perfect world, every baby is wanted and planned.*** I have spoken with many mothers of twins who always wanted twins, who even willed their egg to split or prayed for double ovulation. There are mothers who have lost one or both twins and have subsequently conceived another set. It is ideal if parents are both aware and desirous of a conception during the sexual act. Conscious planned conception in the context of meditation and visualization may take many months. Parents using ART often visualize or pray for success with each cycle.

2. **Ensure optimum nutrition, exercise, and family harmony.** Aside from good nutrition and regular exercise, clear communication between the partners is important prior to conception as well as throughout the pregnancy and after.

3. **Be aware of your family history, especially as it relates to twins and the age of your mother at the time of your conception.** Also significant is the time when a woman reaches the same age her mother was when she or the next sibling after her was born. Plan conceptions and births so that they occur at times other than anniversaries of miscarriages and stillbirths in the family.

*Overall, U.S. women currently average a total of 3.2 pregnancies each, of which only 1.8 are "wanted" by the woman. Research in 1994 by Bustan and Coker showed that babies who were unplanned were twice as likely to die in the first twenty-eight days of life than those who were planned. In a multiple pregnancy, the extra baby or babies are, with rare exceptions, always unplanned. The number of births that are wanted by the mother is closely associated with her level of education.

I knew from the ultrasound that the upper baby was a girl. The gender of the other baby was not identified. Throughout the pregnancy, I used to stroke the top of my belly, talking and humming to Sarah. After the birth, I immediately felt a strong bond with Sarah, but Susan seemed always whining and demanding, especially needing to be touched a great deal.

4. **Visualize your babies from the beginning.** Begin communication with them as soon as your pregnancy is confirmed. Be open to any dreams, images, hunches, or other dimensions of intuition.

5. **Explore the idea of a soft, relaxed uterus that will yield so that each baby can stretch and turn comfortably.** Keep breathing and envisage your uterus softening with each exhalation. Place your hands on your belly as often as you can and reassure the babies inside that there is enough room, enough oxygen, enough nutrients, enough love and attention for each of them.

   Learn their various positions. Ask your midwife or doctor to draw each baby's position on your belly at each prenatal visit. Introduce the babies to the concepts of up, down, right, left, back, and front, and describe their body parts during your conversations with them. When you feel one baby kicking, reassure the other that he or she is safe. Use your hands as well to communicate with each baby. When the father and siblings do this, ask them to state their name each time, for example, "This is your brother Joe," so that the touch, voice, and family relationship are linked.

6. **Affirm the individuality of each twin.** Talk to the babies about sharing. Help them with their identities by referring to them by name. Until you know the genders, make up some special pregnancy names. As psychiatrist Bernabei points out, "More than other people, twins must in each moment live with the problem and the question of identity of the 'I' and of the 'you' and their continuing relation." At no time is this situation more pronounced than during prenatal development. Ultrasound can provide parents with details about the sex, placenta, and sometimes zygosity of their babies before birth. Use this information to bond with each multiple as an individual as well as to talk to them about their special bond.

7. **Remain confident that you will carry your babies to term — however many there are.** Take pride in the power and largesse of your body in responding to the challenge of multiples. Individuals create their own bodily realities; the life of a person is the life of the body. People can learn to control blood flow, pulse rate, blood pressure, and other physiological functions. Visualize and verbalize optimal mental, physical, emotional, and spiritual development for your ba-

bies daily. Meditate on your babies' nutritional, emotional, and spatial needs. Choose the qualities you admire most in yourself and your partner as attributes for your babies to acquire in your visualizations.

8. **Express anxieties, fears, and concerns.** Worries and apprehensions may become self-fulfilling prophecies and lead to complications unless acknowledged and turned around into goals. Each of us brings to pregnancy and birth our own agenda of unfinished psychological business, and this is where personal growth should be centered. For example, let yourself feel afraid to release your fear. Feelings need to be affirmed and explored. Medical professionals often rush to treat symptoms without exploring causes, and the psychological dimension or cause of complications is generally overlooked. (See Louise Hay's *You Can Heal Your Life* and Alice Steadman's *Who's the Matter with Me?*) If you cannot consciously connect with your fears, then hypnosis, applied kinesiology, and dowsing are some techniques that can help.

9. **Keep a journal.** A written record of your thoughts and feelings will help you bond with the multiples as a unit and as individuals, as well as provide them with a wonderful record of their prenatal existence.

Be aware that your babies will remember their experiences before, during, and after birth.

A Healthy Pregnancy Enhances Bonding

Excellent nutrition and carrying your babies to term are important for optimal bonding. A good diet before and after the birth means less fatigue, one of the factors that impairs parenting and predisposes parents to child abuse. Full-time work distracts from your enjoying your pregnancy and often means little time for discovering who is living inside.

Gail S. Krebs, a mother of seven including twins, launched Bloom! The Maternity Wellness Program in 2002 at The Dutch Barn at Kaaterskill Creek, in the Hudson Valley (two hours from Manhattan). The program is for women in early to mid-pregnancy and focuses on proactive strategies: (1) staying well during pregnancy via personalized nutrition and exercise plans; (2) understanding one's personal risk profile versus

When everyone learned I was having twins as a surrogate, they were much more interested and supportive. I guess twins just made the whole arrangement seem way out. People would say, "Now there will be one for the other family and one for you," but that never entered my mind. I wanted the twins to be together.

the standardized risk assessment criteria in current use; and (3) reducing the likelihood of preterm labor, bed rest, "toxemia" of pregnancy and related complications, and Caesarean section. There are group information sessions, one-on-one consultation, massage, and other treats. (See Resources.) Additional locations are planned.

Surrogacy and Adoption Reveal Prenatal Bonds

Mothers who miscarry learn the reality of prenatal bonding in a painful way. Surrogate mothers who are trying *not* to bond nevertheless do so at an unconscious level. One mother who conceived twins and relinquished them to her sister-in-law described to me how she hardly slept the last few weeks of the pregnancy because "there was so little time left to be with them and I didn't want to miss any of it." Another surrogate mother felt relieved to discover that she was carrying twins because she knew that when they went to their adoptive parents, they would have each other. Likewise, mothers who plan to give up a baby for adoption often find they have become surprisingly attached.

A recent study found that the birth weights for singleton pregnancies following IVF-surrogacy and IVF were similar, whereas the birth weights of twins and triplets born from the IVF-surrogates were significantly heavier than those delivered from conventional IVF patients.

In the past, twins were commonly separated by adoption. Mothers were not consulted about whether the twins should be placed together or separated because closed adoptions were anonymous. Today adoption is often open and agencies recognize the bond between multiples and place them together.

I appeared on the *Today* show, NBC's *Newsfront*, and *MSNBC News* in 1999 regarding the case of a white woman who gave birth (after embryo implantation at a reproductive clinic) to twins — one white and the other black. The confusion of embryos led to a custody suit by the black genetic parents. However, the mother who had carried, birthed, and raised the nongenetic "twin" was already deeply attached to both babies, as they were to each other. The judge ruled that the black infant be returned to its genetic parents, and permitted limited visiting privileges for the birth mother. Such bizarre conflicts of parenthood and bonding are unfortunately increasing. Over time, rare mix-ups have occured in the nursery, but with ART, gametes and embryos involve numerous third parties that compound the likelihood of such mishaps.

⬤ Postpartum Bonding

Bonding After Normal Delivery

While almost all quadruplets, and most triplets, are routinely scheduled for Caesarean section in the United States, it is better to birth multiples vaginally unless there is a specific medical problem. The more directly you can experience each stage of pregnancy and birth, especially the hormonal response right after birth, the more secure you feel to trust your instincts. The outpouring of oxytocin — the "love hormone" — is the physiological basis of your attachment to your babies and is strongest right after birth. Odent points out that this crucial phase is often disturbed by the "ritual" of cord-cutting and removing the babies for observation.

A pediatrician, and a nurse for each baby as well as one for you, will be present when you give birth. Most hospitals now encourage contact between parents and offspring immediately after birth. You may want to handle just one baby at a time at first, but to affirm the reality of birthing two babies or more you need to hold them together as soon as you are

It took me many months to feel that I had really attached to each baby. I'm sure it would have been easier if I had held them both right after birth. The nurses want to be helpful and take over much of their care, but it is better if they help you with each baby so the bonding process gets off to a good start.

It was a magical experience to be nursing one baby while laboring with the second.

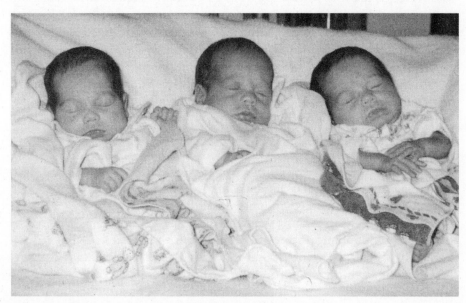

Parents scrutinize for similarities and celebrate the differences.

We simply refused the eye drops and just were overwhelmed by the magnificence of our babies' eyes. They looked so calm and wise!

ready! Remember to photograph them together in your arms as well as individually.

Babies in good health can be placed naked against your skin and may begin nursing at this time. Evolution has prepared mammals for a face-to-face meeting right after birth. Newborns need to make good eye contact with their parents right away and the "windows on the soul" should be clear. (Drops or ointment in the babies' eyes against gonorrhea should be avoided or delayed — hospitals will usually wait twenty-four hours.)

Bonding, for the babies especially, occurs on a continuum from conception to birth. Birth is an event during which hormonal surges and peak emotions facilitate attachment. Ideally, babies experience a smooth transition from life inside to life outside.

Multiple births are considered high-risk, and often hopes and plans can change without warning or time for psychological processing. For example, a new diagnosis or a sudden Caesarean section may cause one or more of your babies to be removed from you for hours or even days after birth. If events happen too fast or without the mother's full understanding, she may withdraw and become less conscious of her actions and feelings, leading to "missing pieces" in her recollection of these important episodes. Uncertainty about the outcome may be a constant pressure and curious onlookers often pose more questions rather than offer help.

Bonding After a Caesarean Section

With an epidural or a spinal anesthetic, mothers can be awake and aware when their babies are delivered surgically. Unfortunately, many Caesarean babies are placed in the intensive care nursery for 24 hours of routine observation.

Thanks to the adaptability of human beings, bonding can and does happen later — it just takes longer. Clearly, you have an advantage when a strong attachment was developed during pregnancy.

Even though time is short when an emergency Caesarean is being set up, it is a valuable opportunity to explain to your babies what is happening and to reassure them that they will be delivered safely and lovingly, if not in the way nature intended. (Chapter 12 explains how the surgery can be made more considerate for the babies.) It's a great help when the staff acknowledge the mother's emotions by allowing her to express disappointment if she had hoped for a vaginal birth.

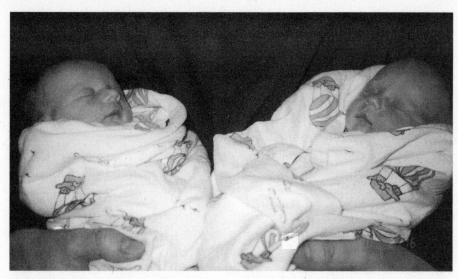

Hold them both *as soon as possible.*

In my experience, mothers of twins who have undergone a Caesarean with this kind of support escape feelings of guilt, resentment, and "unfinished business" that otherwise can linger for months or years. These mothers can move right on with enjoying their babies. Unfortunately, many doctors and nurses are not available or able to support you in the way that you may desire; therefore, consider having a midwife or doula attend you as well.

Breast-feeding boosts a mother's self-esteem after a Caesarean. It is nature's way of continuing the process of bonding, begun prenatally, through hormonal stimulation and physical contact. Stand firm in your determination to do this despite naysayers who will discourage you because you have had a C-section and there are multiples to feed.

The typical hospital nursery interferes in this continuum with its bright fluorescent lights, the crying of other babies, the regrettable separation of multiples from each other, and sometimes even swaddling to prevent movement. Keep your babies with you! If not, at least keep them together, *especially* in the NICU, as soon as their individual equipment permits.

It may be more efficient to focus on the pair or group at the beginning while you sort out their differences and similarities — which every parent of multiples naturally does. Making comparisons and finding physical and personality differences help you to see your babies as separate people. Different schedules and different levels of development make that process easier.

Monozygotic twins take longer to develop as individuals for two reasons. They look alike and they behave very similarly. Sometimes parents themselves cannot distinguish their babies for months without the help of name bracelets, painted nails, or other identifying marks. It helps to use different-colored crib covers and clothes. Begin using the infants' names right away and encourage others to do so. Zazzo found that 10 percent of mothers of MZ twins could not remember which one was given which name and, in a survey by Ricardo Ainslie, 77 percent of mothers of MZ twins mixed them up.

At Home

Frequent physical contact is easily achieved by the family bed and the family bath, by massaging your babies, and by wearing baby carriers (one in front and one in back, or a baby per partner for twins). Super-twins can take turns with carriers and strollers.

Infant equipment such as playpens, swings, and Jolly Jumpers, while very useful at busy times and in emergencies, is designed to separate babies from their mothers. Babies prefer contact with each parent — a human rocking chair. Babies also love to be held while you bounce on a gym ball.

Organize help so you can spend some time alone with each baby — bathing, nursing, playing, and repeating his or her name — as well as with the babies together.

Postpartum Support

New mothers — in the absence of complications — do not need medical care, but they do need rest, nutritious food, and lots of help. It is important that you get that help from the beginning.

A first-class hotel is a better alternative to a hospital when you are all well. The bathroom is close, the sheets are changed daily, and the food will be much better! You will have privacy without inquisitive visitors and intrusive medical assessments. I strongly recommend that you ask family members who want to give a gift to consider giving a hotel stay (postpartum *with* the babies, and two years later *without* them!). Many people have frequent flyer miles with airlines that can be used for hotels and resorts.

Some health insurance companies pay for "mother care" at home if you leave the hospital early. Ideally, expectant parents of multiples will have support from a midwife or doula that continues through at least six weeks postpartum. In the Netherlands, the "kraamverzorgster" attends to the mother and family for eight days.

Mothering the mother is the best way to promote attachment and to establish and maintain breast-feeding.

Complications

A negative birth experience can delay bonding just as a good birth experience promotes your self-esteem and confidence.

A preterm birth interrupts the prenatal bonding phase. In addition, the appearance of premature babies makes bonding difficult because they look vastly different from the parents' idealized image. Preterm babies are usually kept in an isolette and sometimes they need to be rushed to another hospital or even different hospitals.

Hospitalization of One or More Multiples

It is a challenge for parents to bond with an infant in intensive care, as understandably they want to protect themselves in case that baby does not survive. These parents often refer to their baby as "it." But should the baby die, the healthiest process is for the parents to acknowledge deeply their baby's existence, however brief, so that they can let go peacefully. With two or more babies in the NICU, the parents are overwhelmed.

Parents may lack support in the event of death or disability of one or more babies, because outsiders think that any remaining multiple will compensate. If the grieving process is delayed, then so too will be the attachment to the living baby or babies. (Chapter 22 discusses the experience of death in detail.)

Labels such as "premature" and "brain-damaged" or incorrect identification of zygosity can have an impact on the multiples long after birth and can interfere with your attachment to them. Pediatrician Elizabeth Bryan emphasizes that "uncertainty is agonizing and is made worse if the parents feel that something is being hidden. For instance, when the doctor is plainly worried but continues to say that all is well."

Photographs of the baby or babies are essential when they are confined in the NICU. Make sure you have photos of both babies together (they should be in the same isolette together anyway; see Chapter 20).

My triplets came home from the hospital one at a time, and I felt this staggered timing was a great help in allowing me to know and bond to each baby in turn.

The hospital wanted me to take Anne home first. I was afraid that I would bond to her and get used to one baby. If I was going to be taking care of two babies, I wanted to do so from the very beginning. I wanted to be fair to both of them.

Today, with digital cameras and the Internet, photos can be available in minutes for you to regularly monitor your babies' progress. This is an enormous help for parents who have children at home and for whom hospital visits are difficult to organize. Parents can visualize their love and energy going out to their babies when they are physically separated and keep the emotional and spiritual ties strong.

It is ideal if the mother and father can stay in the hospital to provide care and contact. In many facilities, the parents live in at least for a couple of days prior to taking over the care at home.

Shifting Attachment: Preferences

A mother looking after one baby attends to his or her needs without distraction. A mother of twins constantly must choose which one is more upset, which one should be picked up first, which one is hungrier and this forces her to make distinctions.

Multiples often have very different personalities (although MZs are usually similar), and understandably you will feel differently toward each. Feelings are private realities; it is how we express them in our behavior that counts. Parents typically favor one twin over the other at different times, but the favored multiple changes frequently. Understanding this process makes it easier for parents to be spontaneous.

A mother may favor one twin because she feels guilty for having favored the other in the uterus, just as a parent may give more attention to a fussy baby while benignly neglecting the less demanding one. Sometimes one baby comes home while another remains in the hospital. It is far better for a mother to say, "I couldn't hold you after the birth because you needed special care away from me, and I need to hold you right now to make up for that," than to continue to feel distanced from one of her babies.

A parent may pay less attention or feel less attraction to one of the set, or prefer to interact with a baby who is more responsive. Some mothers attach more to the first-born and may experience the second baby as an "extra." In recent years, the emphasis has been on waiting until both twins can be discharged together. Jane Spillman's research in the United Kingdom found that 72 percent of mothers had a favorite twin and for 84 percent of them it was the heavier of the pair.

You can nurse two together but you can only look at one at a time, and you can change only one diaper at a time, so seize these opportunities to connect with one baby. Skin-to-skin and eye contact are important types of "glue" and especially needed if infants are bottle-fed.

Monozygotic twins look identical and may respond similarly to their environment, but there will always be differences. A multiple's position in the uterus may give it an advantage or a disadvantage for nutrition or movement, or touch from the mother. Even in the same home, the effect of the environment after birth is not exactly the same.

Multiples, like all siblings, must learn to take turns, and this concept can be introduced from the very beginning. Some babies seem to understand the situation but others demand to be picked up at the same time!

Parents also sometimes feel that when their love is divided between two babies, each one is getting only half of what a singleton would receive. There are compensating factors, however, such as the special bond between the multiples themselves and the lifelong extra attention from outsiders. Also, parents of twins receive double love in return, and the father is essentially more involved than with a singleton where the mother-baby bond is more exclusive.

The challenge is treating multiples differently yet fairly and if not with the same kind of attention, at least with the same amount! Meeting the needs of each multiple will constantly vary, so let go of unrealistic standards.

Bonding and Gender

In most cases, bonding is easiest with a boy-girl pair and hardest with babies who look alike. However, some parents have strong gender preferences, especially if they already have other children, and these expectations may or may not be fulfilled in their twins. Ideally, disappointment about the sex of the babies can be worked through prenatally, now that technology lets you know the sex. Acknowledge your feelings to permit them to change.

Babies in the uterus can sense conflicts; therefore, it is far better that a mother admit, "At one time I didn't want two more girls, but now I am very happy getting to know you as the special people you are," than for her to suppress negative feelings. Understandably, it is more difficult to love a baby of the less-preferred sex or one with a disability, but it will become easier after the real feelings are addressed. Gender disappointment is very common, and I have led groups for expectant and new parents to address this issue. We explore the reasons why parents have

I resented that Michael took so much time to feed and burp, and cried a lot. Emily was so good, she would wait and smile and I felt terrible that she got so much less attention, when she really deserved it more.

I found it difficult to bond with the unexpected twin, because all through my pregnancy I had related to just one baby.

I had a hard time believing the twins were mine for keeps. I felt I was just baby-sitting them for someone else.

those feelings without judging, and this allows attachment to begin to unfold and flourish.

Guidelines for Optimal Bonding After Birth

1. **Use a sling or baby carrier extensively.** Term as well as preterm babies benefit emotionally and physically from being carried on a parent's body. You will better learn each baby's individual cues about her or his needs and wants with less crying. Slings and Kanga-carriers (for skin-to-skin contact) are listed in Resources.

2. **When your babies start to talk, listen to their memories about their birth and the time before.** Many children spontaneously discuss such memories, but skeptical reactions from adults shut them down. A mother of twins recently told me that she overheard one twin say to the other, "You always kicked me when we were inside Mom," and the other twin admitted, "I remember kicking you a lot. I didn't have much room." Parents can best facilitate such conversations by remaining calmly interested, asking open-ended questions such as "Tell me more," "When did you first feel that?" "How was that for you, Susie, when Tommy was born?" Let them volunteer that it was "warm," "dark," "tight" — whatever — spontaneously rather than using such terms yourself in questions. Be conscious of birth symbols in speech, drawings, and play. (See photo on page 376.)

3. **If you experience complications and interventions, provide a running commentary for your unborn and newborn babies.** They do understand — years later they have been able to quote verbatim conversations that took place in the delivery room! Caesarean babies need additional cuddling, body contact, and massage.

4. **Honor your babies — they are your guides and teachers.** Whether you consciously chose them or not, they chose you as parents!

Bonding with multiples is an initial challenge with exponential rewards. Only families with multiples have the opportunity to experience both the bond between babies and the bond between the unit, and perhaps other siblings too. Each family will have its own challenges and compensations, and pride in the fact that they belong to a very special group.

6
Sharing Space:
Twinship Experiences in Utero

Developments in Prenatal Psychology

The evolving field of prenatal and perinatal psychology offers a wide variety of accounts by children and adults of prenatal memories and preverbal experiences. Psychiatrists such as the late Graham Farrant and Stanislav Grof, author of many books including *Realms of the Human Unconscious*, have compiled impressive clinical evidence of memories going back to implantation and conception.

Neurologists, among others, have argued that memory starts when a child is learning to talk. However, psychiatrist Thomas Verny, author of *The Secret Life of the Unborn Child* and *Tomorrow's Baby*, pointed out that from the sixth month of conception the fetus is sufficiently developed neurologically to receive, process, and encode information. Science has shown us that memory storage is not an exclusive province of the brain. When we think of how much a one-celled creature like an amoeba can do, we realize that human memories can, and do, go back to the single egg and sperm cells which provide the blueprint to create a human being.

If fetal organs and systems function under the direction of the prenatal brain, why not the mind and memory as well? Why *wouldn't* the baby remember early events and emotions? Every mother who looks into the eyes of her newborn knows intuitively that her infant is already an individual with a personality and assumptions about the world. Every maternity nurse knows that each newborn is different.

David Cheek was an obstetrician and hypnotist in San Francisco who scrupulously documented evidence of prenatal and perinatal experiences. Cheek wrote:

Prenatal memories have been presented to me often in workshops by patients and students who had only volunteered to explore their memories of birth. Initially, I was not looking for such memory because I was sure it did not exist. It seemed wise at least to listen to these reports.

David Chamberlain is a California psychologist whose research into concordant (parallel) birth memories of mother and child through hypnosis is presented in his 1998 book, *The Mind of Your Newborn Baby* (3rd ed.). He describes how newborns arrive in the world not just sensing, having emotions, and reacting to their environment but learning, remembering, and communicating. A mother in Germany wrote to Chamberlain that her ten-year-old daughter reported having trouble going to sleep because she feared recurring bad dreams. In the dreams, two girls are running from a menacing shadow, holding hands, both very frightened. She loses her grip and loses sight of the other girl and wakes up afraid, breathing hard, and depressed but with no understanding. Her mother decided to tell her that she once had a twin who was lost eight weeks into the pregnancy, something the child had never been told before. The child reacted calmly to this news and never had the nightmares again.

Ultrasound has revealed sophisticated activity before birth (and in the case of multiples, interactivity, as studied by Alessandra Piontelli in Italy). Twins at 20 weeks easily locate each other and touch each other's face or hold hands! Certain gestures and habits seen at this time persist into their postnatal years. In one case, a brother and sister would play cheek-to-cheek on either side of the dividing membrane. At one year of age, their favorite game was to take positions on opposite sides of a curtain, and begin to laugh and giggle as they touched each other through the curtain.

Chamberlain elaborates:

> Ultrasound observations of behavior in utero, especially among twins, reveal a spectrum of emotions including anger, fear, and affection. Babies appear to react to needles that intrude into the womb with a mixture of shock, withdrawal, and aggression. Studies of pregnant mothers watching upsetting videos suggest that babies can become upset along with their mothers. Several studies have revealed that babies tend to become depressed when their pregnant

mothers are depressed, an effect which begins in the womb and has been measured after birth.

Since memories are behavioral as well as mental, they are held and expressed in specific parts of the body and may be accessed through hypnosis, deep massage like rolfing, energy balancing techniques such as polarity or bioenergetics, craniosacral therapy, primal therapy, visualization, "rebirthing," evocative breathing, and dream exploration. While those who have not witnessed or experienced this kind of age regression are understandably skeptical, the evidence is impressive. Recalled events can often be verified by family members or medical records, and the subject frequently experiences a strong sense of resolution following regression experiences that validate his or her intuition.

Chamberlain and Verny knew about pre- and perinatal memory decades ago but no professional organization was interested. As a result, they founded the Association for Pre- and Perinatal Psychology and Health (APPPAH, www.birthpsychology.com), on whose board I have served. The evidence of prenatal memory is indisputable for the thousand or so members of this and the other two organizations that appreciate the awareness of unborn babies (International Society of Prenatal and Perinatal Psychology and Medicine, and the Society for Reproductive and Infant Psychology). Ongoing investigation deepens our understanding of the physical and psychological dimensions of these early memories and the later effects. Piontelli's studies of unborn twins in *From Fetus to Child* have added important findings to this field of study.

Perhaps our fascination with multiples stems not only from the fact that they were born together but that they shared conception and gestation, as did at least 12 percent of the general population who carry the unconscious memory of a lost twin. Twins can serve as "nature's laboratory" by separately confirming prenatal events for those who doubt preverbal memory. The increasing sophistication of ultrasound will serve to document further the active social life of multiples before birth.

Life Inside

Sharing the uterus with one or more siblings is typically recalled as a struggle for space. Toward the end of pregnancy the uterus is experienced as a cramped environment by most single babies. In an undisturbed intrauterine life, experiences include feelings of cosmic unity and oceanic bliss, while pressure from the uterus provides important tactile stimulation. According to Grof, the twin situation is a disturbance of this ideal intrauterine life and may give rise to experiences of crowding and kicking. When two or more siblings compete for the same resources, there is the potential for a life-or-death struggle. Expectant mothers who understand this will make sure that their dietary intake is sufficient and the existence of each multiple is securely affirmed through exchanges that enhance such bonding.

Generalizations are often made associating behavior with the type of twinning: same-sex twins are thought to be competitive, for example. However, the dynamics of the intrauterine environment, the position of the babies, the tension or relaxation of the uterine and abdominal muscles, plus the birth experience are profound influences.

Dr. Jane Greer, a psychotherapist and twin expert in New York, frequently counsels twins who are experiencing conflicts between the bonds of twinship and the ties of marriage. One of her clients discovered through hypnotherapy that she felt kicked around in the uterus and pushed out during birth. Coincidentally, her twin phoned to say that she was undergoing primal therapy at the same time in another state. Her uterine experience was one of fighting for space and kicking out her sister in order to be born. Both twins confirmed that their prenatal situation was repeated in adult life. The twin who was pushed out at birth fell into relationships where she ultimately felt abused while the other felt she attracted people who wanted to be pushed around.

Dr. Greer also researches and works with twins who have experienced a psychic connection with one another even after the death of one twin.

Such prenatal experiences form *engrams*, or changes in neural tissues and neurotransmitters. These engrams, also known as imprints, are registered in the body prior to the later development of memory involving the cortex of the brain. Imprints set up behavioral patterns that in later life can affect not only the twin relationship but also interaction within the family, the choice of spouse, and other life events.

Italian psychiatrists Bernabei and Levi described a case of male DZ twins, one of whom was successfully treated for hydrocephalus (excess cerebrospinal fluid) while in the womb. The condition was resolved by birth — there were no residual problems and it was never discussed with the twins. However, by the age of seven, the nonaffected twin "assumed the role of doctor and leader," unnecessarily protecting and interpreting for his brother. The "protected" twin clearly resented the role forced on him and when asked to draw pictures of his family drew only his brother with an enormous penis. After a series of discussions with the psychiatrists, the dominant twin explained that he had to protect his brother "because he had a sick head," a comment that clearly reflected prenatal memories.

Farrant in Australia was approached separately by MZ female twins seeking primal therapy. This approach helps patients get in touch with their deepest physical and emotional feelings by guiding them to regress to their first occurrence. Both twins suffered from sexual confusion that had affected their marriages and led to separations. Extraordinarily, they began to develop similar problems independently, although they were not associating closely with each other. During their primal therapy, they relived almost identical experiences. Most striking was their separate yet identical experience of conception. Both recalled two sperm entering one egg at the same time. Both experienced the first sperm pushing the competitor away from the egg, then fertilizing the egg, which split into twins. The brief presence of the second, Y sperm, which would have produced a male child, was sufficient to create their sexual confusion. After therapy, one returned to her husband and the other entered a new and meaningful heterosexual relationship.

Conception, implantation, and birth all present survival issues that are more of a challenge to multiples than to singletons. After the first baby implants in the uterine wall, the wall thickens, which may make it more difficult for the second to implant. As a research project for his higher degrees, Hanspeter Ruch, a twin and clinical psychologist in Switzerland, underwent primal therapy to journey back to life in the womb. He explains how, as the second DZ twin, he experienced implantation as one of "the most traumatic situations in my life," during which he felt "I am not going to make it, I have to die — accompanied by strong physical feelings, wanting to scratch a hole into the wall with my hands."

Once implanted, Ruch says that he experienced life in a soft, tender, warm ocean. This world began to change, however, as he sensed his "kingdom" becoming "limited, even constricted . . . with a sense of something outside of him, far away, yet bumping him . . . sometimes at random, sometimes like a response, a shadow, like two balloons slightly hitting one another." Initially, he felt playful and thought it would be fun to reach out to the shadow, but as he attempted to do so he simply spun around in the fluid. His impression at this stage was of "something in between with no end and no beginning." Later he describes "a kind of a wall . . . many times I touched it, crawled up and down, but I never found an opening." Wanting to reach out to feel "the shadow," he found that his skin and the other's could never touch; there was "always a skin in between" preventing contact.

Disturbances of Ruch's prior oceanic bliss became more frequent, intense, even violent, interrupting his sleep. He became progressively confined, and being kicked and hit in the back made him feel "unprotected and vulnerable." With no possibility of escape, he felt forced to struggle, becoming increasingly angry and frustrated.

"I became more scared and threatened by my brother's presence," he writes. "We started to fight much more, especially if one of us tried to turn. I felt pushed towards the walls, and furiously started kicking and striking out as hard as I possibly could. . . . My warm friend became an enemy and a threat. To survive I had to attack too, had to push him down."

As a result, Ruch always felt a tremendous pressure to compete with his brother in all areas of life. During therapy he associated this competitive drive with his primal struggle in the uterus. When Ruch relived and released the struggle, he became free of this compulsion.

As a psychotherapist, Ruch has observed that the way we are conceived determines the way we are born. For example, in his personal experience, the imprint of the struggle to survive, "to get in" at conception (entering the egg), was further strengthened by a subsequent struggle, to implant in the womb and to enter the world at birth. Such imprints lead to behavior patterns in later life that repeat the primal experience — in this case, one of a struggle *to enter*.

Implantation is not only a powerful psychological aspect of twinning — clinically, many multiples die because of its physiological difficulties. Fertility experts now acknowledge that they spent years perfecting fertilization techniques and embryo retrieval without considering uterine receptivity.

Sharing the uterus with a mate/rival often leads to paradoxical feelings. Another twin remarked, "I can remember times when I would move my body in a way to get more room in the womb, but I wouldn't hold any joy about it inside. I couldn't allow my body to let Claire know about it because if I got more space, it meant that she got less."

Recommendations for Expectant Parents of Twins

This fascinating material on prenatal and perinatal psychology can benefit mothers and babies, although some readers may feel it causes parental guilt about negative experiences babies may go through in the womb. I have counseled mothers, for example, who have made appointments for an abortion and then decided to go ahead with the pregnancy. They wonder what effect their ambivalence may have on their baby or babies. (Incidentally, the discovery of a *twin* pregnancy was the turning point in several cases personally known to me; the mothers felt that two babies were a gift and canceled their scheduled abortions.*) As Chamberlain points out, "Private truths are living history to your child . . . the honest revelation of your inner life is an alchemy that can turn negative feelings into positive ones." I suggest that such mothers explain to their unborn babies exactly how they feel and ask for time and patience as they adjust to the continuation of the pregnancy. Similarly, any negative situation should be explained to the babies to emphasize that they were not the cause of the accident, divorce, job loss, family death, or whatever caused the mother's anxiety.

The Web site www.birthpsychology.com has many interesting articles and studies about the lives of the unborn and how we can make them better.

After birth, twins and other multiples share and develop a special bond, which is discussed in Chapter 18. The effects, both immediate and long-term, of losing a co-twin in utero or soon after birth are explored in Chapter 23.

*The evolving field of pre- and perinatal psychology is sometimes used to pressure women into continuing with an unwanted pregnancy. I support the mother's choice for either.

7
Potential Hazards
of Multiple Pregnancy

Before the recent sharp increase in multiples, women expecting twins (many unknowingly) frequently enjoyed a better diet, kept active, used common sense, and experienced little medical intervention. Many gave birth with a midwife or with a family doctor, even at home. In a multiple pregnancy, the major contributors to mortality and morbidity (illness) are preterm birth (PTB) and low birth weight (LBW) — *prenatal* issues — and these have worsened with each edition of this book despite (or because of) the increasing medicalization of pregnancy and birth and more women having prenatal care!*

The three most frequently reported risk factors in pregnancy — pregnancy-induced hypertension (high blood pressure, or PIH), diabetes, and anemia — rose steadily between 1990 and 2000, by 30 to 40 percent. Problems with either an excess or deficiency of amniotic fluid more than doubled. Acute or chronic lung disease more than tripled during those years (although it affects only 1 percent of women overall). It appears that women are becoming sicker when they have babies.

Medical risks vary with race and ethnicity. For example, Native American and Chinese women have similar high rates of diabetes, 5 percent each. Native American women also have the highest rates of PIH and anemia (also 5 percent) whereas Chinese mothers have the lowest (1 percent). Diabetes ranges from 2 percent for Cuban mothers to 4 percent for those in nearby Puerto Rico. (Most Cuban mothers breast-feed; most Puerto Rican mothers bottle-feed. See Chapter 8 for the link between cow's milk and diabetes.)

*the nocebo effect

Few preventive measures have been advocated over the years. Bed rest, suturing the cervix, and tocolytics and magnesium sulfate to stop preterm contractions have been tried for decades. They are controversial at best and counterproductive at worst. Unfortunately, there is little recognition of the central importance of prenatal nutrition and a balance of sensible activity and rest. Pregnancy and birth remain physiological processes, exaggerated and challenged by multiples, but still natural. (The creation of twins and larger sets by ART are an exception and more complications result.) Measures to improve outcome must be based on better understanding of the physiology of multiple pregnancy in general, and of the placenta in particular, as well as the role of stress hormones arising from the emotional state of the mother.

You will hear — from health care providers, well-meaning friends, and popular literature — of the increased risks (this is the nocebo effect). No wonder parents become anxious as the birth approaches! Statistically it is true that some problems increase with twins, but not all complications occur more frequently in a multiple pregnancy. Also, the samples of women used to generate statistics are biased. Research usually is conducted in large teaching hospitals, which have more high-risk patients with complications, who are often poor or minorities. Twin births at small community hospitals (there are few remaining), birth centers, or at home are never included in such studies.

The existence of successful outcomes is my motivation for writing this book. In this chapter I will discuss nonfatal complications as well as their medical management. (Death is discussed in Chapter 22.) It is my heartfelt responsibility to make as much information as possible available in the event that it should be needed without unduly contributing to the nocebo effect. Again, my priority is exploring ways to *prevent* these complications for which most mothers of multiples will be repeatedly screened, which provokes anxiety as much as reassurance, with or without preventive measures.

Fetal Complications

Preterm Birth (PTB)

A birth before 37 weeks is considered *preterm*. This is by far the major cause of complications and infant death, in both multiples and singletons. Preterm labor is associated with three-quarters of all the perinatal morbidity and mortality in the United States. Although in the year 2000 the overall PTB incidence dropped very slightly from 11.8 percent to 11.6 percent, it has risen fairly steadily over the past two decades and is still much higher than it was in 1980 (7 percent), when I wrote the first edition of *Having Twins*. The annual number of PTBs in the United States has grown to more than 400,000, and some of this is due to the higher component of multiple births and the contribution of ART. The Canadian PTB rate has been increasing gradually, from 6.4 percent of live births in 1981 to 7.1 percent of live births in 1996, with a rate of 6.1 per 100 live singleton and 51.1 per 100 live multiple births.

Differences in newborn behaviors, as well as in predictable effects within the newborn period and within the first two years of life, have been found between full-term and preterm infants. There are also the problems with separation in the neonatal intensive care nursery (NICU), parental coping and bereavement, and postnatal depression, all of which

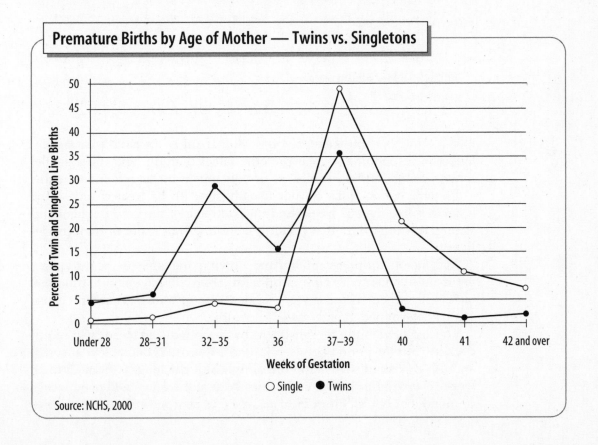

Premature Births by Age of Mother — Twins vs. Singletons

Percent of Twin and Singleton Live Births

Weeks of Gestation

○ Single   ● Twins

Source: NCHS, 2000

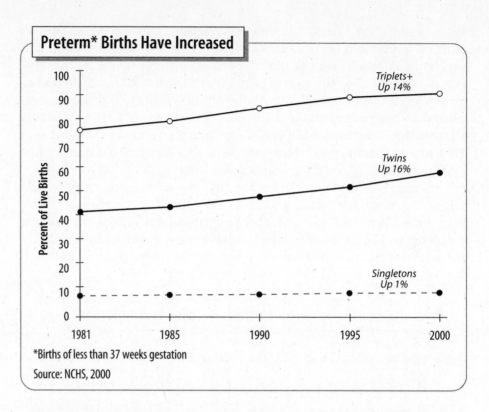

Preterm* Births Have Increased

Triplets+ Up 14%

Twins Up 16%

Singletons Up 1%

Percent of Live Births

*Births of less than 37 weeks gestation

Source: NCHS, 2000

increase rates of abuse and divorce. Mothers of twins have greater challenges in responding to their preterm babies than do mothers of singletons, of course, and the babies are usually much smaller and more fragile.

Preterm contractions do not usually need to be treated unless the woman is less than 32 weeks and the contractions are very frequent and strong. It is important that preterm labor does not result in preterm delivery.

Risk factors for preterm labor are shown in the table on the next page, yet many women who go into preterm labor will have none of the risk factors listed (see Glossary for explanations of terms). When no cause can be determined, it is termed "idiopathic."

The age of viability for newborns has been reduced steadily in recent decades, but the period between 20 and 24 weeks is one of low survival and a high risk of severe and ongoing health challenges. From 25 to 28 weeks is *very early preterm,* and babies born at this stage will need weeks or months in NICU. From 29 to 32 weeks is *very preterm,* and the babies

Risk Factors for Preterm Labor*

Poor nutrition or inadequate hydration

Insufficient omega-3 fatty acids in the diet

Physical trauma, abuse (25 percent of pregnant women suffer domestic violence)

Hard physical labor, tiring travel, standing all day at work

African American ethnicity

Substance abuse — tobacco, alcohol, street drugs

Emotional stress and fear (no partner, unplanned pregnancy, separation or divorce, recent move, geographic and cultural isolation, chronic illness in family, recent death)

Financial stress, unemployment, inadequate housing

Fear of increased body size by term

Fear of birthing two or more babies

Previous preterm delivery

History of preterm labor in the maternal line (for example, mother was preterm herself; preterm birth may be a pattern for several generations)

Low pre-pregnancy weight

*Studies have shown that the mother at highest risk for preterm labor is a black, single teenager who has not completed high school.

Chronic cough (risk of preterm rupture of membranes)

Obesity or underweight

Placental problems — placental abruption, placenta previa, mid-pregnancy vaginal bleeding

TPEH (toxemia/preeclampsia/eclampsia/HELLP)

Infection in the genital tract (mycoplasma, ureaplasma, chlamydia, and other sexually transmitted diseases); severe kidney and urinary tract infections

Congenital anomalies (gastroschisis), congenital heart disease or defect

Fibroids (benign uterine tumors)

Chromosomal anomalies (for example, Down's syndrome)

Uterine anomalies, cervical incompetence

DES exposure

Diabetes mellitus

Oligohydramnios or polyhydramnios (insufficient or excessive amniotic fluid)

Exposure to ionizing radiation (x-rays), anesthetic gases, lead

Motor vehicle accident or other injury

Severe gum disease

Two or more second-trimester abortions

---

still need steroids and much time in NICU, and almost one-fifth do not survive the first year of life. (Very preterm babies accounted for 2 percent of the preterm births in 2000. Many are supertwins.) The risks of early and very early preterm labor are significantly increased in IVF pregnancies, according to a recent study done in Greece.

When I first started to research multiple pregnancy in the 1970s, the saying was "half of twins are premature." Sadly, things have worsened in the three decades since. Preterm birth has steadily increased for two decades for both singletons and multiples. It increased 25 percent between 1981 and 1999. When the first edition of *Having Twins* was published in

1980, the rate was 51 percent; it improved to 49 percent for the second edition, but in 2000 the rate of PTB among twin pregnancies was 57 percent. For triplets the PTB rate in 2000 was 93 percent compared with 10 percent among singletons. On average, twins are born at 35 to 36 weeks, triplets 32 to 33 weeks, and quadruplets around 30 to 31 weeks. Preterm delivery occurs in 35 percent of MZ twins and in 25 percent of DZ twins.

Preterm birth accounts for two-thirds of the deaths of one twin and for 80 percent of cases in which both twins die. Contrast this with 1987 when 57 percent of white twins and 48 percent of black twins *were carried to term* in the United States.

In 1981, the birth certificate in the United States was changed to permit more accurate data collection about gestational age (and thus PTB) by noting the date of the last menstrual period. Unfortunately, information about zygosity is not collected (if this were required, then testing would be routine, as it should be). Nevertheless, trends have not been systematically analyzed by the National Center for Health Statistics, due to lack of resources and interest. An occasional special report focuses on plural pregnancies and their outcome, but I have had to analyze large quantities of raw data from NCHS.

Inducing Preterm Births to Reduce Mortality

Studies in Nova Scotia, Canada, showed the rate of PTB increased from 42 percent (1988–1992) to 48 percent of twin live births (1993–1997). Twin live births born after induction* increased from 4 percent to 9 percent during 1996–1997. However, for babies aged between 34 and 36 weeks, LBW decreased from 18 percent during 1988–1992 to 9 percent. Perinatal mortality rates among pregnancies reaching 34 weeks decreased from 12.9 per 1,000 total births during 1988–1992 to 4.2 per 1,000 total births during 1993–1997.

Twin researcher Emile Papiernik in France observed that induced PTBs (to prevent the death of growth-restricted babies) are as high as 55 percent. For example, when one baby is growing insufficiently or the babies have a blood type incompatibility, the life of one baby may have to be deliberately risked. This means an induced PTB to save the healthier one (usually after the amniotic fluid is sampled to assess lung maturity). He points out:

*when labor is started artificially with the synthetic hormone Pitocin

The rate of preterm births no longer represents spontaneous preterm births, for an increasing proportion of preterm births result from a medical decision to induce labor or schedule a Cesarean delivery.

In France, the PTB rate of 5.4 percent in 1995 increased only to 6.2 percent in 1998.

Isaac Blickstein, another obstetrician specializing in multiples, makes the following valid criticism:

> Given the wide range of false-positive heart rate patterns and the inherent difficulty of interpreting these tracings in twins one may argue that the indicated preterm birth to save the probably distressed fetus will result in a certainly preterm birth of the co-twin.

Hakan Rydhstrom in Sweden found that about 100 twin labors would have to be induced to avoid one fetal death in same-sex twin pregnancies (which are at greater risk).

Every mother of multiples should be aware of the signs and symptoms of preterm labor, listed below, as well as the tests available, described in Chapter 9.

Signs of Preterm Labor That You May Not Recognize

1. Contractions occurring at regular intervals of 15 minutes or less, about 4 or more per hour. The uterus tightens, becomes hard, and peaks — takes a globular shape. Such contractions may cause no discomfort.

2. Menstrual-like cramps, rhythmic or constant, experienced in your lower abdomen.

3. Rhythmic or persistent pressure that may radiate to your thighs.

4. An intuitive feeling that something is wrong.

5. Gas pains, intestinal discomfort, diarrhea.

6. Vaginal discharge of water, mucus, blood.

7. Lower backache, whether it comes and goes or is continuous. It may radiate to your sides or front.

It has generally been accepted that the more babies there are, the earlier they will be born. The "crowding" theory is based on the idea that the uterus delivers the babies when there is no more room inside. But it

My only sign of labor was gas pains. I had been very good with my diet all through pregnancy, but I went to a picnic and had a can of soda pop. I thought that was causing the gas. Several hours later my baby was delivered, ten weeks preterm.

I had to insist that I be monitored. I told the doctor I wouldn't go home until I was convinced that everything was okay.

I felt a bit funny when my labor began, but I thought it was just from the Chinese meal I had eaten.

is not true that twins and triplets "always come early." Singletons weighing more than the combined weight of multiples are successfully carried to term. In one sextuplet pregnancy the combined weight was more than 8 kilograms (at 31 weeks), which is twice the average weight at term for a singleton. A set of quads was born "fully developed . . . in the full time" in Australia over 100 years ago and each one weighed at least 7 pounds — the average weight for a singleton.

Low Birth Weight (LBW)

The amount of weight the babies gain in the uterus is related to their rate of growth as well as the duration of the pregnancy. Both these aspects of development are impaired if the mother is undernourished and if her weight gain is inadequate. The birth weight of the offspring is related to the quality of the mother's diet, her weight gain, and her emotions. It is well known that cortisol, a stress hormone, inhibits fetal growth.

Additional preventable and modifiable personal and social risk factors include poverty, being a single parent, being a teenage parent, little or no prenatal care, living with a violent partner, a generally stressful life, workplace conditions, type and amount of work, smoking, alcohol and other drug use, and limited stress-relief strategies.

Approximately 75 percent of all newborn deaths and illnesses occur in LBW babies. They may also have more serious childhood problems like learning disorders, visual problems, respiratory illnesses, and cerebral palsy.

Birth weight is associated with the weight of the placenta — that crucial organ that transfers nutrients and waste products and manufactures hormones. Growth restriction is measured these days by repeated ultrasound scans rather than measuring the height of the uterus.

Low birth weight is not the same as PTB, although preterm babies, especially multiples, usually weigh less than normal and there has been much confusion between the two definitions. Low birth weight babies have not gained sufficient weight for their level of development. In the United States, the incidence of LBW is 49 percent for twins and 8 percent for singletons. Multiples make up 23 percent (twins, 17 percent) of the LBW statistics. Only about 10 percent of twins weigh more than 7 pounds, the average weight for a newborn singleton.

In the first edition of *Having Twins*, I quoted data from NCHS that showed that 51 percent of twins were below 5 pounds, 8 ounces (less than 2,500 grams, which is the international standard definition of *low*

Twins Weigh Less than Singletons at Birth

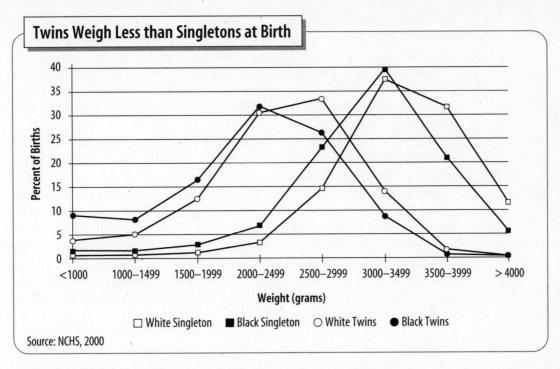

Source: NCHS, 2000

Black Twins Weigh More than White Twins Up to 2500 gms

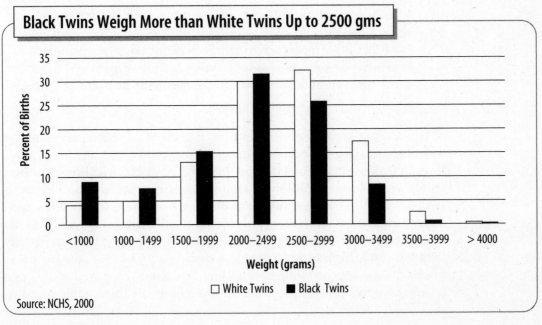

Source: NCHS, 2000

birth weight) and about 11 percent were *very low birth weight* (VLBW), or less than 1500 gms. Put another way, in 1977 twins were 15 percent of LBW infants; now they are 17 percent.

Twins average 5 pounds, 4 ounces (2,400) grams at 37 weeks (average gestational age at birth) and triplets average 4 pounds (1,800 grams) at 33 weeks. Data from 2000 show that 7 percent weigh less than 3 pounds, 5 ounces (1,500 grams).

The incidence of LBW is significantly lower in children born after IVF surrogacy than in those born after IVF for all births, single and multiple, because surrogates are fertile women.

The risk of early death increases as birth weight declines. Unfortunately, the rates of LBW and VLBW infants have been increasing since the 1980s; and twins make up about 12 percent of all infant deaths. During the first year after birth, about 25 percent of all VLBW babies die, compared with 2 percent of babies weighing more than 1,500 grams. Among the survivors with VLBW, 65 percent have severe problems after birth whereas only 0.03 percent of babies weighing more than 2,500 grams die in the first year.

Marsden Wagner, M.D., of the World Health Organization, stated in the *Birth Gazette* in 1989:

> Infant mortality is not a health problem: it is a social problem with health consequences. The first priority for lowering infant mortality in the U.S. is not more obstetricians or pediatricians or hospitals, not even prenatal clinics or well-baby clinics, but rather to provide more social and educational support to families with pregnant women and infants.

Dr. Wagner recommended that the United States focus on smoking, lack of social support, prenatal and postnatal paid maternity leave, other forms of maternity protection on the job, less obstetrical intervention, and increased use of midwives. Countries such as Sweden and Holland, with some of the lowest perinatal mortality and Caesarean rates, have large numbers of midwives involved in maternity care. In 2000, the United States ranked *twenty-fourth* in the world for perinatal mortality, falling in rank from twenty-second a decade ago. In 1988, the incidence of LBW babies in the United States was 7 percent compared with 3 percent in Sweden. Dr. Wagner was consulted for this third edition and regretfully agreed that nothing had improved. In 2000, the overall PTB rate was 12 percent.

Monozygotic twins, despite the fact that they are "identical," often show the greatest disparity in birth weight because of unequal placental function, the most extreme cases occurring with the feto-fetal transfusion syndrome (FFTS, discussed later in this chapter). Monozygotic twins with one chorion have the lowest birth weight. Even with two chorions, 25 percent of DCs have discordant growth, and 29 percent are below the fifth percentile for birth weight. Males usually weigh slightly more than females in twin births, and DZ pairs weigh more than MZ pairs.

The National Institute for Public Health in Japan compiled growth standards for multiples and found that boys were heavier than girls at the fiftieth percentile but quadruplet girls were smaller under 29 weeks yet larger above 30 weeks. For any duration of gestation, twins are born with lower birth weights than singletons, but most catch up by about age three.

TERMINOLOGY: Gestational Age and Weight

Preterm for singletons	Born before 37 weeks
Preterm for multiples	Born between 33 and 35 weeks
Very Preterm (VP)	Born between 29 and 32 weeks
Very early preterm (VEP)	Born between 25 and 28 weeks
Low birth weight (LBW)	Weighing less than 2,500 gms (5 lbs 8 oz)
Very low birth weight (VLBW)	Weighing less than 1,500 gms (3 lbs 5 oz)
Small for gestational age (SGA) Grade I	A 15 percent difference or more between twins
Small for gestational age (SGA) Grade II	A 25 percent difference or more between twins

Intrauterine Growth Restriction (IUGR) and Growth Discordance

One twin may grow more slowly than the other twin (discordant) or both may be growth retarded in comparison with normal rates. Differences in birth weight are usually expressed as a percentage of the weight of the larger twin. A difference of more than 15 percent is more likely to be associated with an infant who is considered *small for gestational age* (SGA). Weight discordance most commonly occurs in MZ twins as a result of FFTS. In DZ twins, some discordance can be expected from their different egg/sperm origins.

The importance of growth can be seen in the following ultrasound evaluation of twin pregnancies recommended by Blickstein. If a difference between the diameters of the babies' heads is more than 5 mm before the thirtieth week, abdominal circumference measurements are made. If the abdominal difference is more than 20 mm, the next step is to estimate the weight of each twin. If a difference of 15 percent or more is found, the discordance is classified as grade I (this occurs in 20 to 25 percent of twin pregnancies). If the difference is greater than 25 percent, it is classified as grade II. Four to 9 percent of LBW twins are grade II SGA and have a perinatal mortality rate almost two and a half times that of infants with smaller differences.

Intrauterine growth retardation (IUGR) is a major cause of stillbirth. Some researchers suggest that individual growth rather than differences between the twins is a better predictor of fetal problems because both twins may be affected by intrauterine growth retardation and the problem of low weight may go unnoticed.

A comparison of males and females and of small and appropriate-size newborns indicated increased risk for males and for infants who are SGA. The stresses associated with IUGR influence central nervous system organization and interfere with temperament development, according to Riese's research at the Louisville Twin Study. In 2001, Riese looked at full-term newborn twins with 15 percent to 47 percent weight differences and suggested that there may be a common cause for minor physical anomalies and discordant weight for twins. Previous research indicates that such twins may be at risk for behavioral problems.

Stress hormones (glucocorticoids) inhibit growth of babies, and negative emotional states are the primary risk factors for cardiovascular disease in adulthood; the restricted fetal growth is an early measurable effect. Opiates such as endorphins, which are released during emotional distress, are also associated with reduced fetal growth. Huttenen and Kearn in Finland showed that adults whose father died when they were in the uterus were more at risk for alcoholism, mental disease, and criminality than those who lost their father during the year following their births. Even the risk of dental cavities at age two is associated with a major maternal stress like bereavement during gestation.

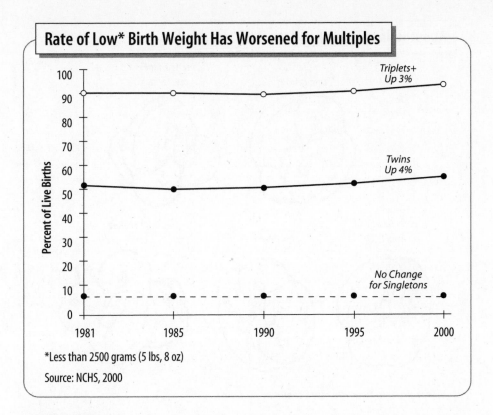

Rate of Low* Birth Weight Has Worsened for Multiples

*Triplets+
Up 3%*

*Twins
Up 4%*

*No Change
for Singletons*

*Less than 2500 grams (5 lbs, 8 oz)

Source: NCHS, 2000

Presentation

Headfirst (vertex) is the easiest way to be born. Babies who present differently may have difficulty. *Breech* presentation, in which a lower part of the body comes first, occurs in about 40 percent of multiple births compared with 3 percent of singleton births. *Transverse lie*, in which the baby's body is horizontal in the pelvis, is very rare, as the uterus accommodates a baby better in the vertical position. A tranverse presentation must be turned to be delivered vaginally (*external version*); otherwise, a Caesarean section is necessary.

Twins present headfirst less than 50 percent of the time. The first twin (Twin A) is in a nonvertex position 20 percent of the time. One is vertex and one breech in about 40 percent of twin births. More commonly, the Twin B is breech. Both present breech about 8 percent of the time. In a small percentage of births, the second twin lies transverse or turns after the birth of the first to present with an arm or a leg or both (*compound* presentation), requiring the obstetrician to turn that baby either exter-

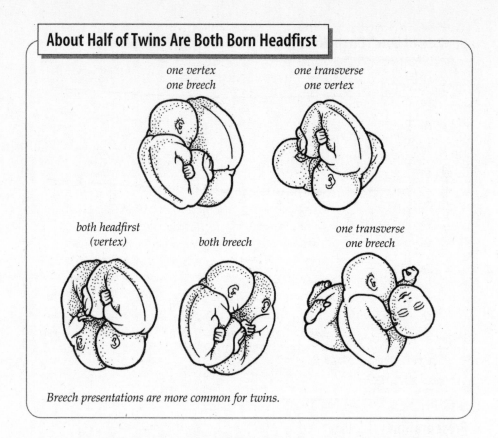

About Half of Twins Are Both Born Headfirst

one vertex
one breech

one transverse
one vertex

both headfirst
(vertex)

both breech

one transverse
one breech

Breech presentations are more common for twins.

nally or internally. Some researchers have found that the larger the difference in birth weight, the greater the likelihood that the heavier twin will be born first. Larger babies do well regardless of method of delivery, whereas LBW infants are much more vulnerable to trauma, even with a Caesarean section.

A breech birth can be hazardous, although some are born spontaneously. Cord prolapse occurs more often with breech presentation: there is room for the lifeline to slip down when the baby's head is not against the open cervix.

The feet or buttocks of a breech baby are delivered first, then the attendant brings down the arms and the head follows last. Sometimes the first twin is delivered vaginally but a Caesarean section is done for the delivery of the second, especially if the obstetrician is not skilled in turning the baby (internal version) or in assisting a vaginal breech birth.

Unfortunately, residents in obstetrics and gynecology in recent years have had little or no training in the manual skills to handle these versions or different presentations and increasingly a Caesarean section is scheduled for such presentations, even for singletons.

Cord Problems

Accidents with the cord, such as compression and trauma, are more likely with a multiple pregnancy, particularly in the rare situation where both twins are in the same sac and the cords can actually become entangled (braiding). Sometimes the cord of one baby is around the neck of the other, and it must be slipped over the head and left intact during delivery. Only 1 to 2 percent of twins share both the chorion and amnion (MCMA) and up to half do not survive, although this rate improves with biweekly ultrasound monitoring and nonstress testing.

Another problem with the cord — velamentous insertion — occurs six times more often in multiple pregnancy. In this condition, the cord is inserted into the membranes instead of directly into the placenta, and bleeding can occur if fetal blood vessels are torn when the membranes rupture. Vaginal bleeding and fluctuations in the fetal heart rate are symptoms of this condition that can be confirmed with ultrasound. In fact, ultrasound evaluation must include implantation sites and cord insertions.

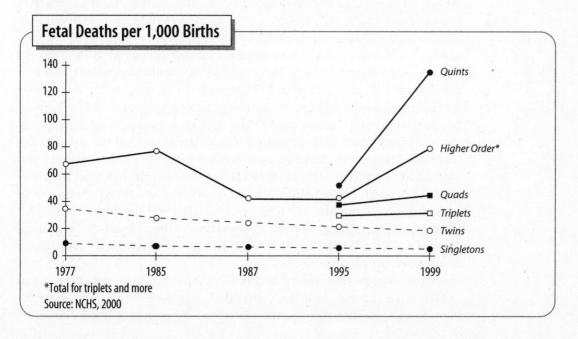

Fetal Deaths per 1,000 Births

*Total for triplets and more
Source: NCHS, 2000

Complications Unique to Multiples

Monochorionic (MC) Placenta

One-fifth of twins share one chorion (MC) and they have five times the rate of late miscarriage and perinatal mortality as DC twins. There is an increased risk of genetic and structural anomalies that require invasive testing and management of any discordant abnormality. About 80 percent of MC placentas have vascular connections between the twins, but each pattern is unique. This results in a wide variety of types, degrees, and timing of clinical problems. The dangers of the MC twin placenta are due mainly to the structure of the blood vessels between the twin cords across the single placenta. If one cord is central and in the best spot, then the other cord is placed in a location more peripheral and less favorable (often velamentous), leading to IUGR and reduced amniotic fluid. This is *not* the same as FFTS, where *simultaneously* the smaller twin has too little fluid (oligohydramnios) and the other twin has too much (polyhydramnios). A twin who is fixed in position against the uterine wall with inadequate fluid is known as the "stuck twin."

Feto-fetal Transfusion Syndrome (FFTS)

About 70 percent of MZ twins are MC. Although the placenta typically manipulates maternal physiology for fetal benefit, about 20 percent of monochorionic diamnionic (MODI/MCDA) twins will share blood vessels in such a way that the amount and direction of blood flow favors the larger recipient twin, at the expense of the donor twin. This FFTS syndrome (previously known as Twin to Twin Transfusion Syndrome — TTTS) can occur in triplets, even trizygotic ones, as reported by Pons in France, where two babies died in the uterus. It is important for parents to understand that the babies are normal; the abnormalities arise in the placenta. Frequently, there are connections between the circulations, but as long as there is equilibrium, FFTS does not result. Unequal distribution of blood and basic nutrients occurs when there is, typically, a one-way shunt from the higher pressure in the artery of the umbilical system of one twin (donor) to the lower pressure in the vein of the umbilical system in the other twin (recipient). Many other types of connections may coexist as well.

Ultrasound can measure blood flow in the umbilical cord and fetus to detect FFTS during pregnancy if different growth rates arouse suspicion. In the absence of abnormalities, if the difference in head diameters is more than 5 mm before the thirtieth week, the cause is probably this syndrome. Ultrasound can reveal discrepancies in the size of amniotic sacs, fetal movements, the size and number of umbilical vessels, as well as edema or congestive heart failure. If the third type of twinning (see Chapter 2) is more common than has been thought, FFTS could be explained by the genetic differences between the two fetuses and a possible reaction from their immune systems.

This syndrome explains the difference in size, weight, and color at birth of twins who are genetically identical. The recipient twin receives extra blood, becomes larger, generates more amniotic fluid, and suffers from circulatory overload and heart failure. The donor twin is smaller, suffers from growth retardation and reduced amniotic fluid, and may die from severe anemia. There are five stages of the syndrome beginning with the imbalance of amniotic fluid between the twins and ending with death.

The reported incidence of the syndrome varies, depending on the interpretations of the placentas and differences in hemoglobin and birth weight. At least 6,000 babies are affected by FFTS every year in the United States and approximately 80 to 100 percent of them will die if untreated. Fifteen to 17 percent of the perinatal mortality of twins is due to this syndrome, which is diagnosed between sixteen to twenty-three weeks. A Japanese study of 133 MZ twins found that in one-quarter of the pregnancies, one twin died from FFTS. Eight of the surviving 33 babies had brain damage and other abnormalities. Machin in Canada gave a rate of 23 percent FFTS for stillborn MC twins.

High amniotic fluid pressures due to the excessive fluid build-up (polyhydramnios) cause preterm labor. Therefore, tapping the excess fluid off at intervals (serial amniocenteses or amnioreduction) can prolong the pregnancy and increase the chance of survival for both babies. Removing up to a quart or more of excess fluid is indicated when the abdominal distention and chest restriction become too uncomfortable for the mother. This helps prevent preterm labor and rupture of the membranes. Amnioreduction is the least invasive and may work (success is indicated by the bladder filling of the donor twin); but if it does not, ablation of the shunts in the placental vessels can be attempted to prevent backflow and/or exsanguination. This is done with a laser (laser coagulation/LC) or with radiofrequency (RFA). Another option is selective termination (sacrificing one of the twins), but that is very risky and the circulations still must be separated.

Even though I am a nurse, I didn't realize that I would have to carry my dead baby inside me until the living baby was born.

Sometimes the death of the donor twin is accompanied by vaginal bleeding, sudden abdominal pain, and leakage of amniotic fluid without the onset of labor. In a pregnancy with polyhydramnios, such signs followed by the mother's reduced girth and increased urine output strongly suggest the demise of one twin and the resolution of the syndrome in the other. Ultrasound can confirm this. When death occurs in early pregnancy, the surviving twin grows to term uneventfully in most cases. The prognosis is less favorable when a twin dies in the latter half of pregnancy; long-term problems in survivors are cardiac and neurological.

There is a special Web site for expectant parents whose babies have this syndrome: www.tttsfoundation.org. The Foundation advocates weekly ultrasounds from 16 weeks until delivery of the babies.

Twin Reversed Arterial Perfusion (TRAP)

This syndrome occurs in 1 percent of MZ pregnancies — one twin is without a heart. The "pump" twin perfuses the circulation of the co-twin. At least 50 percent of the "pump" or donor twins die from congestive heart failure or very early preterm delivery as a consequence of the polyhydramnios. This is the only MC disorder in which a simple ablation of cord or fetal vessels is sufficient because no blood from the twin without a heart perfuses the placenta.

Delivery of the Second Twin

Second twins are not invariably smaller, despite common belief, unless there is a large discrepancy between the babies' weights.

If MZ twins share membranes and placental circulation, birth is riskier and the second twin is delivered immediately should bleeding occur. Another reason for haste in delivering the second twin is to reduce the exposure to the mother's anesthesia. Anesthesia itself leads to complications, such as the need for forceps or vacuum assistance when contractions decrease.

There are reports of intervals of days, weeks, and even months between the births of twins (see Chapter 19). Intervals of an hour or so are acceptable for term babies if the second twin is monitored and the vital signs are stable. Most multiples today, however, are born together by Caesarean section, although no benefit has been shown from surgical delivery.

Maternal Complications

Anemia

Anemia is a condition in which the blood contains a reduced number (volume) of red blood cells or insufficient hemoglobin (which carries oxygen to the tissues) within the red cells. Anemic people suffer from fatigue, faintness, shortness of breath, dizziness, and tingling of the extremities. Exertion increases these symptoms because anemic blood brings insufficient oxygen to the tissues. Typically the skin, mucous membranes in the gums and inner eyelids are pale, and the gums and tongue may be inflamed. Digestion may be poor because of malnutrition, which can lead to irritability. Many women are anemic before pregnancy, especially if they have had inadequate nutrition or heavy menstrual periods. Smoking makes anemia worse.

Although anemia is commonly defined as an iron or folic acid deficiency, it is related to a lack of many nutrients in the diet. All essential vitamins and minerals must be in balance to facilitate absorption of the nutrients. (For a complete discussion of nutrition, see Chapter 8.)

Iron is essential for the formation of adequate hemoglobin. Blood tests measure the level of iron by determining the *hematocrit*, the percentage of red blood cells in the blood (the normal range is 36 to 47 percent) or the hemoglobin levels (the normal range for females is 12 to 16 gm per 100 ml). During pregnancy, both the mother and offspring make greater than usual demands for oxygen, which is transported by hemoglobin.

Several factors decrease levels of hemoglobin in pregnancy; therefore, the hematocrit reading is more reliable. In twin pregnancy, for instance, the mother's blood volume is greatly enlarged (by about 1,500 ml, or about 3 pints) to accommodate two placentas. An increase in the plasma component, which carries the red blood cells in the mother's blood, brings about a physiological condition called *hemodilution*. This is desirable and the hemoglobin levels are adequate but less concentrated in the necessarily expanded blood volume. Hemoglobin in twin pregnancies drops to an average of 10.4 g/dl by twenty weeks. The "thinner" blood can be pumped more easily in compensation for the increased work of the heart. According to Odent, a failure of the hemoglobin concentration to fall below 10.5 g/dl indicates an increased risk of LBW, PTB, and preeclampsia. This "anemia" reflects an ideal maternal adaptation to the needs of the multiples.

Iron deficiency is the most common type of anemia. It is cheaper to prescribe iron supplements than to determine whether someone is actually anemic; but they can do more harm than good. Supplemental iron can be harmful to the bowels and digestive system and it can inhibit the absorption of zinc. Excreted iron turns the stool a blackish color and can cause constipation, already likely in a multiple pregnancy. The most commonly prescribed item in prenatal clinics, it is part of the nocebo effect because its prescription suggests to a woman that her body is malfunctioning.

Women pregnant with twins are told they are likely to develop anemia, although there is no agreed-upon definition of it. Nevertheless, in 2000, it was reported as the third most frequent medical risk factor in all pregnancies (24 per 1,000). A group in Italy stated that anemia is increased in a multiple pregnancy by 40 percent. In contrast, the Scottish Twins Study found no difference in the incidence of anemia between twin and singleton pregnancies when they looked at hemoglobin concentration.

Folic acid, like many other nutrients, is often insufficient in the average diet and, like iron, is depleted from maternal supplies during pregnancy. The protein construction of red blood cells depends on folic acid. Deficiency of this nutrient in animals has been associated with an increase in malformations of the skeletal, circulatory, and nervous systems. Recent research into the prevention of spinal defects with this B vitamin gained widespread publicity, and prenatal vitamins contain additional amounts of folic acid (which is also found in green leafy vegetables, hence its name). Many foods are now fortified with folic acid, which in itself has increased twinning!

A complete blood count will reveal whether the blood cells are small and iron deficient or large and pale from insufficient folic acid in the diet, and appropriate nutritional remedies can be prescribed.

Hypertension (High Blood Pressure)

In a blood pressure reading, the upper or first figure is systolic pressure — the highest pressure attained when the lower chambers of the heart contract to pump blood out to the body. This pressure is lowest during sleep and varies in response to exercise, emotion, and anxiety. The lower or second value is diastolic pressure — the momentary resting pressure during the phase when the heart muscle relaxes. Since the heart actually rests more than it works, diastolic pressure is more important, although smaller changes are observed than with systolic pressure.

Pregnancy-induced hypertension (PIH) is defined by obstetricians as a reading of 140/90 (measured in millimeters of mercury — mm Hg), or a rise of 30/15 over usual readings, taken on two separate occasions with at least an interval of one day. Danger signs of hypertension include headache, visual disturbances, and vomiting. This was the most frequently reported risk factor in the United States for all pregnancies in the year 2000 (39 per 1,000 live births).

Informed obstetricians now realize that a rise in blood pressure in a multiple pregnancy is to be expected. This is functionally associated with extra blood volume and the circulatory demands of extra placentas. One study found that women carrying twins had a lower diastolic pressure in mid-pregnancy but that in the last three months it rose by 50 percent. The conclusion was that a diastolic pressure of 90–95 (accompanied by 20 percent protein or less in the urine) was probably not pathological in a multiple pregnancy. Swelling is the body's way of accommodating the increase in blood volume that is normal in pregnancy and pronounced with multiples. A first-time mother expecting twins has about 18 pints of fluid, depending on the weight of her babies. Mothers of higher-order multiples usually swell even more, although I know of one mother of quadruplets who had no swelling, no proteinuria (see below), and a consistent blood pressure of only 120/80.

The blood volume and nutritional status of a pregnant woman must be assessed before making a diagnosis of hypertension. Calcium is an important part of the diet and, according to the Cochrane Review, can help reduce high blood pressure in pregnancy just like magnesium helps leg cramps. These minerals can be obtained from a good diet because supplements, unless customized and integrated, create imbalances and additional problems.

Several studies confirm that simple gestational hypertension is followed by good perinatal outcomes.

Precautions with the Treatment of High Blood Pressure

Blacks have more high blood pressure, and although many black teenagers have already developed the condition and will continue to have it the rest of their lives, they still require the use of (sea) salt to taste — since their blood volumes must expand, too, as pregnancy advances.

Obese women may be incorrectly diagnosed as hypertensive when a standard-size blood pressure cuff is used to take a reading. When the cuff is too small, additional pressure on the mother's arm reads on the meter as elevated blood pressure. Using a larger cuff prevents this error.

The Importance of Expanded Blood Volume

Weight gain and swelling are normal physiological adaptations to pregnancy, and increase with each multiple in the set. Low protein levels, from inadequate nutrition, cause water to leak out into the tissues from the blood circulation. This condition is worsened if salt is restricted. Diuretics (water pills), if prescribed, actually drive out more fluid. The result is an even more dangerously reduced blood volume that can trigger labor. The woman continues to retain fluid, causing a *sudden* increase in maternal weight and accompanying swelling and puffiness. Blood pressure rises markedly in an attempt to meet the demands of all the organs, particularly the placentas, on the reduced circulation. Women who exhibit these symptoms may be further maltreated with amphetamines to suppress appetite or antihypertensive and sedative drugs to lower their blood pressure. All this medication reaches the babies. If this course of events continues, the woman's urinary output will fall along with her blood volume, and kidney damage may result.

The "roll-over test" can provide information on the blood volume during pregnancy (although false signs can occur). If an expectant mother's blood pressure is lowered when she rolls from her back to her side, the improved reading in that position indicates that the blood volume is subnormal.

Many studies have shown that diets with adequate protein to meet the needs of pregnancy, with salt to taste, can prevent or reverse this syndrome. Sufficient calories must also be added in the diet; otherwise the body will burn the protein building-blocks for fuel, wasting their nutrient value.

Preeclampsia

Insufficient vascularization of the placenta means that there is inadequate blood flow in the later months. Poor development during the critical first four months leads to complex compensatory mechanisms that create the symptoms of the syndrome preeclampsia.

Odent suggests that preeclampsia should be seen as a disease of antioxidant inadequacy, and studies have confirmed this by inducing the disease in rats. Antioxidants are important for certain fatty acids (explained in Chapter 8) and because the brain is 60 percent fat. Arachidonic acid and an omega-3 fatty acid called DHA (docosahexaenoic acid) are the two most important fatty acids. Even when the total levels of these fatty acids fall, the level of DHA remains stable. The price of that stability is a very low level of a parent molecule called EPA (eicosapentaenoic acid), which is the precursor of the whole family of prostaglandins. This imbalance leads to symptoms described below.

According to the most common definitions, preeclampsia is the combination of high blood pressure and the presence of more than 300 mg of protein in the urine per 24 hours (unrelated to urinary tract infection). There are usually other detectable metabolic imbalances as well. Preeclampsia is classified as being mild or severe depending on how high the blood pressure is and the presence of other symptoms. For mild preeclampsia, patients may be watched at home or in the hospital. An intravenous drip of magnesium sulfate (Epsom salts) is used to prevent seizures in patients with severe preeclampsia or they may be delivered immediately. Magnesium sulfate does not treat the disease but is often used when transporting or delivering patients and is sometimes continued for twenty-four hours after delivery.

Instead of this drug therapy, you can (1) increase the amounts of essential nutrients available by consuming sea fish for more omega-3 fatty acids and antioxidants; (2) boost the manufacture of these fatty acids with supplements of zinc, magnesium, and calcium; (3) reduce the amount of transfatty acids, which are artificial molecules found in junk fats (margarine, french fries, fast foods); and (4) reduce stress hormones such as cortisol, which also block the synthesis of the desirable fatty acids.

Eclampsia

The eclamptic patient develops seizures as seen in epilepsy — a life-threatening situation for both mother and baby. Seizures are most likely to occur during and immediately after delivery. Eclampsia is caused by an extremely high blood pressure in combination with fluid retention and vascular problems in the brain. The incidence of this condition declined in the year 2000 (3 per 1,000 of all pregnant women).

A Confusion of Terminology and Symptoms

Toxemia/preeclampsia/eclampsia/HELLP (TPEH) is a combination of symptoms that typically occur after the twentieth week of pregnancy and is not the same as PIH. There are many reasons why blood pressure may be elevated in pregnancy and these need to be differentiated. Thomas Brewer, M.D., explains that metabolic toxemia of late pregnancy (MTLP) is not the commonly believed "toxemia" syndrome, but a distinct entity caused by malnutrition, in particular, protein deficiency leading to liver dysfunction.

The correct medical term for toxemia ("toxic blood") is preeclampsia. The triad of symptoms is: (1) loss of more than 300 mg of protein in the urine in twenty-four hours, (2) high blood pressure, (3) swelling anywhere on the body resulting in *sudden* weight gain, and (4) hyperreflexia. This level of proteinuria indicates kidney problems and shifts "PIH" into the category of "preeclampsia." However, many doctors do not make this distinction between PIH and preeclampsia and use the terms interchangeably. Preeclampsia has been associated with PIH because studies have linked preeclampsia with PIH! The common tendency to confuse preeclampsia with gestational hypertension — which is not associated with proteinuria — is an obstacle to understanding the disease. The three cardinal signs are checked at every prenatal visit because if untreated, seizures, coma, and even death can result. Headaches, nausea, vomiting, changes in vision (spots), and true proteinuria are warning signs.

According to Odent, preeclampsia is probably overdiagnosed by using dipsticks to define proteinuria; and Brewer points out that proteinuria is often from a urinary tract infection, which occurs readily because of hormonal dilatation of the ureters (the tubes between the bladder and kidneys), in addition to pressure from the uterus. Even vaginal infections may give rise to a misleading diagnosis of proteinuria unless one obtains a "clean-catch" urine specimen.

If no protein is found in the urine when the blood pressure is elevated, the condition is classified as mild, but considered more serious if proteinuria, hypertension, and hyperreflexia are present. Diuretics and dietary restriction (typically low salt, low protein, low calorie diets), bed rest, sedatives, and preterm induction of labor for women without protein in their urine are all misplaced, ineffective, and harmful. A mother of quads in France who delivered a surviving set in 1974 developed such serious problems with a salt-restricted diet that her case became the subject of an article in a medical journal.

However, some obstetricians make a reflex diagnosis of one or more of the TPEH syndrome whenever one or more of the "classic" symptoms are present. A mother's blood pressure may be high because she's not eating well — not having enough salt, fluids, or protein to expand her blood volume as needed for pregnancy. Anxiety or "white coat hypertension" can be easily brought on by the nocebo effect. Physical examinations, laboratory testing, hospital admission, and being evaluated for high blood pressure can all raise blood pressure. If the liver is functioning normally and the blood volume is expanded, TPEH is not present.

In 1985, Brewer wrote in his text, *Metabolic Toxemia of Late Pregnancy: A Disease of Malnutrition:*

> In the last fifteen years obstetricians have narrowly focused on the blood pressure of the pregnant woman as being of central concern regardless of her nutritional metabolic status, liver function, blood volume and placental function. If the diastolic blood pressure rises 15 or 20 mm Hg or the systolic rises 20–30 mm Hg, a diagnosis of "pregnancy-induced hypertension" (PIH) is made. All "PIH" is then "managed" the same as if every hypertensive pregnant woman were in jeopardy of convulsions, brain hemorrhage, abruption of the placenta, fetal death, etc.

The HELLP syndrome was first described in the medical literature by Weinstein in the early eighties. The acronym stands for "hemolysis, elevated liver enzymes, low platelets." It is characterized by liver compromise during or after pregnancy, complicated by hypertension and/or preeclampsia. *Hemolysis* means "destruction of red blood cells" and this may cause anemia. Elevated liver enzymes indicate liver damage; and these patients may have pain under the ribs on the right side due to liver swelling. The low platelets occasionally cause bleeding/clotting problems. Feedback from mothers of supertwins indicates that sometimes severe itching may precede this condition (and also the rare condition of acute fatty liver of pregnancy).

About 15 percent of women with preeclampsia will develop this triad of symptoms diagnosed by blood tests for clotting factors, platelet count, liver function, and uric acid. Placental malfunction means malnutrition and possible growth restriction of the babies. In some severe cases, reduced oxygen flow to the fetus (asphyxia) can cause cerebral damage or even death. Blood clots form in maternal blood vessels and can lead to hemorrhage. Besides the liver, other maternal organs such as the kidneys and blood vessels are affected. In severe cases, death results for 1 to 3 percent of mothers and 20 to 35 percent of infants.

Nevertheless, as some French researchers commented, "its precise physiopathological mechanism . . . is still not clearly established." Therefore, treatment remains symptomatic and associated with the treatment of toxemia. Therapies have included low-dose aspirin, calcium supplements, and corticosteroids. A "magic bullet" approach comes too late in the chain of events and ignores the preventive role of optimal nutrition with adequate essential fatty acids.

Nutritional Prevention of TEPH

Since 1929, the nutritional theory has been advanced and TEPH has been eradicated in some centers by thorough and consistent prenatal nutritional counseling. Under ten years of Brewer's guidance, the prenatal clinics in Contra Costa County, California, saw a drop in the incidence of LBW babies from 14 percent to 3 percent and there was not a single case of TEPH. The approach was simply improving the diets of low-income patients. Similarly, Agnes Higgins, a nutritionist at the Montreal Diet Dispensary, showed that for as little as $125 per pregnancy (in the 1970s), the Canadian government could supplement poor women's diets with adequate calories, protein, and other nutrients. Interestingly, the outcome of these births at Higgins's hospital was the same as for private patients at the same hospital and significantly better than the Canadian average. Thus, Higgins showed how to break some effects of the poverty cycle in pregnancy a quarter-century ago.

Inadequate nutrition is not a problem just of low-income groups. Unbalanced and unhealthy diets can be found in the wealthiest families. Often today women work very hard and skip meals, or eat unhealthy snacks on the run as part of their busy, demanding lives.

Santema et al. in the Netherlands found the incidence of preeclampsia was similar in twin (6 percent) and singleton pregnancies (6.5 percent), without a difference in severity or in the occurrence of the HELLP syndrome. They concluded that in twin pregnancy, the incidence of high blood pressure *without* protein in the urine was increased, but *not* preeclampsia *with* proteinuria. Having lived in the Netherlands, I would propose that this is because the Dutch have a more active lifestyle, better nutrition, and a common-sense approach to pregnancy and birth (the majority of births in some areas takes place with midwives at home), followed by domestic help for eight days, supported by government and private health insurance.

Sibai et al. in Tennessee compared women with twin and singleton pregnancies. They found higher rates of gestational hypertension in mothers of twins, too. In addition, there were higher rates of preterm delivery at both less than 37 weeks (51 percent versus 6 percent) and less than 35 weeks (18 percent versus 2 percent.) They also found higher rates of SGA infants (15 percent versus 7 percent). Moreover, when outcomes associated with preeclampsia were compared, women with twin gestations had significantly higher rates of preterm delivery at less than 37 weeks gestation (67 percent versus 20 percent) and less than 35 weeks (35 percent versus 6 percent) and placental abruption (5 percent versus 0.07 percent). In contrast, among women with twin pregnancies, those whose blood pressure remained normal had more *adverse* neonatal outcomes than did those in whom hypertensive complications developed! This observation would support the theory that the heart has to work harder to drive more blood through more placentas, especially with the babies' increasing growth. Where this doesn't happen, the outcome is worse for the babies. Good nutrition allows the blood volume to expand to prevent these complications.

In 2001, Huang looked at 343 cases of twins and one set of triplets in China and found a much lower incidence of PIH — 6 percent. Only 1 percent was complicated with eclampsia. Despite a very low rate of complications (HELLP syndrome of 0.03 percent, one maternal death, and a perinatal mortality of 7.18 per 1,000), the Caesarean section rate was a high 67 percent.* The conclusion was that the incidences of PIH and perinatal death can be reduced by improved prenatal monitoring for prevention, early diagnosis, and treatment. In China, where fewer people own cars or eat fast foods, people are physically active and well-nourished with whole foods.

Physicians monitor, diagnose, and treat, but mothers must commit to prevention.

---

*The overall Caesarean rate in China currently is about 50 percent.

Focus on Fatty Acids and Fish

Essential fatty acids are needed to support vital metabolic functions. Odent described preeclampsia as a maternal-fetal conflict in a 2001 article in the peer-reviewed on-line journal *MedGenMed*. The association of preeclampsia with both high and low birth weight challenges the current belief that reduced uteroplacental blood flow is the single problem in preeclampsia. Preeclampsia, Odent suggests, may be understood as "the price some human beings must pay for having a large brain when they are more or less separated from the sea food chain." The spectacular brain growth spurt during the second half of fetal life is a specifically human trait. Sixty percent of the brain is made of fat, which means that the main nutritional needs are fatty acids. This concept explains the increased risk of preeclampsia in twin pregnancies. By the same token, a case of intrauterine death of a twin was followed by the resolution of the symptoms of preeclampsia: as nutritional needs decreased, the pregnancy continued safely for a further seven weeks.

It is remarkable that the only study that demonstrated highly significant effects of fish oil supplementation on the risk of preeclampsia was conducted in London by the People's League of Health during 1938–1939, when the rates of severe "toxemia" were around 6 percent. This controlled trial was saved from oblivion by Olsen and Secher. The authors randomized 5,644 women to receive or not receive a dietary supplement containing vitamins, minerals, and halibut liver oil from about week twenty of pregnancy. A 31 percent reduction in the incidence of preeclampsia was seen in first-time mothers. Interestingly, no significant effect of treatment was seen with regard to the incidence of hypertension in the absence of edema and proteinuria.

Odent recommends eating ocean fish rich in the fatty acids and minerals that are essential nutrients for the brain (iodine, selenium, zinc) to prevent preeclampsia. Iodine is a major component of thyroid hormones, which are also needed for brain development. This dietary advice conforms with the reduced incidence of preeclampsia in areas where fish is consumed (Iceland, Scandinavia) and the results Odent has observed after encouraging pregnant women to eat sea fish.

Current Research

Trials are taking place in Denver and Los Angeles using omega-3 fatty acids, and Richard Adler, M.D., has proposed a double-blind study of a population of women at high risk for PTB who will be provided with a daily dose of 2.5 grams of molecularly distilled omega-3 essential fatty acids beginning with the thirtieth week of gestation and continuing until delivery.

Researchers at MacGee Women's Research Institute in Pittsburgh are evaluating the role of homocysteine in preterm labor. They have observed a substantial increase in homocysteine in women with preeclampsia compared to women with uncomplicated pregnancies or women with transient hypertension in pregnancy. Methionine is one of the essential amino acids obtained in food. (Animal proteins contain greater amounts of methionine than do plant proteins.) A by-product of methionine metabolism is homocysteine, which is a marker for B vitamin deficiency, especially folic acid (a lack of which has been linked to neural tube defects). High levels of homocysteine are associated with heart disease and osteoporosis. Homocysteine is normally decreased during pregnancy by increased kidney clearance.

Gestational Diabetes (GD)

Sugars and starches in our diet break down into glucose that circulates in the blood or is stored in the liver and muscles. The pancreas secretes insulin to drive glucose into the cells, where it can be used. Hormones in pregnancy reduce the effect of insulin to allow high levels of circulating glucose, which is needed for fetal growth and development, especially during rest at night — which is why blood sugar levels are lower in the morning. It is normal for a pregnant woman's blood sugar levels to rise after eating despite normal or higher levels of insulin.

This "diagnosis" of GD often means a pregnant woman with no symptoms (increase in thirst, amount and frequency of urination, fatigue, and vaginal yeast infections) has laboratory test results similar to those of nonpregnant diabetics. By definition, this "diabetes" ceases when the pregnancy is over. (Clinical diabetes that is diagnosed prenatally and persists after birth is not GD.) It is more likely in women who have a family history of diabetes or who were more than 120 percent of their ideal body weight before pregnancy. In the year 2000, it was the second most frequently reported risk factor for all pregnancies in the United States — 3 percent. The incidence is supposedly two to three times more in mothers of multiples who also show a slower rate of glucose dispersal after a glucose load than mothers of singletons.

Some pregnant women will have blood glucose levels in the true diabetic range either because they had diabetes prior to pregnancy and hadn't been diagnosed or because the metabolic stress of pregnancy was enough to tip them over into the true diabetic range.

Gestational diabetes does not share the risk factors of either type of diabetes. Type I diabetes can cause congenital defects or even death in early pregnancy, but GD manifests after the first trimester when such risks have passed. Type I requires daily insulin whereas Type II is common in overweight people and can often be controlled with diet and exercise. Either type that has existed for a long time before pregnancy can cause damaged blood vessels, high blood pressure, and kidney complications. This is not the case with GD. However, all types of diabetes can mean a larger than normal baby (macrosomia) but multiples rarely achieve normal birth weight!

Henci Goer, author of *The Thinking Woman's Guide to a Better Birth*, points out that GD fails to fulfill any of the criteria for a diagnosis and treatment of a disease. No threshold, observes Goer, has ever been found for the onset or increase of fetal complications below the diagnostic levels of true diabetes. Yet women identified as gestational diabetics will be prescribed restrictive diets, including reduced calorie diets, and have frequent testing for blood-sugar levels, and possibly insulin injections. They will probably have repeated tests to evaluate fetal well-being and an ultrasound scan to estimate fetal weights. These women may have labor induced or even have a planned Caesarean. After birth, a baby may receive heel pricks to measure blood sugar. Based on the results, the baby may be given bottles of sugar water or formula or be removed to the nursery for observation.

Antepartum Hemorrhage and Placental Abruption

Bleeding during the first trimester may be of no consequence. Sometimes there is spotting during implantation in the uterus or from the cervix during intercourse. In contrast, third trimester bleeding can be very serious if associated with placenta previa (0.3 percent of all pregnancies) or abruption (0.6 percent). These conditions are more frequent in older mothers.

Bleeding in pregnancy can result from trauma, or from the placenta lying partially or completely over the cervix (previa) or from its preterm separation from the wall of the uterus (abruption). Bleeding and pain is moderate to severe. Abruption has been linked to malnutrition and smoking; it is rarely seen in well-nourished expectant mothers, and while some studies report an incidence of 13 percent of twin pregnancies, or double the risk compared to a single pregnancy, other studies have found no increase.

Postpartum Hemorrhage (PPH)

This life-threatening event is rarely seen in well-nourished, healthy mothers. Bleeding can occur when the fetal blood vessels are torn or when the membranes rupture from velamentous insertion of the cord. This cord pathology is more common in twins (7 percent) and very common in triplets, and increases the risk of postpartum hemorrhage. It is more frequent in fused placentas — 60 percent of pregnancies with FFTS versus 19 percent of those without the syndrome. However, multiples do not always increase the hazard; there was a case reported in *Lancet* in 1904 of quadruplets born at six and a half months gestational age with no hemorrhage, even though the mother suffered two severe postpartum hemorrhages after two prior singleton pregnancies.

Peripartum Cardiomyopathy (PPCM)

This is a rare form of congestive heart failure that develops in late pregnancy or during the first five months after delivery. It is characterized by a damaged and weakened heart muscle and generally the left ventricle becomes enlarged and unable to pump efficiently. The disorder, of which the cause is unknown, affects approximately 4 out of 10,000 women, most commonly after age thirty. Risk factors include obesity, having a personal or family history of cardiac disorders such as myocarditis, use of certain medications, smoking, alcoholism, multiple pregnancies, being black, and being malnourished. There is a 75 percent chance of survival and a 50 percent chance of a normal lifestyle.

It is often misdiagnosed because symptoms may include difficulty breathing (standing or lying down), fatigue, palpitations, and edema (all of which are common in pregnancy, especially multiple pregnancy), arrhythmia, chest pain, and cough. If you suffer from any of these symptoms during or after pregnancy, and are not recovering from treatments for other complications that may mimic such symptoms, insist on an echocardiogram. If you are refused, seek a second opinion. Prompt treatment is essential to recovery. It includes medications for arrhythmia and high blood pressure, diuretics to remove excess body fluid, and strict rest.

> I found it impossible to be a dedicated new mother at this time because I had to rest and recover. I, as well as many other PPCM survivors, felt robbed of the opportunity to bond with our children at the beginning, but we now realize you can spend the rest of your life bonding.

Karen Berner describes her experience:

I couldn't even think about holding my twin girls after the C-Section. I was so short of breath, panicked and shaking that my only thoughts were "I need to sit up in order to catch my breath." Halfway through the night, I still felt horrible and my ob/gyn was called back in and immediately consulted with a pulmonary specialist and cardiologist. I was diagnosed with PPCM and given a 50–75 percent chance of survival.

My twin daughters were cared for by a mix of family members who came to our rescue. I was devastated that I couldn't be home with them. I stayed on in the cardiac care unit for two weeks.

Massive amounts of fluid needed to be drained from my body, my heart rate was high and irregular, the oxygen level in my blood was low, and I was too weak even to stand up. My husband would come to the hospital at night and lie next to me in the single hospital bed and sleep. That we slept well in that way is testament to the exhaustion that consumed us.

I was finally released from the hospital on the same medications but I needed to sleep at least half the day for quite a while. We bit the financial bullet and hired a full-time nanny, who is now as much a part of our family as our daughters.

Subsequent echocardiograms showed gradual yet steady improvement and today I am fortunate to be considered recovered, although some limitations remain. I still take medication for high blood pressure, watch my salt intake (for fluid retention), should not lift heavy weights, and find that going to high elevation is a difficult transition.

I am still uncomfortable with the fact that I was told I can't have more children. Although I am certain I will not have more children, it makes me sad to have it stated so strongly when I haven't yet said it to myself.

Maternal Preexisting Conditions

A woman already suffering from certain disorders, such as circulatory (heart or kidney) disease, before conceiving multiples will definitely be considered high risk (which means the *potential* for something to go wrong) and will be very carefully monitored during the pregnancy. She will likely have a scheduled Caesarean section.

Smoking

The harmful effects of cigarette smoking on general health are well known. Smoking impairs protein and carbohydrate metabolism and poses an even greater hazard if the mother's diet is poor. By interfering with placental function, smoking can cause miscarriage and disturb fetal respiration and metabolism, and it results in offspring who weigh less than those of nonsmoking mothers. Nicotine narrows blood vessels, which limits the amount of oxygen reaching the developing organs. Carbon monoxide, another compound in smoke, also reduces the amount of oxygen carried by the blood.

Women who weigh less than 95 pounds at the beginning of pregnancy and who smoke during pregnancy are at substantially increased risk for delivering LBW offspring. In the year 2000, the incidence of LBW babies born to smokers was two-thirds higher than that for nonsmokers. Twelve percent of the births to smokers (compared with 7 percent of the births to nonsmokers) were LBW. Smoking is linked to PTB and increases the chance of fetal death by 50 percent. As well, there are negative consequences for the babies' future health and development.

Smoking may be responsible for more than half the cases of gum disease in adults. A significant study of 200 pregnant women has shown that women with gum disease affecting more than 30 percent of the mouth are more likely to deliver a preterm, LBW baby. Everyone should floss as well as brush daily and ideally use a Waterpik spray.

Women who smoke are less likely to breast-feed their babies and are at higher risk for many heart and lung diseases. While smoking in the United States is decreasing, female smokers and especially teenage smokers are on the increase. (Abroad it is even worse.) In the United States during 2000, smoking during pregnancy declined to 12 percent — a 37 percent drop since 1989. The highest rates were among those aged eighteen to twenty-four. Thirty-one percent of non-Hispanic white teenagers smoked compared to 3 percent of Mexican teenagers. College educated women have the lowest rate — 2 percent compared with 25 percent among women who have not completed high school.

Nonsmokers must stay away from cigarette smoke; fortunately the United States leads the world with increasing smoke-free areas. Second-

I had smoked two packs a day for ten years, but the day I found out I was having twins, I stopped completely.

From the minute I was pregnant, I suddenly could not stand even the smell of coffee. I guess your body tells you what you don't need.

hand smoke is known to contain at least 4,000 chemicals. At least fifty of these chemicals cause cancer. As well, infants exposed to secondhand smoke are more at risk for respiratory illnesses.

If you smoke and have trouble quitting, you will need a smoking-cessation program; and despite the fact that smoking diminishes appetite, you must take in extra nutrients to compensate.

Polyhydramnios

The medical term for an excess of amniotic fluid within the uterus is *polyhydramnios*, or simply *hydramnios*. It occurs in about 4 percent of twin pregnancies. Normally, about two quarts of fluid develop within the amniotic sac in a singleton pregnancy, providing an environment in which the fetus is free to move and is buffered from bumps and jolts. More amniotic fluid is required for two or more babies. Although excess fluid can occur for no apparent reason, it may be associated with fetal or maternal problems. A number of congenital abnormalities, especially vascular ones, cause this condition, and it often occurs with diabetes.

Fetal Disability: Congenital Anomalies, Defects, and Disease

Many abnormalities can be detected by prenatal tests, such as ultrasound, amniocentesis, and chorionic villus and fetal blood sampling, which are all described in Chapter 9.

The more common problems include hydrocephalus ("water on the brain"), anencephaly ("no brain"), myelomeningocoele (brain and spinal cord membranes bulging), achondroplasia (cartilage deficiencies) and other dwarfism, spina bifida (openings in the spinal column), exomphalos (protrusion of abdominal contents), duodenal atresia (narrowing of the duodenum, a part of the intestines), fetal hydrops (excess fluid), and cardiovascular, kidney, and chromosomal defects. With advances in technology, conditions such as cleft lips/palate, congenital cardiac abnormalities, and Down's syndrome are more readily recognized.* Markers such as fetal *nuchal translucency* (the skin folds at the back of the neck are translucent) can detect chromosomal aberrations and abnormal fetuses.

*Down's syndrome is a genetic disorder in which the child's mental and physical development are retarded. It is associated with congenital abnormalities, especially of the heart. Persons affected by Down's syndrome may develop a characteristic mongoloid appearance.

Single umbilical arteries are also more frequent in twins, but usually it is only the smaller baby that is affected. The pediatrician should be aware of any case of a single umbilical artery because other anomalies may be present.

Despite the difficulty in defining and collecting data, it is agreed that the incidence of malformations is increased in twins, especially MZ twins and same-sex twins of both zygosities. Monochorionic twins have a greater incidence of anomalies than DC twins do. The most recent report from the NCHS analyzed live births in 1973–1974 and reported that the incidence of congenital anomalies was 18 percent higher in multiples. Spellacy's 1990 study of thirteen hospitals in the Chicago area found that malformations occurred three times more often among twins (especially MZ). It is not understood whether a common factor predisposes offspring to both MZ twinning and anomalies or whether anomalies result from some deviation during the splitting of the embryo that results in MZ twins. Strangely, anomalies such as cardiac malformation in twins, even in MZ ones, are more commonly present in one twin only (discordance). Chromosomal events during fertilization can cause only one twin to have a particular disease such as muscular dystrophy or Down's syndrome.

Some rare anomalies such as conjoined twinning and acardia are unique to twins. Acardia is congenital absence of the heart, a condition that occurs in about 1 percent of MZ twins, either from failure of the heart to develop at all or from atrophy owing to circulation anomalies.

Conjoined twins (sometimes referred to as Siamese twins) occur in about 1 in 200 MZ pregnancies from a later division in the second week after fertilization. A Japanese study of conjoined twins found an incidence of 10 per million births, and they occurred most among mothers over 40 who had several children. Conjoined twins are always joined at identical sites and are classified according to the site of the union. Seventy percent are attached at the chest, a condition often associated with congenital heart disease. Some twins live their lives joined together, as did the famous Cheng and Ang from Siam. Surgical division is attempted where possible. A set of twins born in Paris in 1974 was joined at the head. Fourteen years and 26 operations later, the girls were declared perfectly normal by their surgeon!

Heart anomalies comprise the largest category of congenital malformations. According to Elizabeth Bryan, a cardiac malformation will affect one or both of the pair in about one in fifty of all twin pregnancies.

Bryan pooled two studies and noted that both twins were affected in only 8 percent of MZ pairs and 4.4 percent of DZ pairs. The twin who pumps the blood in the latter situation often develops cardiac failure; this condition can now be seen with ultrasound and treated prenatally.

Pathological closure of the esophagus (passage from throat to stomach) occurs up to five times more often in twins, but both twins are affected only 5 percent of the time. Many common anomalies, such as clubfoot and excess fingers or toes (polydactyly), are less serious. Twins were shown to have a lower incidence of congenital dislocation of the hip and Down's syndrome, in the government's 1973–1974 report. The risk of lethal malformation in twins, according to Doherty, is 1.9 percent, falling with increased maternal age. Lethal malformations cause about 8 percent of twin deaths but 18 percent of singleton deaths.

Most malformations occur early in the pregnancy, although problems can develop in later pregnancy from FFTS or compression of the babies. Pressure on normal body parts from crowding can cause skull and facial asymmetry, torticollis (wry neck), and foot defects. However, since MZ twins have clubfoot and congenital dislocation of the hip at least ten times more frequently than DZ twins do, other causes are involved.

The causes of birth defects are not only genetic but include malnutrition, smoking, alcohol and other substance abuse, infectious diseases, and environmental hazards. The same environmental influences may affect each twin differently because of gender, individual vulnerability, or slightly different age in a DZ pair.

Nutrition's role in birth defects was made clear to the public when the addition of folic acid to cereals and other foods reduced the incidence of spina bifida. Multiple pregnancies make enormous nutritional demands on the mother, and if these are not met, physical and mental impairment of the babies is likely. Low birth weight babies have more congenital abnormalities than normal birth weight babies. In the 1973–1974 government study, babies weighing 5 pounds, 8 ounces or less had about two and a half times as many birth defects as heavier babies. The lowest rate of anomalies was associated with birth weights over 7 pounds, 12 ounces.

Birth defects were more common among the offspring of diabetic mothers and multiples born to women who became pregnant within a year after giving birth. Male infants have 41 percent more defects than females. A 1988 study by Khoury found that almost 25 percent of malformed infants had IUGR, compared with 10 percent of normal infants. The frequency of IUGR increased with the increasing number of defects;

for example, 20 percent of the infants with two defects had IUGR, compared with 60 percent of infants with nine or more defects.

Women with less income and education had a higher incidence of children with birth defects, which can be attributed to inadequate diet, poorer hygiene, greater occurrence of infectious disease, and little or no prenatal care. The lowest incidence of infant congenital defects was found among women who had completed college or postgraduate education.

Couples with a family history of anomalies, or mothers over a certain age, can seek genetic counseling (the age varies among counseling facilities but is usually late thirties to over forty). It is now possible to detect most anomalies prenatally. Choosing genetic counseling and screening, however, may lead to another dilemma — the decision whether to have an abortion. For couples who would not undergo an abortion under any circumstances, prenatal diagnoses may still be helpful for planning their future.

Cerebral Palsy

Insufficient oxygen to the brain during pregnancy or birth can result in cerebral palsy, with varying degrees of physical and mental impairment. Brain damage observed in infancy may have its origin in prenatal malnutrition but cerebral palsy is not progressive. It is a symptom and has no single or common cause.

Cerebral palsy is the most common motor disability in childhood. Its incidence is increased fortyfold for preterm babies but it is also increasing in term babies: sixfold for twins and twentyfold for triplets, according to research in the United Kingdom. In the United States, the incidence of cerebral palsy in twins is approximately five times higher and for triplets seventeen times higher than in singletons. The risk of at least one child being born with cerebral palsy has been estimated at 1 to 5 percent for twins, 8 percent for triplets, and almost 50 percent for quadruplets.

Lower gestational age, lower birth weight, and being a twin all independently increase the risk of cerebral palsy in twin pregnancies. Gestational age is more important than birth weight in cerebral palsy. However, VLBW infants make up one-third of cases of cerebral palsy and 10 percent of cases of mental retardation, although children with cerebral palsy frequently have normal intelligence. Babies weighing less than 1,000 grams (2 pounds, 3 ounces) have cerebral palsy or mental retardation at the rate of 200 per 1,000. Between 1,000 and 1,500 grams (2 pounds, 3 ounces to 3 pounds, 4 ounces) the incidence declines by half, and in newborns weighing more than 2,500 grams (5 pounds, 8 ounces) it is only 2 per 1,000.

Twenty percent of surviving twins have neurological problems. FFTS carries a 25 percent risk of a neurodevelopmental problem. When one twin has died, the risk of cerebral palsy is ten to twenty times greater in the survivor.

Rydhstrom in Sweden found that the incidence of cerebral palsy had not declined with a tenfold increase in Caesarean deliveries.

A study in Western Australia found that intellectual deficit was associated with major defects and IUGR, whereas cerebral palsy with normal intelligence was associated with neither. Prematurity was found to be a key factor in a study in Liverpool, England, and same-sex twins had a higher incidence of brain impairment.

Despite inconsistencies in evaluating and reporting complications, it is clear that women pregnant with multiples are at greater risk for complications. Commit yourself to prevention with due diligence — focus on excellent nutrition, adequate rest, sensible exercise, positive thinking, and self-care. Always keep in mind the many mothers of twins and triplets who carry healthy, normal-weight babies to term without any problems at all. Make them your models!

8
How to Give Your Babies the Best Chance with Optimal Nutrition

My research for the first edition of *Having Twins* made it clear that maternal nutrition and weight gain were key factors for optimal outcome in a multiple pregnancy, just as they are for a singleton pregnancy. In the decades since, the importance of nutrition has become more and more accepted, and it is rare today to hear of a physician who restricts weight gain and salt intake in pregnancy. Organizations such as the American College of Obstetricians and Gynecologists (ACOG) recommend that for women of low body mass index (BMI), the gain be 25–40 pounds; for average BMI, 25–35 pounds; and for high BMI, 15–25 pounds.* The NCHS reported that the median weight gain for a mother of a singleton in 2002 was 30.5 pounds, and noted its correlation with birth weight.

Unfortunately, nutrition has not been a priority in the curriculum of medical schools in the United States and the average physician practicing today received very little exposure to the subject. Thus, it is not surprising that the medical profession still claims that the causes of premature labor and preeclampsia are unknown. Yet a half-century ago, the close relation between diet, fetal condition, and birth weight had been acknowledged — an adequate diet reduced fetal death by one-third, according to Bourne and Williams in 1948.

Food is man's [sic] most intimate contact, far more intimate than copulation. What you eat goes right inside you, is absorbed directly into the bloodstream and carried into every cell in the body, including, most importantly from the point of view of mental health and behavior, the brain cells.

— Richard Mackarness,
Not All in the Mind

---

*A Body Mass Index between 25 and 29.9 is overweight, and greater than or equal to 30 is obese, as defined by the World Health Organization (WHO). To calculate your BMI, go to the Web site www.consumer.gov/weight-loss/bmi.htm or use this formula:
1. Divide your weight in pounds by 2.2 to get kilograms.
2. Divide your height in inches by 39.4 to get meters. Multiple this number by itself.
3. Divide the result of step one by the result of step 2 to get your BMI.

Since 1950, Thomas Brewer, M.D., with Gail Brewer Krebs later, has written, lectured, and campaigned tirelessly for improved nutrition in pregnancy, especially to prevent toxemia/preeclampsia/eclampsia/HELLP (TPEH) and improve birth weight. During a twelve-year period in the prenatal clinics of Contra Costa County in California under Brewer's direction, with more than 25,000 pregnant women, there was not a single case of this disease. Daily intake of 3,100 calories and 140–150 grams of protein for a twin pregnancy, recommended by the Brewers and other nutritionally aware obstetricians, has generally resulted in term babies weighing at least 7 pounds. Gail Krebs herself had twins and they weighed 9 pounds, 3 ounces and 8 pounds, 9 ounces when they were born a few days past their due date. I interviewed many women for this book who delivered 7- to 9-pound twins. Larger babies have a better chance of survival as well as better intellectual and physical development. (Statistically, multiples through age three to four weigh less than singletons of the same age.) The heaviest twins born, according to the 2002 *Guinness Book of World Records*, was a set of twins in Arkansas in 1924 that totaled 27 pounds, 12 ounces. The runner-up was a pair of twins born in England in 1884, weighing a total of 25 pounds, 8 ounces.

The clinical work of Dr. Brewer as well as Agnes Higgins of the Montreal Diet Dispensary reinforced the importance of good nutrition in pregnancy. Mothers expecting twins ate for three and gained 50 to 60 pounds. Higgins found that adequate protein and calorie intakes were "markers" for the general level of a woman's nutrition. She recommended 500 extra calories and 30 extra grams of protein daily per baby, added to a baseline of 2,400 to 2,600 calories per day for the mother. For women with multiple pregnancies who were nutritionally at risk because of poor social conditions or poverty, the Higgins Nutrition Intervention Program was very successful. After controlling for confounding variables, the twins in Higgins's program compared with the control group weighed an average of 80 grams more, had a 25 percent lower rate of LBW, a 50 percent lower rate of VLBW, and a 30 percent lower rate of PTB.

The *Brewer Pregnancy Hotline* by Gail Krebs was published in 2001 and is also on-line as an eBook. You can reach Dr. Brewer at the Pregnancy Hotline number 802-388-0276; he provides record review, counseling for a current pregnancy, and interfaces with care providers, medical professionals, and parents, free of charge.

The Multiples Clinic in Ann Arbor, Michigan, founded by Barbara Luke, offered a nutrition-based program that resulted in birth weights up to 35 percent more than the average twin, triplet, and quadruplet and far fewer complications. Luke built a University Consortium on Multiple Births (with a membership of nine universities in the United States involved in research to improve multiple birth outcomes). Every year they publish large studies, showing the importance of prevention — good prenatal care and abundant protein and calories. The improved birth outcomes have a ripple effect through early childhood. Follow-up studies have been done through age three and will be extended further. Luke, now at the University of Miami, is applying for a grant from NIH to randomize her program to five university sites around the country. Her research is in line with the Barker hypothesis — that is, how babies grow before they are born influences their lifelong risks for many chronic diseases, including hypertension, diabetes, and cardiovascular disease. Luke's ultimate goal is to use randomized trials to change the standard of care for women pregnant with multiples, including guaranteed growth and developmental follow-up for all children of multiple pregnancies.

All the above-mentioned programs provide adequate protein and calories, but regrettably a great proportion come from dairy products. These are cheap (heavily subsidized), convenient, and very familiar (from lobbying and advertising). However, the evidence shows that consuming any form of dairy products has risks (see below). Diet gurus who abstain from dairy products manifest superior health and appearance; for example, the youthful vitality of Neal Barnard, M.D., endorses his vegan lifestyle.

Mothers themselves, fortunately, are increasingly aware of the importance of nutrition. *Twins* magazine published a Toronto study in which more than 400 pregnant women were divided into three groups according to their diets. The mothers who received an average of 92 grams of protein daily fared best, with an average labor five hours shorter than that of the group with a poor diet. The less-nourished women had more cases of anemia, toxemia, and threatened abortions. That group also experienced 3.4 percent stillbirths and 6 percent miscarriages compared with zero in the better diet group. Almost four times as many babies were born preterm to the mothers with a poor diet, and the babies were more often sick.

The evidence supporting good nutrition in pregnancy continues to mount, yet the national incidence of PTB and LBW babies keeps *increasing*. (I believe this is because mothers who have optimal nutrition are in the minority, and the adverse effects of stress and bed rest have not been recognized.) Luckily, your diet is something over which you have total control. Nutrition and exercise are prenatal care that only you can do; your doctor or midwife evaluates and treats. You are the one who has to eat optimally for three or more, drink plenty of fluids, reduce stress, rest frequently, and be sensible about your physical activities and workload.

Eating is a life-sustaining activity that we engage in several times a day — therefore it behooves all of us to be informed about nutrition, a topic on which the research doubles every two years or so. In this chapter, I hope to whet your appetite to learn more and explore new foods, and I have assembled important technical information for health care providers.

The Limitations of Numbers

Mothers who pushed themselves to eat beyond their appetite for the sake of their babies' health were always glad they did. Nevertheless, quality is more important than counting grams and micrograms. It is impossible to determine a magic number to suit all mothers, and even then the value of a given food is influenced by soil quality, fertilizers, pesticides, harvesting, preparation, processing, shipping, storage, preparation, cooking, and combining with other foods. People vary in the way their bodies metabolize food; lifestyle also influences food consumption. On the other hand, the ideal "nutrition by intuition" is difficult in a society where so many women have eating disorders to some degree. Anorexia and bulimia are very common in our culture and it's a challenge for women who find themselves pregnant to suddenly eat for two, three, or more.

The recently updated recommendations are now called Recommended Daily Dietary Intakes (RDDIs) and comprise amounts from the 1989 Recommended Daily Allowances (RDAs) as well as the 2000 Dietary Reference Intakes (DRIs). These are different from the reference values for food labels established by the U.S. Food and Drug Administration, creating a confusing array of systems and numbers. These are amounts that will keep a population free from a deficiency of an essential vitamin, mineral, or other nutrient and were developed only after widespread food processing caused deficiency diseases. What is *optimal* for each person's individual metabolism and lifestyle is not addressed at all.

Some women are able to remain steadfast despite a strong nocebo influence from their doctors:

> I was 5'3" and weighed 107 pounds when I became pregnant with my sons in 1985. My obstetrician suggested I prepare for a May delivery, although my due date was August 1! I'd had two previous healthy pregnancies, delivering large (over 9 pounds each) healthy singletons each time, following Adele Davis's early nutritional guidelines. I asked my doctor why I should think about so early a delivery. He said the odds were against anyone my size successfully carrying twins to term. He couldn't have given me a better incentive, and it was in researching what I could do to prove him wrong that I came across the Brewer nutritional guidelines. I'd gained 33 pounds with each of my singletons so I told him I planned to gain 66 pounds with twins. He was a little appalled, and didn't think I'd be able to do it. I didn't actually gain 66 pounds; I think I weighed 166 when I finally went into labor; my boys were actually late (born on August 13) and everyone in the delivery room (except me) was stunned when they weighed 8 pounds, 2 ounces, and 7 pounds, 14 ounces, for a total of 16 pounds of baby. They were the biggest twins my doctor had ever delivered. They are 16 now and both a little over 6 feet tall.

Weight Gain

In 1889, the Norriss quads were born in Australia and weighed about 7 pounds each (for a total combined birth weight of around 12,700 gm, or almost 28 pounds). This makes them the heaviest set recorded to date, but unfortunately they died in early infancy from "conditions of poverty . . . diarrhea." One wonders how Mrs. Norriss in such an economic situation was able to obtain the nutrients to produce such impressive birth weights! This thirty-four-year-old mother had already birthed a set of twins who also died.

Wide ranges of weight gain have been observed in pregnancies with healthy outcomes. Midwife Jeannine Parvati Baker is a vegan who gained only 20 pounds with her twins, who were conceived and born in

My twins weighed 7 1/2 pounds and 8 1/2 pounds, although I gained only 28 pounds. We live on a farm and I was as plump before the pregnancy as I am now.

I ate good food all through my pregnancy. Was I hungry! I used to wake before six A.M. and have to get something to eat. Then I would go back to sleep. I couldn't keep my eyes open — just like a newborn babe after he eats.

I was unable to eat all the recommended foods and calories due to abdominal space constraints and acid reflux after even the tiniest meal. I liquified foods in the blender to make them easier and faster to digest — this helped a little. Also, I found separating carbohydrates and protein and eating fruit completely apart from all other food helped with acid reflux because it speeded up digestion. In the end, I gained 35 pounds, the same as with my singleton, who weighed 4.5 kg (9.9 pounds). Max and Charlotte were born at 37 weeks weighing 2.5 kg (5 pounds) and 2.8 kg (6 pounds). After three months of breastfeeding they reached the 97th and 75th percentiles of their growth charts.

— Conner Middelmann

Every night my husband would make me a plate of sliced turkey with raw apples, carrots, or green peppers. He would wrap it in plastic and put it by the bed. When I got up to go to the bathroom — at least three times a night — I would eat a little off the plate. No one can really understand how tough a job it is to eat like that when I was so full of babies. I was convinced that the only way to have a healthy home birth with twins was to have a term birth.

the same bed, weighing at least 5 pounds each. Thirty years later, they are tall, strong and healthy.

Older, heavier, and taller mothers do best with a multiple pregnancy, and they are the ones who typically conceive multiples. How much weight gain is desirable for a woman expecting two or more? Forty to 50 pounds on average for mothers of twins, 55–70 for those carrying triplets, and 65–80 for quadruplets. In addition to the weight of each additional baby, there is the weight from the placentas, amniotic fluid, necessary maternal fat storage, and blood volume.

Gain Weight Early

Unlike with singletons, mothers of multiples show the greatest weight gain in early (before twenty weeks) and late pregnancy. Animals that hibernate consume enough to see them through the winter (and shiver to keep their muscles active); similarly, you need a head start so that your babies have excellent reserves when their growth becomes rapid and your stomach capacity and physical activity levels become more and more reduced. Marilyn Riese's study of full-term newborn twins with 15 percent to 47 percent weight differences found that the *weight discordance within these twin pairs began in the first four months of fetal life.*

The larger the set of multiples, the earlier you need to gain weight, as much as 50 pounds by six months for a mother of quads. This means eating constantly, at least every couple of hours. Your babies are growing around the clock and you will find yourself waking up at night to snack. Although the babies grow more slowly in the first few months than later in pregnancy, mothers have a great need for energy in the first trimester to fuel the transition from the nonpregnant state and to develop powerful placentas.

Gain weight early in the pregnancy to build up your reserves for when the babies grow rapidly later. The placenta is still developing until the sixteenth week.

Pre-pregnancy weight is significant. If you were underweight before the pregnancy, you need to add the missing pounds to your goal of weight to be gained; otherwise, there is a risk of miscarriage or slow-growing and preterm babies. For the same reason, smokers and those who underwent ART need extra weight in the beginning.

Women with a high BMI may have normal to large single babies even

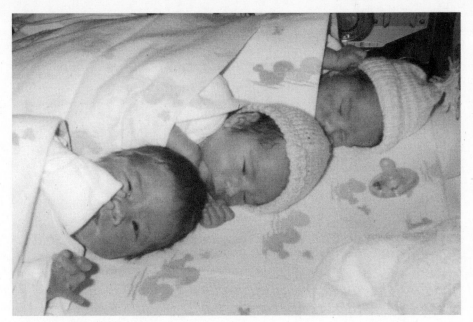

Just after birth, triplets weighing 5 lbs., 2 oz., 5 lbs., 11 oz., and 5 lbs., 13 oz., born to a 42-year-old mother.

As well as improving my diet with more whole grains and green leafy vegetables, I started cooking with iron pans when I was pregnant. My hemoglobin increased so I didn't need any iron supplements.

I ate a tremendous amount of good food during my pregnancy and I felt great. My appetite was just unbelievable, which is actually what led my doctor to suspect twins.

I found while carrying triplets that I would have double meals, like one dinner at six o'clock and another one at nine.

if they gain little weight during the pregnancy. Nonetheless, overweight women are often the most malnourished, and they must eat well during pregnancy. Dieting to lose weight during pregnancy and nursing is dangerous. It is a paradox in the United States, where obesity is so common, that women and some doctors look askance at a gain of 50 or more pounds during the childbearing year. Your babies' health depends on your weight gain! You create your babies from what you eat; a builder could not construct a house without all the right materials.

While some women are ravenous in the first trimester, others feel nauseated and may vomit, sometimes a lot. Major hormonal changes affecting your respiratory and cardiovascular systems cause understandable fatigue. Eating small amounts helps to keep blood sugar levels stable and prevent "morning sickness," which may occur at any time of the day when blood sugar levels are low. Keep rice cakes or whole wheat crackers handy to maintain normal blood sugar levels and avoid high-glycemic foods (such as bananas and white bread), which can upset them. Fresh grated ginger added to food or made with boiling water into

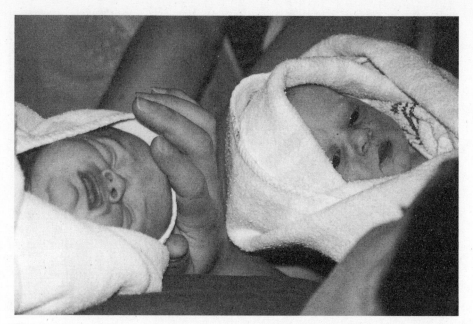

The size and health of these newborns pay tribute to their mother's weight gain.

a tea can relieve nausea, as can tiny amounts of umeboshi plum (a Japanese ingredient available from health food stores). Anti-nausea wristbands that stimulate an acupuncture point to prevent seasickness bring relief to some mothers. Often women themselves find something that relieves nausea, such as ginger ale, Popsicles, or sucking sour candy. A 2002 update from the Cochrane Database showed pyridoxine (vitamin B_6) helps to reduce the severity of nausea. Traditional acupuncture is effective in treating nausea and vomiting in pregnant women, according to a 2002 article in *Birth*.

Excessive vomiting in pregnancy, called *hyperemesis gravidarum*, occurs in 3 to 5 percent of twin pregnancies and may require hospital admission and intravenous hydration and nutrition. Usually in such cases, there is something very serious going on in the woman's life. I knew a woman who kept being readmitted because of the stress of her husband being in jail for shooting her father, who had sexually abused her during her youth. Symptoms must be explored to understand and resolve them on a symbolic level as well.

It is easier to eat more small meals through the day and through the night if you wake up. This keeps your blood sugar more stable and you will feel better in the morning. Small frequent meals will be necessary when your stomach is crowded into a smaller space. If you have difficulty eating enough food or have persistent nausea or obsessive cravings, you need help. (See Resources.)

 ## The Loss of Whole Foods

Processing and refining of many food products enables them to last longer without spoiling, but valuable nutrients are removed. Refining separates the protein, fiber, minerals, and vitamins from the whole food. Grains are stripped of the bran and germ (which are sold as health supplements). Wheat flour must be enriched to compensate for the loss of nutrients during processing. Excessive intake of refined starches and sugars can be harmful and have resulted in Syndrome X (which includes increased risk for obesity, high blood pressure, and diabetes). The average American receives 25 percent of his or her calories from refined sugar and 45 percent from fat. These altered substances become a double liability because the body must release stored nutrients to metabolize them.

The lack of fiber in the standard American diet is well-known, and not only does it cause constipation (already a common annoyance in pregnancy), it is linked to colon cancer and other serious diseases.

In just the past few years, supermarkets have begun to offer an impressive range of natural and organic foods. This makes it easy to choose whole foods from the beginning of the food chain rather than industrialized preparations that come in expensive packaging. How can "dead" food be good for growing new lives? You and your babies will do best eating food close to its natural condition.

 ## What Is Good Nutrition?

Nutrition is an immensely complex subject; opinions are diverse and contradictory and eating habits are ingrained. There are people who are overweight, eat junk food, smoke and drink alcohol daily and yet, like Winston Churchill, live to their nineties. How can Zen monks live on brown rice and water for years and not suffer any vitamin deficiencies? But when it comes to eating for our preborn babies, we need to find out what is best, not just what we can get by on.

The essential foods are:

- 20 or more minerals

- 13 vitamins

- 9 amino acids

- 2 essential fatty acids (EFAs)*

- energy (starch/glucose)

It is an interesting exercise, at least once during your pregnancy, to keep a record of your food intake for several days and to analyze your diet using the *Nutritive Value of Foods* guide or some of the on-line tables listed in the Resources.

Making the right food choices is just the first step. We may expect foods to contain a certain type and amount of nutrients, but much will be lost if the foods become stale or are overcooked. The nutritive value of a food is frequently enhanced or diminished when combined with other foods. Citrus fruits will cause starches to ferment in your stomach; thus, orange juice and toast should be eaten apart. Proteins and starches are best eaten separately, as well. Raw food requires more digestion and is best eaten before activity. Melons should always be eaten alone.

The American Heart Association, the American Cancer Society, and the U.S. Surgeon General have all warned the public about the association of a poor diet with conditions such as heart disease, colon cancer, hypertension, diabetes, and obesity, to name just a few, and they recommend that dietary intake of red meats, sugar, and fried and processed foods be greatly reduced. Animal products are nevertheless heavily promoted by the meat and dairy industries but they are unwholesome and polluted unless they are free-range and organically raised.

*Essential fatty acids LNA (linolenic acid) and LA (linoleic acid) must be obtained from food sources. They govern every life process in the body, including oxygen transport and formation of prostaglandins to regulate tension in the arteries and thus blood pressure. Both are involved in the secretion of all glands and in the formation of the brain during fetal development. During pregnancy, the child draws EFAs from the mother's body to build its brain, which is over 60 percent fat and very rich in both omega-3 and omega-6 derivatives. The placenta contains receptors that ensure that these EFAs are transported from the mother to the baby. No such receptors are found for the nonessential monounsaturated and saturated fatty acids.

Do Americans Care About Their Diet?

Four out of the ten leading causes of death in the United States are from poor diet (and lack of exercise), yet a Healthy Eating Index (HEI) study done by the U.S. Department of Agriculture (USDA) in the years 1994–1996 showed that people were generally unconcerned. Only 23 percent wanted to improve their diet, 37 percent were not interested, and 40 percent thought their diet needed no improvement. The total score was 64 out of 100 — fruits being the least consumed. The majority of all respondents agreed that their snacks were unhealthy. Dairy intake score was lowest (4.6) among those who were interested in improving their diets. Those who were unconcerned thought healthful eating was too complicated.

Some people, when they give up red meat, unfortunately substitute more dairy products — which have been linked to at least 45 diseases according to Frank Oski. High blood pressure, abnormal elevation of cholesterol, and obesity are occurring in ever-younger children. The problems with fat have been well publicized; greasy plates mean greasy arteries. Americans are eating less fat now but unfortunately more refined carbohydrates, which are stored as fat and cause diabetes and cardiovascular diseases.

John Robbins's *Diet for a New America* is an enlightening journey through our food supply. With the shocking background information he provides, you will be inspired to make some changes in your diet. *Fat Land* by Greg Critser and *Fast Food Nation* by Eric Schlosser are similar exposés that everyone who eats should read.

Your levels of weight and nourishment prior to pregnancy will influence the weight of your offspring (and, in some ethnic groups, the likelihood of twinning). The mental and physical health of your babies will be determined by your prenatal nutrition, and this is the time to make positive changes for the diet of the entire family.

Pregnancy is the ideal time to commit the whole family to a healthier lifestyle.

Toward Healthier Sources of Food

The nutrition section of any bookstore displays the wide range of different theories. There are various types of vegetarian diets (vegan — no animal products; lacto — with dairy products; ova — eggs are eaten; lacto-ovo — both eggs and dairy products). Some schools of thought push raw fruits and vegetables for the enzymes; others feel strongly that both these foodstuffs should be cooked (which destroys enzymes) as in macrobiotic food preparation.

I have found the most helpful discussions of nutrition tend to be written not by dieticians or academics but by cooks! *Food and Healing* by Annemarie Colbin is excellent and one of the abundant titles available today. The ever-increasing number of different cookbooks indicates that dietary habits of the American population are changing, and for the better. Sales of organic products grew at an average annual rate of 42 percent from 1992 to 1997, and organics are expected to be a $20 billion business by 2005. Four out of ten consumers buy some organic food, according to a Rodale Press survey. Despite this, only a small percentage of Americans shops regularly for health food. Even that statement is bizarre: should not all food be healthful?!

It is better to spend your time obtaining a wide range of healthy ingredients and learning how to prepare them than bothering to weigh and measure serving sizes. If you choose only high-quality foods and get the majority of your calories from complex carbohydrates (vegetables, fruits, grains) rather than refined foods and sugars, you will be in good shape. You need healthy fats, too, for your brain and the development of your babies' brains, and I will discuss later the dangerous fats that have resulted from industrialized food.

Eat from the farm, not from the factory.

Add Calories!

Studies show that caloric intake in the presence of high protein helps prevent low-birth-weight babies and infant death. Placental weight is consistently higher in groups of women who consumed supplemental calories. Choose fresh and dried fruits (Nature's fast food) instead of cheeseburgers, fries, other greasy fast foods, and sweet confections that provide only calories.

Protein, fat, and carbohydrate — the three major components of common foods — all contain calories: 1 gram of protein or carbohydrate provides 4 calories and 1 gram of fat provides more than twice as many — 9 calories.

Protein

The word *protein* comes from a Greek word meaning "of primary importance."* This nutrient is needed for hormones, antibodies, and enzymes as well as construction, maintenance, and repair of tissues, including the muscle of the uterus, the placenta, and your babies. Getting the right amount of protein each day is essential because this nutrient is not stored in the body like fats and carbohydrates. The usual recommendation is 0.8 grams of protein per kilogram of body weight, which has a buffer of 25–50 percent because it is set for populations and not individuals.

For the adult nonpregnant female, the RDDI is 2,200 calories and 50 grams of protein, or about 9 percent of calories as protein. Most of the common plant foods provide more than 10 percent of calories as protein. Vegetarians eat up to 15 percent of calories as protein, but people who eat animal flesh consume much more. During pregnancy, about 20 percent of your calories should be from protein of the highest quality.

How much extra protein is needed during pregnancy? For a single pregnancy, the current RDDI is 10 extra grams of protein and 300 extra calories per day: a total of 2,500 calories and 60 grams of protein. There are no official guidelines for mothers expecting twins, but experienced clinicians generally use 100–150 percent of these guidelines, as do training athletes.

Luke recommends 176 grams of protein and 3,500 calories for twins, 200 grams of protein and 4,000 calories for triplets, and 225 grams of protein and 4,500 calories for quadruplets. This is similar to Higgins's increments of 30 grams of protein and 500 calories per baby.

Frequent intake of protein is needed as babies grow around the clock. Eat protein with every meal and always eat some after physical exertion. According to the Harvard University Women's Health Information Web site in 2002, a single baby weighing 3,300 grams at 40 weeks has used 925 grams of protein. They calculated the protein requirement to be 6 grams a day in the first trimester, increasing to 11 grams in the last trimester.

---

*Protein quality used to be evaluated by the protein efficiency ratio (PER) which was determined using the (faster) growth rate of rats that also had higher amino acid needs. This has been replaced by the Protein Digestibility Corrected Amino Acid Score (PDCAAS). For example, if egg white and beef rate a "1" then soy protein is .99, kidney beans .68, pinto beans .57, rolled oats .57, whole wheat .40, and lentils .51.

This kind of information for singletons has little relevance for multiples, where *early* growth of both babies and placenta is so important. The placenta grows until the fourth month and viability is around the sixth month (although younger babies have survived). These landmarks must be reached with optimal nutrition and weight gain, and before the progressive decrease in stomach size as the babies grow. Luke recommends that a mother of twins gain at least 24 pounds by twenty-four weeks (an easy number to remember); a mother of triplets should gain at least 36 pounds, and 50 pounds when there are quadruplets.

Sources of Protein

Protein is broken down by the body into amino acids. There are twenty-two amino acids, nine of which are considered essential because, unlike the others, the liver cannot manufacture or convert them. They must be obtained from the diet. Animal protein contains all the essentials, which is why meat, fish, fowl, and eggs have been considered classic protein sources.

A major problem with animal protein is its source. It was different when families lived on the farm and raised their own uncaged livestock. Today most people consume the unhealthy meat of diseased, confined animals that are fed slaughterhouse waste, antibiotics, pesticides, and herbicides as well as sex hormones to stimulate growth. Also, livestock are generally slaughtered under unsanitary conditions that further reduce food quality, as described in *Fast Food Nation*.

Poultry has less fat content than meat, but if it is commercially raised it is unwholesome. The spread of feces during slaughter and processing contributes to the high content of salmonella (which can cause food poisoning). Although food poisoning is rarely lethal, up to one-third of the United States population suffers from it each year.

While fish are usually free from many of these hazards, they may come from polluted waters, and labeling of their origin is not required. However, the ocean has suffered less from industrialization than the land. You always know when fish is fresh: it has absolutely no odor. If you live near a coast, you can ask when the fish was caught.

Eggs are a whole food but commercial hens are dosed with antibiotics and hormones, fed processed granules, kept in tiny cages, and debeaked because otherwise they would kill each other because of the stress related to immobility from overcrowding. The eggs laid by such chickens are higher in cholesterol than those of free-range chickens, lack essential fatty acids, and taste very inferior to natural eggs.

Health food stores and increasingly supermarkets carry meat and poultry products that are raised naturally and eggs from free-range chickens. Kosher poultry is also raised free from drugs. Such products are worth the extra price for the health of you and your family.

Protein is also available from many other sources (see the chart on the following pages) that do not have the liabilities of animal protein, such as high fat and toxins. The average protein level in legumes (beans, lentils, etc.) is 27 percent; in nuts and seeds, 13 percent; and in grains, 12 percent; thus, plant foods can supply the recommended daily amount of protein as long as the overall energy requirements are met with carbohydrates and fats. It was once thought that various plant foods had to be eaten together to get their full protein value, known as protein combining or protein complementing. Intentional combining is not necessary and protein needs are easily met as long as the diet contains a variety of grains, legumes, seeds, nuts, tofu and other soy-based products, and vegetables.*

Beans and whole grains are excellent sources of protein. However, most of us were not raised on such foods and we need to learn how to cook them so they are digestible and appetizing. They are easy to store because they do not require refrigeration, and they can be bought in bulk, which is a big consideration for a busy mother of multiples. If you cook them ahead of time, rice can be kept for five days in the refrigerator and legumes for about three days, or for weeks in the freezer.

People tend to categorize "protein foods" without realizing how universal this structural material is. Protein enables plants as well as animals to grow upright and if you keep this in mind, the sources are not so "hidden." Most fruits contain 1 gram of protein, such as a peach, pear, apple, and a cup of pineapple or watermelon. Likewise, vegetables are a source of protein. There is 1 gram in a carrot and in a cup of lettuce. Two grams can be found in a cup of spring onions, tomatoes, or tomato juice; 3 grams in a cup of cooked butternut squash; up to 5 grams in a baked potato; and 8 grams in a cup of frozen peas. A taco shell and a cup of

---

*According to the USDA, in 2002, 74 percent of America's soybeans were grown from genetically modified beans and one-third of America's corn crop will be genetically modified. Monsanto conveniently manufactures seeds that can survive Monsanto's pesticide (Roundup). Search for organic soybeans.

popcorn also contain 1 gram of protein. One tablespoon of wheat germ contains 2 grams, as does a glass of orange juice. A tablespoon of peanut butter has 4 grams of protein. One cup of soymilk has 7 grams of protein (compared with cow's milk, which has 8 grams). Three tablespoons of flaxseed (28 grams) gives 5 grams protein and is an excellent laxative (soak overnight in water or grind) and high in omega-3 EFAs.

You will notice in the chart below the high nutrient value of the leafy green vegetables, such as kale, collards, and mustard greens. Take frozen packets to work and heat up for a snack in a toaster oven (see http://www.healthfree.com/paa/paa0001.htm for the many hazards of microwave cooking). I selected a range of whole foods to demonstrate their protein and calorie content, adding any bonus nutrient such as calcium and iron.

Protein and Calorie Content of Selected Foods

NAME	MEASURE	PROTEIN (GM)	CALORIES	BONUS NUTRIENT
Egg, hard boiled	1 cup	17	211	1.6 mg iron
Cod, baked, broiled	3 oz	20	89	
Halibut, baked, broiled	3 oz	23	119	
Oysters, raw	1 cup	17	169	16.5 mg iron
Sardines, in oil	3 oz can	21	177	325 mg calcium
Tuna, solid white	3 oz can	20	109	12 mg calcium
Apricot nectar (canned)	1 cup	1	141	18 mg iron
Avocado (California)	1 oz	1	50	
Banana	1, approx. 7 in	1	109	467 mg potassium
Cherries, sour red, canned, pitted	1 cup	2	88	3.3 mg iron 1,840 IU Vitamin A
Dates, chopped, pitted	1 cup	4	490	2 mg iron 57 mg calcium 13.4 gm fiber 1161 mg potassium
Pink grapefruit, raw juice	1 cup	1	114	1,087 IU Vitamin A

NAME	MEASURE	PROTEIN (GM)	CALORIES	BONUS NUTRIENT
Mango	1 whole	1	135	8,061 IU Vitamin A
Cantaloupe	1 cup	1	56	5,158 IU Vitamin A
Prunes, stewed	1 cup	3	265	75 mg calcium 2.8 mg iron
Raisins	1 cup, loose	5	435	1,089 IU potassium 3 mg iron 71 mg calcium
Bagel, enriched	1 x 4 in	9	245	32 mg iron 66 mg calcium
Bread, cracked wheat, enriched	1 slice	2	65	
Pita	6.5 in	5	165	52 mg calcium
Corn grits, Cream of Wheat	1 cup	3	145	
Oatmeal, regular	1 cup	6	145	
Granola	3/4 cup	6	248	41 mg calcium
Raisin Bran, Total	1 cup	6	186	238 mg calcium 18 mg iron
Bulgur, cooked (as in tabouleh)	1 cup	6	151	49 mg calcium 25.6 gm fiber
Oatmeal cookie	1	2	113	
Croutons, seasoned	1 cup	4	186	
English muffin, enriched	1 muffin	4	134	99 mg calcium
Granola bar	1 hard, plain	3	134	
Pecan pie	1 slice	5	452	
Rice, brown, long grain	1 cup	5	216	
Rice, wild	1 cup	7	166	
Spaghetti, enriched	1 cup	7	197	
Beans, navy	1 cup	15	258	127 mg calcium
Hazelnuts (filberts)	1 cup	17	722	131 mg calcium 5.4 mg iron
Pistachio nuts	1 cup	6	161	

NAME	MEASURE	PROTEIN (GM)	CALORIES	BONUS NUTRIENT
Lentils	1 cup, cooked	18	230	
Soybeans, dry, cooked	1 cup	29	298	175 mg calcium, 8.8 mg iron 10.3 gm fiber
Soybeans, green, cooked	1 cup	22	254	261 mg calcium 4.5 mg iron
Beef, lean and fat	3 oz	23	234	
Lamb chop, lean loin	3 oz	21	269	
Veggie burger	1 patty	14	91	87 mg calcium
Burrito, bean and meat	1	11	255	
Turkey, light and dark	1 cup`	41	238	
Green pea soup	1 cup	9	165	
Baby limas	1 cup	12	189	50 mg calcium 10.8 gm fiber
Broccoli, raw	1 cup	3	25	42 mg calcium
Brussel sprouts, frozen	1 cup	6	65	37 mg calcium
Collards, frozen	1 cup	5	61	357 mg calcium
Dandelion greens, cooked	1 cup	2	35	147 mg calcium 12,285 IU Vitamin A
Kale, frozen	1 cup	4	39	8,260 IU Vitamin A 179 mg calcium

An Interactive Healthy Eating Index is available from the Center for Nutrition Policy and Promotion (http://www.usda.gov/cnpp/). You can submit your foods for analysis and store the information on-line for up to thirty days. Further information on nutrients in foods can be found at http://www.nutritionfocus.com and www.networks.com, where you can sort more than 1,000 foods alphabetically by fat, protein, or calorie content.

Carbohydrates

Extra calories are required to support your body's increased workload in a multiple pregnancy. If you do not consume sufficient wholesome, complex carbohydrates, instead of using protein as the essential construction material for the babies, placentas, and uterus, your body will burn fat and even protein for fuel (and the ketones that are thus produced can be measured in your urine).

Carbohydrate consumption increases your basal metabolic rate (BMR, the number of calories you burn at rest) to maintain the functions of vital organs. Also, carbohydrates promote the anabolic properties (building-up) of the hormone insulin, which is important for protein metabolism. Increasing the percentage of calories from carbohydrates improves the efficiency of protein metabolism, even without changing the amount of protein in the diet.

Carbohydrates are the most abundant foodstuff in the diet, and the two forms that supply fuel are sugars and starches. Sugars are generally present in fruits; starches are found in vegetables and grains.

Sugars in fruits are simple carbohydrates that give quick energy. In contrast, whole grains such as brown rice, oats, buckwheat, barley, millet, and corn are complex carbohydrates that slowly release energy in the body. Grains also contain protein, B vitamins, iron, and other nutrients. Soaking grains improves their digestibility and nutritional value.

The maintenance of blood sugar levels is very important, especially for brain function, and this is achieved through complex carbohydrates that are digested slowly. Fruit, which contains fructose, a simple carbohydrate, still takes time for digestion whereas other simple sugars, such as table sugar (sucrose, a refined chemical with no nutritive value), are absorbed immediately. Such quick assimilation causes the rush of energy that typically follows eating candy, pastry, syrups, honey, or other sweet "pick-up" foods. Unfortunately, this high-energy state soon passes and is replaced by low energy as blood sugar levels drop. Although people vary in their resistance to these hypoglycemic attacks, weakness, irritability, and anxiety result. The vicious cycle also strains the pancreas, which secretes insulin to force the excess glucose into the cells. When the cells can take no more, the excess is stored as fat and if this situation becomes chronic, diabetes will result. According to George Blackburn, M.D., at Harvard, 85 percent of Americans have some degree of insulin resistance and about 25 percent are diabetic. This portion of the population is distributed on a bell curve, with Native Americans, Mexican Americans, Polynesian Islanders, and African Americans being the most impacted. See www.elizabethnoble.com/healthtests for a test that can determine if a person is at risk for diabetes (and other degenerative diseases).

Metabolism of sugar drains your body of nutrients, vitamins, and minerals. Like salt, sugar (such as high fructose corn syrup), is often added to canned and processed foods. Sodas and juice drinks are loaded with sugar in various forms. For example, one can of Pepsi contains eight teaspoons of sugar. Sugar contributes about 25 percent of the calories in the typical American diet and most Americans eat more than their weight in sugar each year.

Your dietary goal, especially in pregnancy, is to eat more complex carbohydrates in their less processed, more natural form. One-third to one-half of your diet should be whole grains.

Balancing Protein and Calories

It is important to balance your intake of protein and calories. Carbohydrates cannot be made from fat, but they can from protein, which has undesirable side effects of uric acid and ammonia production that strain the kidneys. You must have enough calories for energy needs and thus spare protein for your multiple pregnancy. Excess calories actually improve protein digestibility and an extra 700 to 1,000 calories can spare protein by 30 and 50 percent respectively.

One cup of rice and a half cup of beans, so common around the world, supplies a favorable ratio of 28 calories for each gram of protein. When one eats candy, jam, and other sweet foods, several hundred calories are taken in with very little or no protein. One then goes into debt for many nutrients, as well as protein.

Fats and Oils

Fats supply more than twice the energy (calories) per gram than do carbohydrates and protein. Fat-soluble vitamins A, D, E, and K, and EFAs for cell metabolism, are also carried in fats and oils. Fats digest slowly, give a "filling" feeling, and are well absorbed. Cooking and salad oils, butter, margarine, shortening, and mayonnaise contain fat, but fats vary from essential to toxic. Fat, a major part of animal flesh, is where environmental poisons are concentrated, making it wise to choose organic animal products. Meat contains approximately fourteen times more pesticides than do plant foods, and dairy products contain five times more.

It is recommended that fats make up no more than 25 to 30 percent of one's daily total calorie intake. The issue, however, is not the amount of fat as much as the type.

The industrialization of our food has created "transfatty acids." The typical American diet not only lacks adequate EFAs but is loaded with undesirable forms of fat as well. Refining increases the shelf life of oils, as it does for grains, but strips down the nutritive value. Americans each eat about 10 pounds of altered fat substances each year! Transfats become incorporated into our body, and in addition to the harm they cause, they block the absorption of EFAs. As their name implies, EFAs are not used for fuel and energy but for vital body functions. Insufficient EFAs have been linked to depression, attention deficit disorder/attention deficit hyperactivity disorder (ADD/ADHD), learning disabilities, chronic degenerative diseases (e.g. fibromyalgia, chronic fatigue), inflammatory, autoimmune, and collagen diseases, as well as neurological diseases like multiple sclerosis. Women suffer these problems much more frequently than men, whose EFAs are not depleted by "baby brain-building" during pregnancy. Each subsequent child fetus gets fewer EFAs and further depletes the mother unless she augments her diet. By the same token, this explains why younger children have far more developmental and behavioral problems than older children, especially in large families in which the children are born close together.

The prevalence of eating disorders among lipophobic young women on low fat or fat-free diets is associated with the increased use of mood altering drugs like Prozac® and Zoloft®. Omega-3 fatty acids are important for brain chemicals, serotonin and dopamine, that affect moods. Many women start their pregnancies already deficient in omega-3 fatty acids and each baby will deplete their stores.

The challenge is to cut down the amount of unhealthy saturated and unsaturated fats as well as to increase your sources of EFAs. They are needed by every cell of your body and your babies' bodies, especially the cell walls, and for the absorption of trace minerals that activate a large number of enzymes. The fat-soluble vitamins E and K also require EFAs for their metabolism.

Balancing Omega-3 and Omega-6 Fatty Acids

Both these EFAs use the same enzymes to convert into end products that influence body function; therefore, too much of one will further diminish the other. There is much discussion about the ideal ratio, but everyone seems to agree that the modern diet has too many omega-6s and not enough omega-3s. Livestock and farmed fish today are fed foods very different from what sustained them in the wild, so they contribute few omega-3s to the human diet.

Udo Erasmus, in *Fats that Kill, Fats that Heal*, recommends a 2:1 ratio but others, like Christiane Northrup, M.D., think you should aim for 6:1. About 150 years ago, the ratio was 4:2; today it is 20–25:1. The most important EFA (omega-3) is often lacking in the diet and is best obtained by eating wild-caught salmon, mackerel, and the more affordable small fish such as sardines, pilchards, anchovies, and herring. Chewing pumpkin seeds, walnuts, soybeans — even grape seeds — is an easy way to obtain omega-6 fatty acids but most people's diets have too many already.

There is a major difference between the omega-3 of the land food chain (flaxseed oil, perilla oil, etc.) and the omega-3 of the seafood chain. Although many people supplement, it is better to eat fish, because the important components (DHA and EPA) are preformed in the seafood chain only.

Seafood is also rich in antioxidants such as selenium and iodine, a major component of thyroid hormones. Selenium and iodine, like EFAs, are needed for brain development. Magnesium, calcium, and zinc are involved in the body's use of omega-3 (catalysts) and have been explored as preventive agents for preterm labor.

Sources of DHA:

- salmon
- mackerel
- sardines
- anchovies
- eggs
- dark leafy green vegetables
- DHA or fish oil capsules

Consumption of fish was found in Danish research to be a strong influence in reducing PTB and LBW. Likewise, these complications are rare in the Faroe islands, Greenland, and Japan because of fish consumption. The omega-3 fatty acids can stop preterm labor contractions and prevent eclampsia. (A 15 percent increase in the ratio of omega-3 to omega-6 was associated with a 46 percent reduction in the risk of preeclampsia.)

Theoretically, the most direct way to prevent preeclampsia and preterm labor would be to consume ocean fish rich in omega-3 fatty acids and minerals that are essential nutrients for the brain (iodine, selenium, zinc) and that tend to be more scarce these days in land food. This conforms with the geographical variations in the rates of preeclampsia and preterm labor, and with the results achieved after Odent encouraged his own pregnant clients to eat ocean fish. Fish oil supplementation should not be confused with the consumption of sea fish because of the EFAs that are preformed in fish, plus the mechanics of processing fish oil puts it higher on the food chain and at risk for more pollution. Consuming the actual fish rather than capsules also involves the intake of high quality proteins and a good balance in minerals. Furthermore, when people eat fish they automatically reduce the amount of other kinds of protein, such as meat and dairy. The Japanese eat ten times more fish than Americans and rank high by any criterion of health.

Nuts and seeds contain oils and should be stored in the refrigerator because they turn rancid quickly. Often rancidity is disguised with salting and roasting, oiling, and flavorings. Peanuts (actually a legume — a pea) frequently harbor a carcinogenic mold; Valencia peanuts are more resistant to the mold than other types. It is possible to buy mixed nuts in bulk on-line. Put them in smaller bags and store them in the freezer until you are ready to eat them.

Households in former times obtained fresh oil frequently but no longer with today's mass storage and handling. Raw, natural oils readily become rancid because they are unsaturated; that is, gaps exist in the molecular chain (which in saturated or hydrogenated fats would be filled with hydrogen molecules, making them solid, like margarine and lard). Oxygen fills these gaps and the subsequent changes in the molecular structure cause the oil to smell and taste bad as well as reducing its value. When the fatty acids become oxidized like this, free radicals are formed. Free radicals have been associated with cardiovascular disease, cancer, arthritis, and premature aging. Antioxidants (such as vitamins E and C) counteract free radicals but are often insufficient in the diet.

In health food stores you can find flax, hemp, pumpkin, soy, and walnut oils that contain both EFAs. They should be used for dressings on salads, a baked potato, or pasta — heated oils are damaged oils. Olive oil (although healthy for other reasons) is low in EFAs and is less damaged during cooking. Make sure that the olive oil you use is extra-virgin, unrefined, and cold-pressed. Light, oxygen, and heat destroy the EFAs in oils; look for oil in opaque containers.

Fried foods tend to increase heartburn in pregnancy. Eat baked or broiled foods, choose leaner cuts of meat, remove the skin of chicken, and avoid dairy products to lower the intake of unhealthy fat.

Meat or saturated fat consumption has remained constant in the past hundred years. What has gone up, however, is consumption of margarine and other transfatty acids; lifeless, packaged dietary junk;

Every tired body lacks calcium.
— Bernard Jensen

Be assured that much of the publicity referring to the health benefits
of dairy products is commercially
motivated. . . . Although the real
reason for the advertising campaign
is to reduce the surplus, the ads attempt to convince you to buy milk
for its many so-called health benefits.
— Harvey Diamond, *Fit for Life*

processed vegetable oils; pasteurized/homogenized milk; commercially
raised livestock; corn syrup and refined sugar. These, along with exposure
to a growing number of environmental poisons, are the real culprits in the
modern epidemics of cancer, heart disease, and other chronic illnesses.

Minerals

In addition to protein, carbohydrates, and fats, your body requires vitamins
and minerals. Minerals include potassium, chloride, sodium, calcium, phosphorus, iron, zinc, iodine, magnesium, and traces of copper, manganese, flu-
oride, molybdenum, selenium, chromium, and cobalt. RDDIs are given for
calcium, phosphorus, iodine, iron, magnesium, and zinc, but for the rest
there is insufficient information on which to base allowances. I concentrate
here on calcium, magnesium, iron, sodium, and zinc, because opinions regarding their roles in health and disease vary widely.

Calcium

Calcium is the most abundant mineral in the body and is the main component of bones and teeth. It helps the functioning of the heart, muscles,
and nerves and plays a major role in blood clotting after bleeding. Inactivity tends to deplete the skeleton of calcium, which is why old or
bedridden people incur fractures easily and why bed rest is harmful.
Calcium intake must be adequate, particularly during the last two
months of pregnancy, because more than half the calcium required will
be deposited in the fetal bones at that time. It is simplistic to take calcium
supplements, even those that come with magnesium and zinc. It is much
better to choose foods that have an abundance of calcium, such as leafy
green vegetables (see the table).

News for Milkaholics!

Milk, cheese, yogurt, and other dairy products immediately spring to
mind when calcium is mentioned. Dietitians who term them "nature's
perfect food" are deplorably unaware of the extensive contrary evidence
that can be found, for example, at http://www.notmilk.com. A lengthy
expose of the hazards of cow's milk was featured in an article by breast
cancer surgeon Robert Kradjian, M.D., in *The New York Times Sunday Magazine* (October 6, 2002). Few would ever drink milk after reading his
well-referenced article! The book *Milk: A–Z* is a very readable summary
of medical studies showing 26 diseases linked to milk.

While the average American eats more than 350 pounds of dairy produce a year, milk is not part of the typical Eastern diet. A high percent-

age of all ethnic groups have trouble digesting lactose because, after about the age of four, we naturally lose the ability to secrete the enzymes lactase and rennin. There are countless "lactose free" products in stores today because milk intolerance can interfere with calcium absorption and the digestion of other foods as well as lead to malnutrition. Milk combines poorly with other foods and forms curds in the stomach. If you can digest milk, you are "lactase persistent," which is unusual. However, the more serious problems with milk are its proteins and hormones (inherent and added), discussed below.

Milk is not a natural source of the vitamins A and D that "fortify" milk. In many areas they must be added *by law*. Often the amount is not well-regulated and an excess of these two fat-soluble vitamins can contribute to toxicity as well as calcium loss and osteoporosis.

Your best source of vitamin A is foods high in beta-carotene, which the body uses to produce vitamin A. Vitamin D is actually a hormone. The vitamins A and D produced by your own body, not those of another animal or from a genetically engineered substitute, are necessary for your own vital functions. Your body makes vitamin D when your skin is exposed to sunlight. An average of 15 minutes of sunlight per day on the hands and face is enough for the necessary amount of vitamin D, but in the absence of adequate sun exposure, supplementation is advised, through fortified soymilk or 20 mg supplements. In his book, *Vegetarian and Vegan Nutrition*, George Eisman, M.A., M.Sc., R.D., writes:

> It has since been discovered that the Vitamin D necessary to absorb the calcium moving down the intestine must already have been in the bloodstream for a while; what is present with calcium (in milk) is useless at that stage. Vitamin D is part of the mechanism to break bone down so that it can then stretch and grow. Thus an overdose of D can eventually lead to osteoporosis.

Thirty-eight years ago, the *Journal of Pediatrics* reported that "consuming as little as 45 micrograms of Vitamin D-3 in young children has resulted in signs of overdose." Vitamin D is toxic in overdose. Testing of forty-two milk samples found only 12 percent within the expected range. Testing of ten samples of infant formula revealed that seven contained twice the amount of vitamin D as was reported on the label, according to the *New England Journal of Medicine* in 1992.

As well as synthetic vitamin D, additives to milk include iodine (from disinfectants used to clean cows' udders, milking machines, and storage tanks) and dioxins if the milk comes in a chlorine-bleached carton. (The common use of corn as a filler in beverage cartons often causes allergies as well.) Since 1994, Bst (Bovine somatotropin), a synthetic hormone manufactured by Monsanto, has been given to cows in the United States. (See *Milk: The Deadly Poison* by Robert Cohen for the full story.) Experiments with feeding calves the processed cow's milk sold to humans caused them to become sick and die. Most adults today no longer give their pets milk because the animals get diarrhea and other sicknesses.

Milk is also mucus-forming, often causing pimples, acne, phlegm, and allergies. This "liquid meat" is sometimes produced under unhygienic conditions, as was seen in the 1985 accidental cross-connection in Chicago between raw and pasteurized milk that resulted in a violent salmonella outbreak that killed four and made an estimated 150,000 ill. In 1999, coliform bacteria was detected in 62 percent of bulk tank milk. As I write this, Wal-Mart is recalling its Danish Havarti cheese because of listeria contamination (which survives pasteurization). Cows are routinely fed antibiotics to cut down on these problems and antibiotics are detectable in one out of three cartons of milk.

Northrup (www.drnorthrup.com) has observed that many cases of breast cysts, endometriosis, uterine fibroids, and vaginal discharges can be reversed or substantially improved by eliminating dairy products. Breast cancer incidence (and twinning) is highest in Holland and Denmark and very low in Japan, and these contrasts parallel each nation's consumption of dairy products. Research published by The Physicians Committee for Responsible Medicine has shown that dairy product consumption is linked to breast and ovarian cancer. Dairy products were never part of the Japanese diet until introduced by Americans after World War II. A decade later the first cases of breast cancer appeared.

Formerly we were taught "milk is one of the four food groups and the major source of calcium." However, the amount of phosphorus in pasteurized milk can impair the body's absorption of calcium. Animals much larger than humans, for example the elephant, develop their bone structure not from drinking the milk of another species but from eating a vegetarian diet — leaves, grass, and vegetables.

Consumption of animal foods that contain high levels of protein and phosphorus acidify the blood. Calcium is then leached from bones to alkalinize the acidity. This is a major cause of osteoporosis, which is increasing in both women and men. Osteoporosis begins slowly (a "pediatric disease with geriatric consequences"); therefore, pregnancy is a good time to become aware that milk may not be the ideal source of calcium.

Cheese and yogurt are concentrated, and thus worse, forms of milk. They are high in methionine, which breaks down to homocysteine (now being researched as a cause of preterm labor). It takes ten pounds of milk to make one pound of cheese and Americans today each consume more than thirty-one pounds each year, consumption having tripled in the past twenty years.

Dr. T. Colin Campbell of the Oxford-Cornell-Chinese study showed that no animal products are needed to prevent osteoporosis and its incidence is much lower in vegetarians. Ironically, osteoporosis tends to occur in countries where calcium intake is highest, most of it coming from dairy products.

Rates of hip fracture among different populations is one way researchers measure the prevalence of osteoporosis. One such study of ten nations revealed that as calcium intake increased, so did the number of hip fractures. The blacks in South Africa have the lowest rate of hip fractures, yet their calcium intake is about one-tenth of what the United States government recommends. In a twelve-year Harvard study of 78,000 women, those who drank milk three times a day actually broke more bones than women who rarely drank milk. Similarly, a 1994 study of elderly men and women in Australia, showed that those with the highest dairy product consumption had approximately double the risk of hip fracture compared with those with the lowest consumption.

What might milk do to your babies' bones?

Would they or you want to nurse from a cow's udder?

The Physicians Committee for Responsible Medicine filed a petition with the Federal Trade Commission (FTC) requesting an *Investigation of Health Claims Made in and Omissions of Material Facts from Milk Mustache Advertisements* by the National Fluid Milk Processor Promotion Board, the Milk Industry Foundation, and the International Dairy Foods Association. The FTC turned the petition over to the USDA — the same government agency responsible for disseminating the ads in the first place! Although the Agriculture Research Service's scientific review raised concerns about the false and misleading nature of many of the health claims made in the challenged milk mustache ads, the FTC ended its almost two-year investigation by declining to take action on the petition.

Yet the American Dietetic Association endorses the National Dairy Council! Most of the free brochures made available in prenatal/

Most people are not interested in new ideas, but prefer to have their own opinions validated.

One of the bonuses of our starting to eat sea vegetables is that our two older children, who never liked milk, just relish them.

menopause/osteoporosis clinics are provided by national or state Dairy Boards to promote their products!

The Women, Infants and Children (WIC) supplemental food program is the largest purchaser of formula in the United States and provides pregnant and postpartum women and children up to the age of five with lots of dairy products; it is organized by the Department of Agriculture and also helps to take care of the dairy product surplus. By the same token, WIC offers no protein substitute for milk and cheese for women who might be vegans.

Unfortunately, we are so accustomed to the promotion of dairy products as healthful that it seems like heresy to expose the truth. Pregnant women and nursing mothers are usually exhorted to drink *extra* milk for both the protein and calcium content. (A lactating woman does not need to drink milk to make milk, although high fluid intake, preferably pure water, is essential.)

Milk substitutes are becoming more available in regular supermarkets because of public demand. They are made from soy, rice, almond, tofu, and millet. You can also make your own grain milks for just pennies; see http://www.soytoy.com. Whole wheat pancakes and sauces can be made with soy milk, and soups can be "creamed" by blending in some soft tofu or rolled oats.

Excellent Sources of Calcium

Dark leafy green vegetables, such as kale and collards, mustard, and turnip greens provide calcium that is well absorbed. A single cup of broccoli contains almost a fourth of the RDDI of calcium. You can see in the table below that arugula has up to seven times as much calcium as dairy products and about three times more than broccoli. Also known as rocket or rocquette, it has a delicious nutty taste and has recently appeared in gourmet restaurants. Yet, arugula, like mustard greens and kale, is very hardy and will self-seed and survive even in cold winters like those in New England. (You can order it from www.diamondorganics.com.) Dandelion greens, also high in calcium and delicious in soups, stews, and salad, grow free on lawns!

The Benefits of Sea Vegetables

Sea vegetables contain the highest calcium levels of all foods and abundant minerals, trace elements, and vitamins. Hijiki, for example, contains ten times more calcium than a comparable volume of cheese, milk, or other dairy food. It is also high in iron, protein, and vitamins A, D, B_1,

Calcium Content of Certain Foods

FOOD	AMOUNT	MILLIGRAMS OF CALCIUM PER 100 CALORIES.	FOOD	AMOUNT	MILLIGRAMS OF CALCIUM PER 100 CALORIES.
Arugula	1 cup	1,300	American cheese	1 cup	160
Watercress	1 cup	800	Kelp (Seaweed)	1 cup	170
Turnip greens	1 cup	650	Mustard Greens	1 cup	150
Collard greens	1 cup	548	Wakame (Seaweed)	1 cup	150
Mustard greens	1 cup	490	Blackstrap Molasses	1 tbs	140
Spinach	1 cup	450	Amaranth	1 cup	140
Broccoli	1 cup	387	Great Northern Beans	1 cup	140
Collard Greens	1 cup	355	Dried Figs	5 figs	135
Bok Choy	1 cup	250	Vegetarian Baked Beans	1 cup	130
Swiss cheese	1 cup	250	Navy Beans	1 cup	130
Milk (2-percent)	1 cup	245	Corn Tortilla	1 tortilla	120
Green onions	1 cup	240	Fortified Orange Juice	6 ounces	120
Okra	1 cup	213	Kidney Beans	1 cup	115
Turnip Greens	1 cup	200	Black Beans	1 cup	105
Kale	1 cup	200	Okra	1 cup	90
Cabbage	1 cup	196	Acorn Squash	1 cup	90
Whole milk	1 cup	190	Pinto Beans	1 cup	85
Broccoli	1 cup	180	Tofu	1 cup	130
Cheddar cheese	1 cup	179	Soybeans	1 cup	175

Mineral Content of Sea Vegetables in mg per 100 grams

SEA VEGETABLE	CALCIUM	IRON	IODINE	POTASSIUM
Agar-agar	567	6.3	0.2	0
Dulse	296	150.0	8.0	8,060
Hijiki	1,400	30.0	0	0
Irish moss	885	8.9	0	0
Kelp	1,093	100.0	150.0	5,273
Nori (green and red)	470	23.0	0	0

Source: Sara Shannon, *Diet for an Atomic Age*.

Toward the end of my pregnancy when my twins were huge, I used to blend the high-protein powder sold in health food stores into a shake with fruit. It was quick to prepare and delicious.

and B$_{12}$. Seaweed (dried) comes from Maine and Japan and is sold in health food stores. Agar functions like gelatin and is easy to use in desserts. Wakame and dulse can be added to soups. Strips of kombu placed on the bottom of a pan of beans will prevent them from sticking as they cook and will add minerals and nutrients to the meal. Seaweed granules are available with other spices (garlic, ginger, or cayenne) to season food as a salt substitute. Seaweed, after soaking to soften it and remove excess salt, can be sauteed with other vegetables (and some grated ginger and soy sauce), baked, stir-fried, steamed, and eaten with salads — they are a most versatile and delicious food. I put ginger and seaweed (both very alkalinizing) together with my customized supplements in a fruit smoothie every morning.

Individuals with thyroid dysfunction should consult their physicians before adding sea vegetables to their diet because some have high iodine content. Lawrence Wood, M.D., author of *Your Thyroid*, considers the basic American diet already too high in iodine. Excess iodine results from milk consumption, use of iodates as dough oxidizers in making bread, and the (often excessive) use of iodized table salt.

For almost everyone, sea vegetables are a safe and healthy addition to the diet and a better source of many essential micronutrients than land-grown foods. Further information about sea vegetables can be found in Evelyn McConnaughey's *Sea Vegetables: Harvesting Guide and Cookbook* and in any macrobiotic cookbook.

Magnesium

This mineral is important for nerves and digestion and is known as the "relaxer." It is also a laxative, as you may find out if you are taking too much in supplements. When women are in preterm labor, magnesium sulfate (Epsom salts) is pumped in through an IV to relax the uterus. Magnesium is found in corn, figs, barley, sea vegetables, and beans.

Iron

The transport of oxygen requires iron. Although the amount needed is comparatively small, adequate amounts are vital and anemia is relatively common in women and men, despite the amount of meat consumed by the average American. (Iron deficiency anemia rates are similar in vegetarians and non-vegetarians. The higher vitamin C content of vegetarian diets may improve iron absorption.)

Together with protein, iron forms hemoglobin in the red blood cells to bind with oxygen. Hemoglobin gives the blood in arteries a bright red

Iron Content in Various Foods in mg per 100 grams

(3 1/2 oz. or 1/2 cup)

WHOLE CEREAL GRAINS	
Millet	6.8
Soba (buckwheat noodle)	5
Oats	4.6
Buckwheat	3.1
Brown rice	1.6

BEANS	
Soybeans	8.4
Chickpea	6.9
Lentils	6.8
Azuki	4.8

VEGETABLES (RAW)	
Swiss chard	3.2
Dandelion greens	3.1
Kale	2.2

Source: U.S. Department of Agriculture and Michio Kushi and Aveline Kushi, *Macrobiotic Pregnancy and Care of the Newborn*.

SEA VEGETABLES	
Hijiki	29
Wakame	13
Nori	12
Arame	12
Dulse	6.3

SEEDS AND NUTS	
Pumpkin seeds	11.2
Sesame seeds	10.5
Sunflower seeds	7.1
Walnuts	3.1

MEAT AND POULTRY	
Beef	2.5–2.7
Chicken	1.6
Eggs	1.3

DAIRY FOODS	
(not recommended but added for comparison)	
Cheddar cheese	1
Whole milk	Trace

color; the blood in the veins is darker because its oxygen has been given up. Protein, folic acid, vitamins B_{12} and C, plus trace elements such as copper and cobalt, are also required for the production of red blood cells.

Menstruation is usually blamed for iron deficiencies in women, but more typically the cause is the modern diet. Iron deficiency may manifest itself in early pregnancy in loss of appetite (which hinders the cure), weakness, fatigue, skin eruptions, bronchitis, hemorrhages, asthma, and hair loss.

Additional iron is needed for both the mother's and the babies' circulations, and a store of iron for the babies' postpartum life must be laid down as well. With two or more babies, the requirements are increased proportionately. Furthermore, in the last weeks of pregnancy, each fetus doubles its own iron requirements; babies born preterm are often anemic because the liver is too immature to store sufficient iron. Low iron levels in mothers expecting multiples, however, usually indicate *high* levels of storage in the babies' livers.

What appears to be anemia in a multiple pregnancy may be the result of the increased plasma volume in the circulation, which dilutes the quantity of red blood cells. A simple check is to stretch open your hands and look at the color of the lines — they should be deep pink to reddish, as should the mucous membranes of your lower eyelid.

Getting enough iron is not simply a matter of dietary intake — its absorption is critical. Foods containing vitamin C and protein help iron absorption when they are eaten at the same meal. Some iron will be obtained from iron cookware. Liver and meat directly supply heme iron (both protein and iron), which has long been advised as a remedy for anemia. However, liver and meat are high in toxic components such as hormones, pesticides, and antibiotics unless you have an organic source.

Excess iron from supplements is excreted from the body and turns the stool black. Iron capsules may cause constipation and occasionally vomiting, and can deplete the body of other nutrients, such as zinc. Also, routine prescriptions of iron and other supplements may mask more complex and serious dietary deficiencies, so any use of supplements needs to be monitored carefully (see information on metabolic testing in the section "Testing and Customization"). The average Chinese adult, who shows no evidence of anemia, consumes twice as much iron as the average American does, mainly from vegetables. Sources of iron include legumes, tofu, green leafy vegetables, dried fruit, whole grains, iron-fortified cereals and breads, prunes, and blackstrap molasses.

Chlorophyll, a blood-builder, is high in iron and potassium; it can be obtained in tablets as well as leafy green vegetables. For example, there is eighty times more chlorophyll in dark green or red leaf lettuces than iceberg (leave that type on the shelf). Both play a role in the development of new tissue, and the production of cells is greatly accelerated in a multiple pregnancy. Brown skin pigmentation, especially on the faces of women who take oral contraceptives or who are pregnant, may be related to folic acid deficiency. After the publicity about the preventive role of folic acid against neural tube defects, it is now added to many foods.* Vegetarian women typically have higher intakes than non-vegetarians.

*Its supposed role in preventing neural tube defects like spina bifida was published in *Lancet* and the *New England Journal of Medicine* in 1991 and 1992, followed by massive public health campaigns. However, the British Isles Network of Congenital Anomalies register showed that it was between 1980 and 1985 that there was a significant drop in neural tube defects and the graph remained flat after 1985. Odent postulates that the development of supermarkets, which meant easy access to a greater variety of food, occurred in Europe during that drop.

Vitamin B_{12} and folic acid (found in bright green foliage, hence its name) are also important in the prevention of anemia. Vitamin B_{12} is needed only in minute amounts (4 micrograms per day in a singleton pregnancy), and it is supplied by oatmeal, whole grains, sea vegetables, eggs, and fish. Tempeh, made from fermented soybeans, provides 2–4 micrograms per 100 grams. If small amounts of animal food are included in a vegetarian diet occasionally or supplements are taken, vitamin B_{12} deficiency can be avoided. The American Dietetic Association recommends that pregnant and lactating vegans supplement 2.0 micrograms and 2.6 micrograms, respectively, of vitamin B_{12} daily.

Sodium (Salt)

This mineral is indispensable for good health. It keeps the stomach wall alkaline to secrete enough hydrochloric acid for digestion. Okra and celery are excellent sources of sodium along with strawberries, apples, and most fruits.

There is no RDDI for sodium; recommended amounts range from 500 mg to 2,400 mg (about a teaspoonful), according to the Food and Nutrition Board.

In contrast, the typical American diet has 1 to 3 teaspoons a day, and those who eat many canned and processed foods and drink artificially softened water are taking in about 4 teaspoons of sodium daily. Salt appetite is determined by habits, especially those formed in early childhood. There is plenty of sodium in milk, cheese, processed meats, canned vegetables, snack foods like potato chips and nuts (unless unsalted), and many baked goods.

The Dangers of Salt Restriction

Salt restriction during pregnancy limits the normal expansion of the blood volume, with disastrous consequences. Placental development may be slowed, with the formation of dead tissue (infarcts) reducing the transfer of nutrients to the babies. Sometimes the placenta will separate from the wall of the uterus (abruption), causing bleeding and cutting off oxygen to the babies.

When salt is restricted below the body's requirements, the kidney reacts by releasing a hormone, rennin, into the bloodstream. Rennin influences other hormones that in turn cause the small arteries to constrict. This raises the blood pressure because the same amount of blood is being pumped with the same force but through a smaller opening.

Understandably, obstetricians worry about high blood pressure because it accompanies the dangerous pregnancy syndrome of toxemia/ preeclampsia/eclampsia/HELLP. However, a low-sodium diet can cause hypertension where there was none before.

Restriction of salt also reduces the mother's food choices, and makes the permitted foods less palatable. Her appetite wanes, so by eating less she becomes more malnourished. As her intake of protein falls, her liver becomes less able to manufacture circulating serum proteins, such as albumin. When albumin levels fall, water is lost from her circulation in the area surrounding the cells (interstitial space). Ironically, this can give false assurance that other substances in the blood, such as iron, are present in adequate levels (and mask anemia). Fluid lost from the bloodstream in this way shows up as generalized swelling of tissues (edema).

Edema caused by this fall in albumin levels is abnormal, a sign of the dreaded disease. It will increase as long as the woman's body is malnourished. Her kidneys excrete less water in the urine as they try to conserve salt and water within normal limits. However, the reabsorbed water cannot be held in the bloodstream since albumin levels are too low, so it leaks out into the tissues. The result is rapid swelling and added pounds that imperil the babies' development and even life.

Sodium is essential not only for the fetus but for the amniotic fluid as well. Requirements increase with the demands made by maternal tissue, muscle function, digestive system, and blood circulation. Cravings for salty foods such as olives and pickles, the subject of many pregnancy jokes, are often a response to a biological need and point to a dietary imbalance. Sodium helps the fluid balance.

During pregnancy the blood volume increases — 100 percent or more in the case of multiples. Adequate fluid levels must be maintained so that sufficient blood volume can perfuse each placenta. (A helpful guide is that your urine should be pale yellow, excluding vitamin tints.) That means that expectant mothers of twins should drink at least sixteen 8-ounce glasses a day including teas, soups, and other liquids. More than 80 percent of the body, 75 percent of the brain, and even 25 percent of our bones is water! You may want to fill three jugs every morning to make it simpler to estimate. (This will be a good routine to establish for nursing when you will need to ensure a high fluid intake as well.)

When the level of circulating blood does not meet the demands of pregnancy, particularly in a multiple pregnancy, a serious state of inadequate blood volume (hypovolemia) results. In addition to limiting the function of the placentas, low blood volume predisposes the mother to dehydration and preterm labor.

Commercial salt has several additives, including iodine, whereas evaporated sea salt (usually from France and found in health food stores) does not and contains a host of other natural minerals as well. Use sea salt to taste.

Zinc

Essential for more than 100 enzymes involved in protein synthesis and growth, zinc is very important in pregnancy. Oral contraceptives and iron supplements deplete zinc from the body. It is found in whole grains (especially the germ and bran), eggs, cereals, legumes, and nuts.

Vitamin and Mineral Supplements

For the doctor or midwife, routine prescription of one-size-fits-all iron and vitamins is much simpler and quicker than an in-depth session of nutritional history and counseling. Supplements can be used therapeutically as well as preventively. People who swallow large doses of megavitamins and other supplements from health food stores are moving into the realm of pharmacology. They risk overdose, secondary depletion of other nutrients, and potential interaction with medications they might be taking. Many people wrongly believe that the more vitamins one takes, the better. Some vitamins, such as A and D, if taken in excess can be stored in the body and actually reach toxic levels; they also can cause birth defects. Others, such as vitamin C, are water soluble, and excesses are passed out in the urine.

Testing and Customization of Supplements

This wave of the future has arrived: determining micronutrition according to your own biochemisty. People do not readily fit into charts — it is better to investigate a person's individual nutritional requirements and customize the supplements.

The Vegatest (now evolved into the Electrodermal System — EDS) picks up preclinical illness (that is, cellular changes that occur before a diagnosis is made) and can determine individual vitamin and mineral needs, food allergies, stressed internal organs, toxins, and so on. It was developed by visionary Helmut Schimmel, M.D., D.M.D., in Germany. This noninvasive biofeedback measurement is ideal for pregnancy. After a specific deficiency has been determined, remedial doses are prescribed using the same biofeedback system. This test is available in Australia, Great Britain, and Europe but difficult to find in the United States where our "managed don't care" system is still oriented toward treating instead of preventing disease.

A biofeedback device that taps into your "living systems" information network, the Vegatest picks up signals from the connective tissue, which triggers information about specific body functions and can determine toxins blocking the absorption of nutrients. Symptoms do not exist in isolation — they are part of a constellation of causes and effects stemming from a primary source or event. When we treat only symptoms, we do not address the cause of the problem. The one-on-one testing to diagnose problems and customize solutions at the preclinical level is expensive. (Some practitioners will simply hook you up to a computer, which is not the same at all.) Stuart Zoll, a doctor of Oriental Medicine and director of the Center for Preventive Medicine in Boca Raton, Florida, and author of *The Bridge Between Acupuncture and Modern Bio Energetic Medicine*, is one of the nation's foremost practitioners and can refer you to skilled testers in other areas. (See Resources.)

Metabolic testing used to be a privilege of elite athletes and the rich, requiring a physician to order the analyses. However, today various in-home tests enable you to benefit from customized vitamins and supplements. The lab kits collect various body fluids to be tested by MetaMetrix Laboratories in Atlanta. The results are sent to Douglas Labs, a formulary in Pittsburgh, Pennsylvania, where, for example, your daily dose of vitamins, minerals, amino acids, and other supplements will be scientifically selected from up to fifty-five nutrients. Cellophane packets containing your daily supply of capsules are then auto-shipped to you each month through the mail. Your body gets exactly what you need, which ends the expense and waste of guesswork. You can find out more about this high-quality, low-cost program by visiting www.elizabethnoble.com/healthtests.

Many excellent prenatal vitamins are now available, but you have to choose with care. Doctors will often recommend a prenatal supplement, and some even prescribe them, but the quality can vary dramatically. Look for a prenatal formula that is in capsules because tablets are much harder to digest and typically use fillers like cellulose (cardboard) and chalk. Some are even coated with shellac. Make sure the supplements are free from additives, sugar, and artificial color. The highest quality supplements will be properly mixed so that the ingredients are evenly distributed and manufactured to United States Pharmacopia (USP) standards, the highest in the industry. Look for calcium, magnesium, and other minerals that are chelated to amino acids for maximum absorption. Quality supplements may have nutrient amounts that vary significantly from the RDDIs. Most will be significantly higher, while a few ingredients may be lower, to create optimal balance. Obtain your prenatal vitamins from someone knowledgeable, whose opinion you trust, or contact me (info@elizabethnoble.com) for recommendations.

There are also some excellent nutritional supplements that provide an easy way to increase intake of nutrient rich "green foods." These capsules containing dehydrated and concentrated powder are derived from a range of green vegetables including broccoli, kale, blue-green algae, and dozens of others. However, to test is best.

Planning Your Diet

A healthy diet consists of a variety of whole foods. Pregnant and lactating mothers of multiples should eat as much as they can, choosing whole grains and vegetables, and legumes or organic animal protein (especially coldwater fish as already discussed). Snack on fruit, nuts, and seeds between meals. Dried fruits such as dates, raisins, prunes, apricots (high in iron), and figs (high in magnesium) can be eaten as is or soaked in water overnight.

Whole Grains

Whole grains include wheat, brown rice, corn, barley, millet, oats, buckwheat, bulgur, quinoa, and rye. These grains come in many forms such as bread, pasta, couscous, cereals, corn grits, and of course, flour. Such complex carbohydrates, together with starchy vegetables like potatoes, should provide half to two-thirds of the calories in your diet. Quinoa, pronounced "keenwa," has all the essential amino acids and cooks in half the time of rice. It is very delicious, as is buckwheat, which makes great pancakes. Bulgur (cracked wheat) turns into tabouleh when parsley, mint, carrots, tomatoes, and some olive oil and lemon juice are added. Various "breads" such as pita pockets (also known as Lebanese or Syrian bread), tortillas, chapattis, and "wraps" are even easier than sandwiches to combine with your favorite protein and salad. Cooked oatmeal (porridge) makes a hearty breakfast. You can add organic soy milk, or just use more water when cooking it.

Vegetables

Choose a mixture of surface, leafy, and root vegetables each day. Surface vegetables include squash, pumpkin, cucumber, peas, beans, zucchini, cauliflower, and celery. Leafy vegetables are bok choy, collard greens, kale, Swiss chard, parsley, watercress, dark green lettuce (e.g., romaine), arugula, dandelion greens, endive, escarole, and broccoli. Root vegetables include carrots, onions, radishes, parsnips, turnips, daikon (long white radish), and potatoes.

The liver is the detoxification center of the body and one-quarter of our blood is in the liver at all times. Two or more servings of green leafy vegetables (especially parsley and dandelion) will help it function well.

Vegetables are the builders, fruits are the cleansers.

Fruits

Fruits make ideal snacks between meals; eat them apart from grains and starchy vegetables because the combination will cause fermentation in the stomach (particularly melons). Fruits can be eaten fresh (when ripe), stewed, or dried. Prunes and dried apricots are a good source of iron. Fresh fruits have high water content, which helps to keep you hydrated and your bowels regular. However, dried fruits will pull water out of your body; therefore, you will need to increase your fluid intake when eating them. (Pure water is best and should be consumed at room temperature. Any kind of cold or iced drinks will cause the glands in your stomach to contract, making less gastric juice available for digestion.)

Legumes

Legumes include soybeans (from which tofu, tempeh, and miso are made), chickpeas (garbanzos), lentils, azuki beans, kidney beans, split peas, pinto beans, lima beans, navy beans, and black-eyed peas. They can be eaten hot or cold. A mixture of kidney beans, lima beans, navy beans, and green and yellow fresh garden beans makes a tasty salad that is very high in protein; add some olive oil, chopped garlic, and spring onions. "Veggie burgers" from various sources are widely available today in supermarkets and can be enjoyed on a whole wheat bun.

Animal Protein

Fresh fish from a fish market is best. It is worth a special trip because supermarket fish is often older and smells and, if farmed, has insufficient omega-3 EFAs. Sardines are an excellent source of calcium as are canned salmon, smelts, and any fish with edible bones. Search for poultry, eggs, and meat that are naturally grown. Eggs with increased omega-3 fatty acids can be bought in most supermarkets.

Fats, Oils

Eat a few tablespoons per day of the best quality, on salads and in dressings. It is just as easy to steam food or to stir-fry it in liquid as to heat (and damage) oils. Fresh bread dipped in olive oil, as offered in upscale Italian restaurants, is just as delicious as bread and butter. Spread avocado or tofu "mayonnaise" on bread or rolls.

Leave on the shelf anything with the label stating "partially hydrogenated" (typical of almost all packaged snack foods including peanut butter). Cottonseed oil is the cheapest and most toxic; it escapes regulation by the FDA because it is not a food! A 1998 article in *Toxicology* warns that "farmers who raise livestock have known for years that cottonseed feedstuffs can disrupt pregnancy and early embryo development in female animals, and can cause sperm immotility and depressed sperm counts in males." Cottonseed oil is used in many processed foods, so check your ingredients carefully.

In addition to pesticides used to kill the boll weevil, cotton plants before harvest are sprayed with strong defoliating chemicals to make the leaves fall off so that it is easier and cleaner to pick. I read a label on a peanut butter jar recently that said "fully saturated cottonseed oil." How fortunate that I was warned, thanks to labeling laws.

Both EFAs can be found in walnuts, fish, flaxseed, soybeans, sesame seeds, sunflower seeds, pumpkin, black currant or primrose oil, amaranth (a grain), oatmeal, lemon balm, and wheat germ oil. However, the best source of omega-3 fatty acids — so important for a healthy pregnancy — is ocean fish.

Bitter Condiments

Beets in apple cider vinegar, artichokes, mustard greens, and other bitter foods stimulate the gastric juices and enhance digestion. We have four different taste zones on our tongues, and the bitter one is underserved.

Desserts

Eat fruits, cooked or fresh, depending on what is in season. For dessert sweeteners, use rice syrup, barley malt, amazake, and pure maple syrup instead of white sugar. You can get the herb stevia, which is many times

The whiter the bread, the bigger the spread, the sooner I'm dead.

The more you fry, the sooner you die.
— Wayne Pickering

sweeter than sugar, as a powder or drops. It does not cause tooth decay or dump empty calories into your body. There are nutritious desserts such as carrot cake, nut tarts, apple pie, and jelled fruits (beware of gelatin allergy, which is common; instead use agar-agar, derived from seaweed to make a gel).

Seeds

These include hulled sesame seeds (which are high in calcium and can be roasted with sea salt to make a delicious condiment called Gomasio to sprinkle over cooked grains), sunflower seeds (toss in a spinach salad to help counteract the oxalic acid, which makes the calcium less absorbable), and pumpkin seeds (which supply EFAs and zinc). Keep jars of these seeds handy to use as garnishes and add to cereals. Flax seeds provide EFAs and prevent constipation (soak overnight).

Nuts

Buy only raw fresh nuts and keep them in the refrigerator or freezer because they become rancid easily. Mixed nuts make great snacks and provide EFAs, calories, and protein. Buy them unsalted and add sea salt to taste.

Snacks

Fruit, raw vegetables, rice cakes, whole grain crackers, unsalted popcorn, trail mix, granola bars, small jars of applesauce, and organic soymilk in aseptic boxes with straws are convenient snacks to carry around.

Tortilla chips with salsa became popular since the last edition of this book. The blue corn chips are very tasty. Fast foods can be nutritious — even MacDonald's has a salad bar now. Try enchiladas, tortillas, chili, corn on the cob, baked potatoes. Stay away from the refined carbohydrates (white flour) and reheated fats. Both are huge culprits in the degenerative diseases plaguing modern life.

Beverages

Choose from pure water, herbal teas (double or triple strength chamomile is good before bed), green, bancha, or twig tea (non-caffeine teas, available from health food stores), fruit and vegetable juice (preferably made fresh).

Eat More! Drink More!

- Eat more courses at a meal: Start with a soup and bread or rolls, then a salad, then the main course, and finish with dessert.

- Eat more snacks between meals.

- Eat seasonal foods as much as possible. Select organic produce that is locally grown. For example, baked turnip and squash is a delicious, very inexpensive dish, satisfying and warming in winter. Contrast this with a winter salad of costly imported iceberg lettuce and hothouse tomatoes, yielding little nutritional value (or taste).

- Mix the colors in your food; the darker the colors, the higher the nutrition. Use yellow and green vegetables every day, especially leafy green vegetables. Choose foods that will offer a variety of tastes — sweet, bitter, and so on.

- Every day eat some raw as well as cooked vegetables, at least 6–8 servings (about one cup per serving).

- Every day eat different fruits, at least 6–8 servings.

- Chew your food well to enhance digestion.

Cooking Hints

Shop for the best-quality food and cook it with skill. Replace any aluminum cookware because this toxic metal has been linked to Alzheimer's and Parkinson's diseases. (For the same reason, buy beverages in glass rather than cans.) Use cast iron, stainless steel, glass, or earthenware cookware. Steam vegetables, and bake and broil rather than fry. (The problem is not the fat because expectant mothers of multiples need calories, but its alteration through heating and the creation of toxic by-products.) Browning destroys nutrients and creates compounds that can cause cancer.

Wash fruits and vegetables with care and cook animal flesh well to destroy bacteria and other harmful microorganisms.

Soups can be eaten several times a day and are ideal for mothers of multiples with diminishing stomach space and high fluid requirements. You can carry soup around in a thermos. Save vegetable stock for soups to use the nutrients leached out during steaming. Miso (a Japanese paste of fermented grains or legumes, which is high in protein, can be kept for a long time in the refrigerator. Simply add miso to your supply of stock, with some sea vegetables, garlic, onions, and ginger to create a nutritious soup.

Blend fruits to make a smoothie to consume more in the semi-liquid form than if you ate the whole fruits. Vitamin, mineral, and protein supplements, ginger, sea vegetables, and other nutrients that you might find unpalatable by themselves can be easily disguised in soups and smoothies. Smoothies retain all the fiber, which you need to keep your intestines moving.

Soak grains and legumes in water overnight to improve cooking and digestibility. Beans in particular need to be well cooked (a stainless steel pressure-cooker helps) and well chewed. Adding herbs such as coriander and cumin improves digestibility and protein availability.

Growing sprouts, parsley, arugula, and basil on your windowsill guarantees some fresh green vegetables in the winter even for city dwellers.

Tofu can be found in various consistencies in the produce section of most supermarkets. Made from soybean curd, this traditional Asian food can be made into dressings, omelets, or dips, and it can be served cubed in soups, vegetable dishes, and spaghetti sauce and is used in "veggieburgers." Silken tofu can be blended into a shake with fruit, wheat germ, and protein powder. Tempeh is another soybean product that lends itself to cubes, slices, and "burgers." Like soy sauce, tempeh and miso are fermented, which renders the soybean more digestible and processes some otherwise harmful substances.

Eat slowly in a calm state of mind. Food is to be appreciated and enjoyed; the French, for example, think a "business lunch" is uncivilized, and in that country a midday break is observed so that families can dine at home together.

Meal Suggestions

The following meals are examples of what foods to eat when animal products, especially dairy, are reduced. Eating habits can take a long time to change, but in the meantime you can make sure you buy animal protein that is organically raised.

An expectant mother of multiples should eat as much as she can in each category. An excellent book of natural food recipes, divided into the four seasons and with helpful instructions to minimize time and maximize efficiency, is *The Book of Whole Meals* by Annemarie Colbin. Additional cookbooks are suggested in Further Reading, and mail-order whole food wholesalers are listed in Resources. Consider joining a food coop to save money, buy in bulk, and get top quality at wholesale prices.

Beverages

Drink pure water, coffee substitutes, herbal teas, juice, or mineral water in warmer weather, and hot cider in colder months (unfortunately many state laws have recently made pasteurization — killing with heat — a requirement). Invest in a blender so you can make the "smoothies" listed below.

PROTEIN DRINK	STARCH DRINK	VEGETABLE DRINK	FRUIT DRINK
Sunflower seeds	Cooked Cereal	Carrots	Pineapple
Cashews	Amasake	Parsley	Ripe banana
Organic Soy Milk	Cinnamon	Celery	Apple juice
		Tomato juice	Kiwi fruit

Breakfast

Fruit

Eat several different kinds whole, as juice (mix the pulp back in!), or in a smoothie. Eat fresh berries and dried fruit like figs, prunes, and dates.

Cereal

You can make your own organic granola: mix rolled oats, raw wheat germ (keeps fresh only for a week in the refrigerator), pumpkin seeds, sesame seeds, sunflower seeds, cinnamon, raisins, sliced almonds, and crushed walnuts. Regular oatmeal or cornmeal is a filling breakfast and if cooked with enough water does not need liquid added (although amasake is a delicious milk substitute). Cook and stir without boiling.

Bread/Muffins

Warm rather than toast bread (burning creates toxins). Use jam sweetened with fruit juice, without added sugar, but better still is tahini (sesame seed butter, which is very high in calcium) or nut butters (soy, almond, cashew). Whole wheat muffins are easy and quick to make. If you buy them, watch out for hydrogenated oil.

For variety and extra nutrients, eat whole wheat pancakes with barley malt, maple syrup, or blackstrap molasses (high in iron).

Protein

Eat eggs (lightly cooked) several times a week. Also sardines or peanut butter.

Morning Snack 1

Whole grain bread (rye or millet causes fewer allergies than wheat does) or rice cakes with tahini or nut butter.

Celery sticks filled with sardines or salmon.

Vegetable or fruit juice. Carrot, beet, and celery juices, separately or mixed, are delicious.

Morning Snack 2

Turkey and avocado wraps with sprouts, watercress, grated carrot.

Jar of applesauce. You can add vanilla or cinnamon. Some applesauce is already combined with other fruits such as apricot or strawberry.

Lunch

Soup

Vegetable, kale and barley, lentil or miso soup (with tofu cubes for added protein and seaweed for extra minerals). Use a crock pot and make up a batch of hearty minestrone soup (containing pasta and as many vegetables as you have to toss in.)

Pasta made with Jerusalem artichoke (e.g., DeBole brand) is delicious and helps stabilize your blood sugar and contributes iron.

Grains

Whole grain rolls, cooked barley, millet or brown rice.

Vegetables

Kale, broccoli, butternut squash in winter.

For salads, mix many different ingredients — two or three kinds of lettuce, sprouts, carrot, cucumber, beets, red and green pepper, mushroom, radish, tomato (vine-ripened and locally grown). Left-over cooked vegetables like broccoli, green beans, asparagus, snow peas, and okra can be tossed in the salad.

Protein

Hummus (made from chickpeas and tahini) goes well with salad in whole grain pita bread.

Afternoon Snack 1

Whole grain crackers or crispbread with mackerel or herring.

Dried fruit and nuts. Dried fruits can be chopped, mixed, and rolled in (freshly grated) coconut.

Herbal tea or grain "coffee."

Afternoon Snack 2

Burrito with black beans, salsa, rice, and avocado.
Mixed seasonal fruits.
Baked potato.

Dinner

Soup

Potato-leek or pumpkin-chicken broth in winter; tomato or asparagus in summer. Gazpacho is a cold soup made with tomatoes, cucumber, peppers, parsley, garlic, and spring onions.

Main course

- Ocean fish with corn, green beans, carrots, Swiss chard.

- Lentil loaf with millet, broccoli, zucchini, parsnips.

- Tempeh with udon (whole wheat) or soba (buckwheat) noodles and mixed vegetables: onion, garlic, carrots, mushrooms, scallions, beans, broccoli, red pepper, snow peas, bean sprouts, endive, ginger. (Stir-fry in stock or water.)

- Beans and brown rice.

- Tofu cubes in spaghetti sauce with whole grain pasta.

- Roasted free-range chicken with potatoes, squash, turnip, parsnip, yams, collard greens, brussel sprouts, and whole wheat stuffing (onions, sage, parsley and celery).

Dessert

- Apples stuffed with raisins and baked with cinnamon tapioca.

- Couscous cake with fruit jelled in agar.

- Stewed apricots and soy "ice cream."

- Fresh fruit.

Non-Nutrients

Substances that deplete the body of vitamins and minerals include alcohol, coffee, sugar, drugs (antibiotics, sleeping pills, street drugs), laxatives, and tobacco. Luckily, pregnant women often develop a strong aversion to many of these harmful substances. Alcohol, pure sugar, and transfats are blocking agents for the EFAs needed by the developing brains and to prevent pregnancy complications. Smokers are advised to take in extra vitamin B_6, B_{12}, and C and bone minerals.

Caffeine and Additives in Beverages

Coffee, black teas, colas, sodas, and other beverages containing caffeine should be reduced and ideally eliminated during pregnancy. High intakes of caffeine (about eight cups a day) have been linked to complications.

Sodas also contain many additives, especially sugar. In hot weather, drinking such sweet liquids leads to dehydration because the sugar pulls fluid out of the circulation. Soft drinks also weaken bones because they contain phosphoric acid, which impairs the absorption of calcium. A study at the Harvard School of Public Health found that women who were athletes in college and who also drank sodas had twice the risk of breaking their first bone after age forty as their female teammates who did not drink sodas.

The long-term effects of chemical sugar substitutes in pregnancy are not known. When in doubt, leave them out. However, against great resistance from the sugar industry and the FDA, the herb stevia is now available as a sweetener (in health food stores).

Dilute fruit juice with filtered water. If you do not have a good source of drinking water, bottled water with a slice of lime or lemon is refreshing.

Alcohol

Consumption of alcohol by expectant mothers, according to the March of Dimes, is the third most common cause of mental retardation in newborns in some areas of the United States. It has not been established how little is safe, but the amounts are reduced with each study. It is known that as little as 10 grams of alcohol (one drink) per day leads to a small but significant decrease in birth weight. Too much alcohol during pregnancy can cause serious, long-lasting effects on the child. Typical signs of the fetal alcohol syndrome include physical and mental defects such as a small body and brain, poor coordination, and deficient attention span. The appearance of such a child may be characteristic — narrow eyes and a short nose with a low bridge. Heart defects and behavioral problems have also been observed. Nonalcoholic beer and wine, cider (plain and sparkling), and grape juice can be substituted.

Drugs

Any kind of drugs — street narcotics, over-the-counter medications, prescription drugs (check carefully for risk during pregnancy) — put your babies at risk. Before you take nasal sprays, cough medicine, antihista-mines, sedatives, painkillers, sleeping pills, salves, ointments, and so on, ask to see the package insert, which contains information about the drug's actions, side effects, and contraindications. If you do not have the insert, consult the Physicians' Desk Reference at the pharmacy or your local library.

If you have a special condition for which your doctor prescribes a drug, the dosage may be critical in pregnancy. Follow the instructions carefully. It may be possible to do without the medication or to try an alternative therapy such as homeopathy, meditation, or visualization. An excellent guide is *Prescription for Nutritional Healing*, by James F. Balch, M.D., and Phyllis Balch, C.N.C. Just because a drug has been approved by the FDA and prescribed by your physician does not mean it is safe for your unborn babies. Thousands of people die from prescription drug use every year. Mothers found out, many years later, that DES (diethyl-stilbestrol — a drug used in the 1950s to prevent miscarriage) led to problems in their female offspring. Tetracycline (which causes staining of the offspring's permanent teeth) was another medication that was once thought harmless during pregnancy.

Radiation

Dental or other X-rays should only be done if the benefit outweighs the risks. Sit at least 20 feet from color television sets and stand away from a microwave oven. Other household appliances that produce low levels of radiation include alarm systems, paging devices, remote-control garage door openers, and cellular phones. Electric blankets and water bed heaters have been associated with miscarriages. Computers with the old-fashioned screens, like a TV monitor, emit radiation from the cathode ray tube; the safer flat screens of liquid crystal generally do not. If you live near high-voltage power lines or a nuclear power plant, increase your intake of sea vegetables and miso. The calcium, iodine, and sodium alginate in sea vegetables help remove radioactive substances from the body.

Household Products and Environmental Toxins

Paint, solvents, glues, stains, pesticides, herbicides, and harsh cleaning compounds have various degrees of toxicity. Natural detergents are available in health food stores and on-line.

Arsenic is in 90 percent of chicken feed and the hormone DES is given to 80 percent of beef and lamb feed in the United States. Heavy metals can be absorbed by the body; check the blood vessels under your tongue (the veins should be thin and light-colored) or have a hair analysis to reveal any toxicity.

Make Time for Yourself and Your Babies' Needs

The enormous success of the fast-food industry has shown how difficult it is for busy working people to take the time for a good diet, to shop for the most healthful foods, and to prepare them in the most nutritious way. The availability, convenience, and low price of dietary junk (most of it could not be called "food") is very seductive, especially to children. Yet the growth of health food stores and the proliferation of healthful foods (many of them convenience items) in conventional supermarkets, plus specialized books and magazines, also show that increasing numbers of people care about what they eat. It takes time and commitment to change one's diet. Since we are what we eat (and so will your babies be), it is certainly worth the effort. Eating can be an avenue for creativity, growth, change, and increased body awareness.

Exercise, rest, and relaxation are also important for physiological and psychological well-being. Physical activity allows nutrients to be more efficiently digested and circulated, which alleviates many of the discomforts of pregnancy. Chapter 10 examines the significance of exercise and relaxation in a healthy pregnancy and preparation for birth.

9
Prenatal Care and Screening Tests

The best prenatal care is what you do for yourself to achieve optimal outcome. This self-care is so important that I have devoted three chapters to it, one on nutrition (Chapter 8), one on preparation for birth with exercise, rest, and education (Chapter 10), and this chapter, which focuses on the surveillance offered by the medical establishment.

The detection of a multiple pregnancy has become reliable with the routine use of ultrasound. Without ultrasound, more than two-thirds of women suspect a twin pregnancy because of increased size and weight. Some are aware of more fetal movement or even separate movement. The earlier you know you are pregnant with two or more, the better, to allow you time to adjust to the news and make adequate logistical and psychological preparations. Yet despite increasingly earlier diagnosis of multiple pregnancy in recent years, outcomes have worsened!

A twin pregnancy is frequently associated with exaggeration and earlier onset of the customary signs and normal discomforts of the pregnant state — what medical texts used to call a "high suspicion index." The uterus may be very large for the stage of pregnancy, assuming an accurate menstrual history. Marked weight gain is another indicator, particularly at the beginning and end of pregnancy (rather than at the middle, as is characteristic of singleton pregnancies). Before the routine use of ultrasound, 37 percent of respondents to a 1987 survey by *Twins* magazine suspected they were carrying multiples because of their weight and abdominal size. Physical changes are always more apparent in subsequent pregnancies than during the first, but growth is much faster in the early weeks for multiples than for a singleton.

Although an earlier detection of multiples has not been translated into significant improvements in outcome, the continuing high perinatal mortality rate associated with all orders of multiple pregnancy is a legitimate reason to perform additional studies in sub-groups with multiple gestation and varying chorionicity.

— Birgit Arabin and Jim van Eyck

My twins were my only pregnancy, so I have nothing else for comparison but I never would have guessed I was carrying twins. I had none of the typical symptoms.

Weight Gain

The mother's weight gain relates to her baby's weight gain, so a woman carrying twins may gain up to twice what she would if carrying one baby. This is a necessary and healthy sign. A *Twins* magazine survey found that weight gains ranged from less than 30 pounds (the national average for a singleton) to more than 80 pounds. Most mothers, especially those who breast-fed, quickly lost the extra weight after birth. Nutrition and weight gain are of vital importance for the future mental and physical development of your babies, for your own physical requirements, and for the successful outcome of the pregnancy. Formerly, twins detected during pregnancy were heavier than those who were not because for several decades the obstetric fashion was to restrict weight gain. Standards of weight gain vary among cultures, ethnic groups, and health care providers; therefore, mothers should trust their appetite and common sense.

At each prenatal visit your doctor or midwife may measure the distance from your pubic bone to the top of your uterus, a measurement known as the *fundal height*. Guidelines exist for normal distances at each stage of development. With twins, the fundus may reach your rib cage by thirty weeks and your uterus will be similar in size to a singleton pregnancy six to eight weeks further along (triplets up to three months, quads even four months). Other providers just rely on ultrasound to track the babies' development.

The extra stretching that occurs with a multiple pregnancy, in addition to higher levels of circulating hormones that soften your tissues, predisposes to stretching of the center seam between your abdominal muscles (*diastasis recti*). You may notice a peaking or bulging in the midline of your abdominal wall, which develops as muscles and connective tissue expand to accommodate your extra baby or babies. If a woman's abdominal muscles are poorly supportive and she experiences severe backache, a corset such as the Baby Hugger® (an all-cotton support designed by a physical therapist, www.babyhugger.com) may help. With higher-order multiples, especially for women of small frames, supportive garments may provide welcome comfort (see Resources for additional styles).

With the medicalization of pregnancy and birth, plus increasing litigation, "prenatal diagnostics" and "fetal surveillance" have become ever more routine. Some, like ultrasound, have been around for decades and others are recent, such as fetal fibronectin. If you have a family history of a disease, or poor outcome in a previous pregnancy, some of these tests may be warranted, but they can compound the nocebo effect.

Screening Tests

Human Chorionic Gonadotropin (HCG)

The hormone HCG, which is secreted by the outer placental membrane, maintains the fertilized egg in early pregnancy until it can develop sufficient hormones for its own survival. In a multiple pregnancy there are higher levels of HCG, which can be measured in the mother's blood or urine. The hormone human placental lactogen (HPL) is a monitor of placental function and is associated with your weight. Low levels of this hormone during pregnancy have been linked to LBW and shorter newborns. In triplet pregnancies, levels of HPL are even higher, as one would expect.

Maternal Serum Alpha-fetoprotein Test (MSAFP)

Maternal serum alpha-fetoprotein testing is done between 15 and 20 weeks and detects about 65 percent of all twin pregnancies. This blood test measures a specific protein, alpha-fetoprotein (AFP), which is made by each baby and circulates in the mother's bloodstream. Elevated levels of the protein may indicate multiples because more babies manufacture more AFP. It can also signal a neural tube defect, such as spina bifida or anencephaly, or it can simply indicate that you are just further along in the pregnancy. Corrections for maternal weight, diabetes mellitus, and race, as well as multiple pregnancy, are necessary.

The median value for twins is approximately 2.5 times the median for singletons. Most providers will do further testing and ultrasound for any value of 1.5 times this median. Virtually all uncomplicated twin pregnancies have an AFP level above the median for singletons. However, the normal range for singletons extends quite high, and production of AFP differs for MZ and DZ pregnancies because AFP represents a total, not a score for each baby. This can cause much anxiety for expectant parents and many physicians consider the test unhelpful. Low levels, on the other hand, may indicate increased risk of Down's syndrome. The purpose of this test is to identify those with sufficient risk to warrant amniocentesis (about 1 to 2 percent of those screened). This screening technique detects about 80 percent of fetuses with open spina bifida and 90 percent with anencephaly.

Laboratories vary in their reliability with this test, largely owing to differences in classifying the stage of pregnancy. One pregnant woman submitted identical samples to three different laboratories and received three different results! Nevertheless, this test is recommended by ACOG for all pregnant women. California was the first of several states to require physicians to offer the MSAFP test. Recently, MSAFP has been computed with acetylcholinesterase for greater accuracy.

Follow-up diagnostic tests such as ultrasound and amniocentesis may put your mind at rest about the nature of your pregnancy if there is a query about the MSAFP test (if you agree to have it). Ultrasound for low levels of AFP may show that the dates are wrong or that the pregnancy is less than 16 to 18 weeks. Ultrasound for elevated levels may show that the pregnancy is past eighteen weeks. The simple facts are that biochemical screening is inadequate for twins and unavailable for higher-order multiples so invasive procedures such as amniocentesis and chorionic villus sampling (CVS) are done.

Amniocentesis

Amniocentesis may be recommended if AFP and HCG levels indicate risk factors or if you have a history of genetic defects in your family. Confirming the sex of each fetus is important because some genetic diseases, such as hemophilia and the Duchenne type of muscular dystrophy, are gender specific.

This prenatal screening procedure involves inserting a needle through the mother's abdomen into the uterus and withdrawing a sample of amniotic fluid to examine fetal cells. The purpose of an amnio varies with the stage of the pregnancy. Between the fourteenth and eighteenth weeks it can uncover genetic defects or biochemical problems. In later pregnancy, amniocentesis is done to draw off excess fluid caused by certain conditions.

Amniocentesis is most commonly done to detect Down's syndrome if the mother is older than thirty-five. The recommended age has been continually lowered since amniocentesis became available in the 1970s. Down's syndrome, also known as trisomy 21, occurs when three copies of the number 21 chromosome are made instead of two. This condition causes mental and physical retardation. The mother's age is not the only factor involved because it occurs in the offspring of younger mothers, too.

Not all anomalies can be detected through amniocentesis. A normal amniocentesis does not guarantee a normal baby at birth; it simply indicates whether a baby has the condition for which it was tested. The test costs at least $1,500 in the United States and carries a risk of miscarriage.

Amniocentesis can detect recessive diseases such as Tay-Sachs, sickle-cell anemia, and cystic fibrosis. Such diseases occur when both parents carry the same recessive gene and pass it on to the same offspring. Because the twins of older women are more often DZ, the risk that both twins will have a recessive disease is only 6 percent. If both the father and mother carry the same recessive gene, they have a 25 percent chance of having a baby who receives both recessive genes and hence the condition. They have a 25 percent chance of having a baby who is not affected and is not a carrier. They also have a 50 percent chance of having a baby who is not affected but, like the parents, is a carrier. Certain recessive disorders occur more often among particular ethnic groups such as Ashkenazi Jews (Tay-Sachs disease), blacks (sickle-cell anemia), those from the southern Mediterranean (thalassemia), and Caucasians (cystic fibrosis).

While providing relief for some, amniocentesis, like all genetic screening, can have stressful repercussions, especially if the results are inconclusive. The need for further testing understandably raises anxiety levels. Finding a serious problem with one or more babies leads to the dilemma of whether to abort both babies or choose "selective birth" in the case of one affected multiple. The first case of selective birth occurred in Sweden in 1978, when one member of a pair was diagnosed with Hurler's syndrome, an enzyme deficiency. Prenatal screening has thus thrust on parents an emotionally wrenching decision — whether one's child or children should live or die.

Barbara Katz Rothman in *The Tentative Pregnancy* interviewed women who consented to amniocentesis and those who refused it. She found that this test delayed the mother's awareness of fetal movement — an understandable form of psychological protection until she is reassured by the results (which can take up to two weeks). Babies become very quiet for up to several days after the procedure.

The procedure can be more challenging with a multiple pregnancy, because each sac must be sampled. With sophisticated ultrasound machines, however, the dividing membrane can be seen. If you decide on amniocentesis, search for a doctor who is experienced in performing the procedure with multiples. In the year 2000, only 2.4 percent of all pregnant women in the United States had an amnio, and the rate is declining as the use of other tests increases.

Chorionic Villus Sampling (CVS)

Chorionic villus sampling is a genetic test that can be done earlier in the pregnancy than amniocentesis but requires much more skill of the practitioner. The chorions are located with ultrasound at their point of attachment to the placentas. Fetal cells are sampled in the tiny projections called villi, through the abdomen or vagina, usually between 10 and 13 weeks of gestation. If the placentas appear to be fused, the sampling is done at opposite ends. Diagnostic errors are 4–6 percent.

The advantage of the earlier CVS over amniocentesis is that termination of pregnancy, if chosen, is less traumatic in the first trimester than in the second. According to the Cochrane Review, the increase in miscarriages after CVS, compared with amniocentesis, appears to be procedure-related. Second trimester amniocentesis seems safer than CVS. Therefore, the benefit of earlier diagnosis with CVS must be set against the increased risk of pregnancy loss.

Fetal Fibronectin Test (fFn)

Fetal fibronectin is a protein found in the membranes and amniotic fluid. It attaches the membranes to the uterus and by twenty-two weeks is no longer released into the vagina because the membranes are normally sealed. Detecting fFn between 24 and 34 weeks in the vaginal secretions has been used to help determine the risk of delivery. Higher-order multiple pregnancies show fFn more frequently than do those of twins or singletons, which can mean the pregnancy is shortened by about three weeks.

Now FDA-approved, the fFn test assesses the risk of PTB both for those who are showing signs of preterm labor and for those who may not have symptoms. The procedure is like a Pap smear and involves swabbing secretions in the vagina and cervix with a cotton swab to examine them for fibronectin. The results can be available within an hour. High-risk women without symptoms can be tested as early as twenty-two weeks gestation or before, and retested at two-week intervals or as appropriate. A negative test is reassuring because it means a much greater chance of carrying to term. A positive fFn will mean closer observation and the possibility of bed rest, hospitalization, and prescription of antibiotics or corticosteroids as infection may be present.

Of women with a negative fFn, only one in thirteen will deliver before 37 weeks but if the test is positive, one out of two will deliver preterm. The fFn test may reduce admissions for preterm labor symptoms, which means lower medical costs — a shorter or avoided hospital stay and decreased use of medications to stop contractions. "The clinical implications of a positive test result have not been evaluated fully because *no obstetric intervention has been shown to decrease the risk of PTB.*" (ACOG Compendium, 2003, italics mine).

Ultrasound (US)

Sound waves at a frequency beyond the range of human hearing are used for identification and measurement in many fields. The technology was first used to follow submarines, find shipwrecks, and measure the depth of lakes and oceans. Also known as sonography, echography, B-scans, or Doppler, US procedures are now commonly used in medicine.

Many obstetricians perform US in their offices, and malpractice insurance in many jurisdictions requires one or more ultrasound per pregnancy. Ultrasound is highly diagnostic and in the year 2000 it was used in 67 percent of pregnancies. You can get prints or even video footage of your unborn babies. These images show how your babies develop and motivate you to modify your lifestyle to enhance their health. A gallery of US scans of twins can be seen on http://pregnancy.about.com/library/ultrasounds/bltwinusindex.htm.

For a US scan, a transducer is moved over your abdomen to create a "window on the womb." Sound waves are passed through body surfaces at different angles and are deflected by the different densities of body tissues. These echoes are amplified and displayed on a screen as white dots outlined against a black background. Repetitive arrays of ultrasound beams scan each baby and the different reflections form a picture on the monitor screen. Real-time scanners provide a continual picture of the moving babies that is captured on videotape.

Vaginal ultrasound (transvaginal sonography — TVS), which does not require a full bladder as abdominal ultrasound does, is more accurate in the first few weeks. This technique is also used to assess the length of the cervix and is considered more reliable than a vaginal exam to predict preterm labor (until the cervix is 3 to 4 cm dilated and almost completely effaced). TVS can also detect "funneling" of the cervix that

I had an ultrasound with a specialist who told me I looked perfect and then wanted me to have an ultrasound every week! They harassed me when I didn't want to do tests (AFP, glucose).

When we saw two little babies on the screen, we were awed by the miracle of their creation and humbled by our own inability to determine our lives.

My first scan showed twins, but in later pregnancy I had a follow-up scan that revealed triplets. People often ask me what my husband said when he heard the news and I tell them the truth — nothing!

My doctor wanted me to have an ultrasound because he suspected twins. I refused, right to the end. It wasn't the test itself, but I knew that I'd be rated as high risk. I wanted to feel in control of my own normal pregnancy.

Ultrasound Gives a "Window on the Womb"

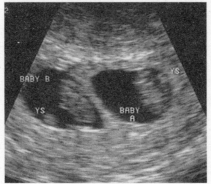

The lower twin is termed Baby A.

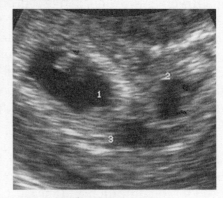

Triplets at 27 weeks.

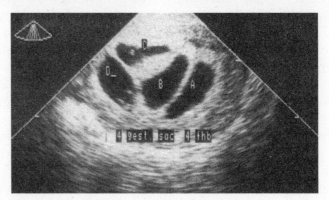

Quadruplets at 8 weeks.

may increase when the mother moves from a lying to standing position, which is considered a risk factor for preterm labor.

The first signs (the gestational sac) can be detected by US as early as four and a half weeks and heartbeats usually by seven weeks. The circulatory systems, gestational age, size, and growth of the babies can also be assessed. The position of the placentas can be determined, along with the presentation of the babies. Many structural abnormalities can be reliably diagnosed before 20 weeks.

For determining the age of your babies, ultrasound in early pregnancy is accurate within seven days during the first three months. At the end of the second trimester, accuracy for age falls within a range of two weeks, and in the last trimester, three weeks. Using the date of your last menstrual period and the calendar is as accurate as ultrasound, a 1977 study from Denmark found!

In addition to the detection of multiple pregnancy and diagnosis of anomalies, ultrasound is used to guide the needle during amniocentesis, CVS, percutaneous umbilical blood sampling, and in fetal therapy. The babies' heartbeats in pregnancy and during labor are monitored by ultrasound, too. This monitoring can be continuous (fetal monitor) or the pulsed Doptone may be used from time to time.

There is no evidence that routine ultrasound in the second or third trimester improves outcome in a total group of pregnancies, according to the Cochrane Review, which also concluded that it is unclear to what extent ultrasound may be valuable in multiple gestation. Its benefit will depend upon the individual cases. For example, MC twins are usually scanned every two weeks, starting before 18 to 20 weeks, when the clinical problems may occur.

Prenatal Measurements with Ultrasound

Determining the progress of growth within the uterus may predict an outcome for twins, although it may not change it. In early pregnancy, the length from the crown to rump can be measured between 7 and 13 weeks and gives an estimation of the gestational age to within three to four days of the last menstrual period. The biparietal diameter between the two sides of the head is measured after 13 weeks. It increases from about 2 cm at 13 weeks to about 10 cm at term.

Different babies of the same weight can have different head sizes; therefore, dating in the later part of pregnancy is generally considered unreliable and it is less helpful for twins because after the thirtieth week their growth rate may decline if the mother is not well nourished. Investigators have called for special scales for twin skull measurements, and in Aberdeen, Scotland, such scales have been developed. However, standard measurements of the length of thigh bones or abdominal circumference growth charts can be used to predict the stage of growth for twins (ACOG Compendium, 2003). The femur length measures the longest bone in the body and indicates the longitudinal growth of the fetus. It increases from about 2 cm at 14 weeks to about 8 cm at term. The abdominal circumference is the most important measurement in late pregnancy to assess size and weight rather than age. The weight of the baby at any stage can be estimated using equations containing the bi-parietal diameter, femur length, and abdominal circumference.

Uses of Ultrasound

- Confirmation of pregnancy

- Estimated due date (gestational age)

- Development and growth of each baby

- Evaluation of health of babies by monitoring fetal movements, breathing

- Measurement of the nuchal skin fold for risk for Down's syndrome

- Sex, in most cases

- Presence of anomalies, such as the feto-fetal transfusion syndrome

- Placenta: location and function

- Number of membranes (chorionicity)

- Amount of amniotic fluid

- Evaluation after vaginal bleeding, changes in fetal movement

- Problems such as intrauterine death

- Presentation and position of the babies

- Diagnosis of uterine and pelvic abnormalities such as fibroids, bicornuate uterus (two compartments)

Serial measurements monitor the growth of babies. The first scan is generally done at about seven to eight weeks (especially after ART) to confirm the pregnancy and viability of the babies, and to measure the crown-to-rump length for determining the due date. A scan at around 13 to 14 weeks can measure the nuchal skin fold thickness to evaluate the risk for Down's syndrome. This is not widely used nor has its efficacy in higher-order multiples been adequately studied. Between 18 to 20 weeks, ultrasound is used to check for any congenital malformations and to determine placental position. After the sixth month of pregnancy, scans are typically done every three to four weeks, so you may be offered up to five or more during the pregnancy. The total number of scans will vary depending on whether a previous scan has detected anything that requires follow-up.

However, a 1998 study from Germany found that only 58 of 193 growth-restricted fetuses were diagnosed before birth. Worse, 45 were diagnosed as being growth restricted in error! Despite an average of 4.7 scans, the problems of only 28 of the 72 severely growth-restricted babies were detected before birth. The admission rate to the NICU was three times higher for the diagnosed babies because the pregnancy was two to three weeks shorter due to elective early delivery.

Doppler Ultrasound

This technology assesses vascular function in cases of IUGR. Color flow mapping shows the babies' blood vessels in a real time scan with different colors representing the direction of the blood flow. Another recent development is the Power Doppler (Doppler angiography). It uses amplitude information from Doppler signals rather than speed of flow to visualize slower circulation in smaller blood vessels. Doppler evaluations, which emit more power than a conventional 2-D scan, can be performed abdominally or vaginally. Most useful in cases of heart anomalies, they are typically done at 24 weeks. The Cochrane Review concluded that Doppler US "appears" to improve outcome and reduce perinatal deaths.

Color Imaging and 3-D Ultrasound

"Chroma" scans allow the technician to select color hues and assign them to the shades of gray for better visualization.

The quality of 3-D images depends on operator skill, the amount of fluid around each baby, its position, and degree of maternal obesity. You can view some images and movies on the Web site of Dr. Joseph Woo (http://www.ob-ultrasound.net/).

What About Safety?

It has been more than three decades since ultrasound was first used on pregnant women. Unlike X-rays (which also were considered safe when they were used in pregnancy), no ionizing irradiation occurs with ultrasound. The use of high intensity sound waves, however, is associated with cavitation (formation of bubbles), and heating can occur with prolonged exposure in laboratory situations. This technology has raced ahead and powerful new machines have been developed without a review of their safety and efficacy, unlike the studies required to approve the use of new drugs.

A study of more than 2,800 women in Australia compared the half receiving five ultrasound exams with the half receiving only one during

After many years of infertility I was finally pregnant. It might have been a coincidence that my membranes ruptured the day after I had my first ultrasound scan, and I lost the babies.

pregnancy. The former had significantly higher IUGR and LBW babies than the group having only one scan. (Numerous studies over the years found similar results concerning pregnant rats, mice, and monkeys.) The study concluded that repeated ultrasounds should be limited to cases where the information was clinically indicated.

Three studies confirmed increases in left-handedness among offspring exposed to prenatal ultrasound, an issue discussed at an international conference in Edinburgh in January 2002; the findings were published in the journal *Epidemiology*. Boys exposed prenatally to ultrasound were found to have a 30 percent increased risk of left-handedness. A study published by the Canadian Medical Association revealed that children with delayed speech were about twice as likely to have been exposed to prenatal ultrasound. This is data from a different perspective, delayed speech being a developmentally defined symptom-complex rather than a pathological or organic syndrome. The researchers warn against routine ultrasound exams and comment that the current popularity of ultrasound could cause this developmental delay in an entire generation of children, with enormous implications for public health.

British midwife Beverley Lawrence Beech listed many disturbing side effects of ultrasound in an article in *Midwifery Today*. She quotes one small and two large statistically significant studies showing an increase in miscarriages from scans and an increase in fetal deaths from Doppler exposure. Beech also points out that exposure varies so much among machines that it is not possible to say if these studies represent greater risks for everyone. One study showed that an ultrasound diagnosis of placenta previa in 250 cases out of 4,000 women scanned did more harm than good. Only four actually were found to have this condition at birth! Worse, all 250 had Caesareans, at the end of an undoubtedly highly anxious pregnancy. Four cases of placenta previa also occurred among the unscanned women in the study and no difference in outcome existed between the two groups. (The uterus stretches as the pregnancy progresses. This well-intentioned screening is yet another example of the nocebo effect with surgical consequences.)

In a Norwegian study, ultrasound detection of serious defects not only did not benefit the babies but also decreased their survival rate. In the diagnosed group, 77 percent survived but among those whose defects were not detected until after birth, 96 percent lived. There were three deaths out of the 13 babies diagnosed prenatally and all were delivered by Caesarean section, but of the twenty-three undiagnosed and vaginally delivered babies, only one died.

It becomes increasingly difficult to find a control group that has not been exposed to ultrasound; and continued vigilance is necessary, particularly in the use of pulsed Doppler in the first trimester. No technology is foolproof and operator skill and machine reliability vary widely. Establishment of chorionicity is important, as explained in Chapter 2, but repeat ultrasounds should be used only for a valid medical reason, not just for information-gathering. Parents and their doctors understandably enjoy watching the private lives of unborn babies. However, in order to limit exposure to this technology, always ask your doctor what information she or he hopes to gain from the ultrasound and how that might change your plan of care.

Fetal Heart Rate Surveillance

External fetal monitors (EFM) using ultrasound are placed on the mother's abdomen during pregnancy and labor to evaluate the babies' heart rates.

Nonstress Test (NST)

The NST is done in the last trimester, when preterm labor, fetal distress, or overdue birth (which is rare with twins) is anticipated. It may be done as early as the eighteenth week, although it is usually begun at 30 weeks and repeated three to seven days later.

The test can also be used to determine whether abdominal pain is caused by labor contractions (which NST will detect) or by other problems unrelated to labor such as gas, intestinal problems, appendicitis, or kidney infections.

Three transducers are strapped to the mother's abdomen to record the activity of the twins' hearts (one monitor per baby), and the results are printed. If two machines are not available, each baby is monitored separately. The third transducer registers contractions.

The babies' heart rates should maintain a healthy variability, changed only by sleep or drugs. This is known as a *reactive NST* and if observed twice a week indicates all is well. In contrast, a *nonreactive NST*, which according to O'Grady occurs in about 20 percent of twins, is associated with problems such as cord entanglement, diabetes, oxygen deprivation, PIH, IUGR, newborns with depressed vital signs, and even death after birth.

If the babies are sleeping, vibratory acoustic stimulation (VAS) may be applied to awaken them and stimulate heart rate and movement. This stimulation is also being used to study the development and maturity of the central nervous system of the fetus. Unborn babies respond to VAS with increased heart rate, movement, and startle responses, which vary with gestational age.

After activity, the fetal heart rate should go up 15 beats per minute or more. If it does not reach this level, the test may be repeated soon. An absence of variability — low baseline and low spikes — is a worrisome sign. Deceleration (slowing) of the heart rate that is late, early, or variable relative to a contraction can signify fetal distress. Late decelerations are the most ominous, indicating serious fetal distress. Fetal movement followed by acceleration is a good sign.

There are two kinds of variabilities. A heart rate that changes constantly within the normal range (an irregular saw-tooth pattern) is a healthy sign. However, decelerations that vary or show inconsistent shape and timing are abnormal. This may mean a problem with the umbilical cord. Variable decelerations lead to the next test.

Contraction Stress Test (CST)

The CST determines the babies' ability to tolerate uterine contractions. An EFM is applied when the pregnant woman feels contractions at the rate of about three within ten minutes. The contractions may be spontaneous or the physician may have the woman stimulate contractions so the test can be performed. Contractions can be induced by manual breast and nipple stimulation or by use of an electric breast pump. If these techniques do not succeed in causing contractions, the oxytocin challenge test (described next) can be done.

Repeated late decelerations suggest utero-placental insufficiency and chronic fetal distress. Caesarean section will be done when one or more babies are distressed.

Both the NST and CST may give false positive results, which means that a healthy fetus may erroneously be judged to be at risk, leading to an unnecessary Caesarean section. A false negative result — an apparently normal test when the baby in fact is at risk — also can occur. Parents must know that no technology is perfect.

While the NST and CST can be done in a doctor's office, the following test, the oxytocin challenge test, is almost always done in the hospital.

Oxytocin Challenge Test (OCT)

The oxytocin challenge test involves the intravenous administration of Pitocin, a synthetic form of the hormone oxytocin, which the pituitary gland produces to cause contractions. Although the test induces uterine contractions, the possibility of the mother going into labor is slight unless she is at term. The purpose of the test, as for the CST, is to make sure that each baby can take the stress of contractions without decelerations. A *positive* result on the OCT is *unfavorable*. Severe decelerations in one or both twins are ominous and Caesarean section may be considered.

While variability and accelerations of the fetal rate are significant with both the stress tests, the absence of decelerations is more important. Always, slowing of the heart rate indicates fetal distress.

The OCT may take hours to complete because it is started with a minimum dose of Pitocin and the dose is increased only every half hour or so until three contractions occur in ten minutes. Many obstetricians allow their patients to sit, stand, and walk, all of which are much preferable to lying on the back. Other physicians feel that the OCT is too cumbersome and not appropriate for multiples because of their high risk for preterm delivery.

Biophysical Profile (BPP)

The Biophysical Profile, started at 32 to 34 weeks, evaluates five variables of fetal health: heart rate activity, respiration, body movements, muscle tone, and amniotic fluid volume. Sometimes the placenta is graded as part of the Biophysical Profile; grade 3 is mature (term). High-risk patients (including those who are past their due date and insulin-dependent diabetics) are normally tested twice a week.

Heart rate activity is monitored by the NST test, and the rest of the parameters are assessed with ultrasound. Lack of oxygen affects an unborn baby's heart rate reactivity, movement, and muscle tone. A score of 4 or less on the tests is usually considered pathological and immediate delivery is indicated, except for babies of less than 28 weeks gestation. A score of 2 indicates high risk and 0 indicates absent or abnormal activity. If the score is 6 or more, the test may be repeated the next day, which may be too late or too early, and thus some physicians have suggested immediate further testing. A score of 8 or more is considered normal and indicates that the baby is in good condition. False positives are possible, however, and they may lead to unnecessary interventions and maternal and fetal complications.

Some doctors feel that decisions should be based on the individual components (amniotic fluid, fetal movement) rather than a profile or composite score. Controversy also exists over the normal amount of amniotic fluid and assessment of fetal movements such as trunk versus limb action.

Fetal Movement (FM)

The mother's assessment of FM is part of the BPP, and many doctors consider her observations more reliable than other single variables of the BPP. She can detect and report any change in activity level; diminished movements may mean a baby is in trouble. Most unborn babies don't sleep for more than an hour and they are usually most active after a meal.

The mother checks for movement at a particular time, typically three times a week, using a "kick chart." Samueloff found that expectant mothers of multiples experienced an average of 774 movements per day at the peak period of gestation — about 27 weeks. These FMs were calculated for a 24-hour period based on the number of movements that mothers counted three times a day for 30 minutes. By the time of delivery, the average number of FMs had declined to 224. If the mother is given a steroid drug to promote the babies' lung maturity, there will be a marked decrease in fetal activity for a day or so after.

In early and mid-pregnancy, fetal activity is often more pronounced in a multiple pregnancy than in a singleton pregnancy, but movement gradually declines toward term because of the decreased space available in the uterus. When you know the characteristics of each baby, you will be aware of any sudden decrease in activity. Your involvement is more important than the actual methodology. Chapter 6 describes ways to communicate with the babies in the uterus; the more you do this, the more skilled you will become in recognizing each one's individual movements.

Screening for Gestational Diabetes (GD)

In 1993, Professor R. J. Jarrett, in an article in the *British Medical Journal* ("Gestational Diabetes; A Non-Entity?"), advised that transient changes in glucose metabolism in pregnancy do not call for classification as pathology. This condition "fails the major tests . . . suitable for a screening programme."

Nevertheless, your urine usually will be checked for the presence of glucose at each prenatal visit. Additional tests include fasting blood sugar, one-hour glucose, a two-hour post-prandial blood sugar, a random blood sugar, hemoglobin A1C, and the oral glucose tolerance test (OGTT) — usually considered "definitive."

For the OGTT, you will be asked to fast for 10 to 12 hours and then drink 50–100 gms of glucose (*Glucola*). Blood samples are taken prior to and at hourly intervals afterward up to three hours. However, the fasting itself may cause decreased carbohydrate intolerance ("starvation diabetes"), which is also decreased by inactivity so that bed rest, regrettably so common in multiple pregnancies, may also lead to false positive results (and serious nocebo effects in which treatment is undertaken for a nonexistent disease). A sudden flood of highly concentrated glucose is most unphysiological, especially as complex carbohydrates are recommended throughout the day to maintain even blood sugar levels.

Neither the screening test nor OGTT are reliable because they may vary when repeated in the same person. In addition, blood glucose values rise as pregnancy advances, but no adjustments are made for this. This means you could "fail" a test in week 28 that you would have "passed" had you taken it in week 24.

A Guide to Effective Care in Pregnancy and Childbirth by Murray Enkin, M.D., et al. includes under "Forms of Care Unlikely to Be Beneficial" both screening and treatment (insulin and diet therapy). Nevertheless, the dietary advice given for GD is sound and helps 80 percent of women with GD to "normalize" their blood sugar:

- Reduce simple sugars.

- Increase complex carbohydrates and protein at each meal.

- Eat small meals frequently, at least six per day.

- Eat foods in their natural state (e.g., fruit rather than juice, oatmeal rather than processed cereals, avoiding convenience foods with their often added sugars and fats).

- Avoid milk (it contains simple sugars).

- Walk or exercise after a meal.

The quality and regularity of nutrition are at issue. Any reduction in calories or limitation of food intake is harmful in a multiple pregnancy where mothers are challenged to eat enough for two or more.

All these screening tests, except ultrasound and amniocentesis, have been developed since I wrote the first edition of *Having Twins*. Prior to their development, more mothers carried healthy, normal-birth-weight

The doctor of the future will prescribe no medicine but will interest
his patients in the care of the
human frame, in diet and the cause
and prevention of disease.
— Thomas Edison

babies to term. Tests can be useful when indicated, but keep in mind that procedures for investigating and monitoring high-risk patients tend to get used more and more for those women of lower risk because technology always expands as far as the resources will stretch. The problem is that many tests are misunderstood and misused. Fetal surveillance, as we have seen, often finds a problem that in fact doesn't exist (high false positive rates). Frequently growth curves and other parameters derived from singletons are used to assess the health of multiples. Test results can be affected by stress hormones, too, as mothers understandably become anxious about both the procedures and the outcomes.

In the United States in particular, obstetricians are forced to practice "defensive medicine" in a highly litigious society that obliges them to adhere to out-of-date "guidelines" and "standards of care" whether they are beneficial, useless, or harmful. Prevalence implies endorsement and busy doctors do not always have the time to stay current and base their practices on the latest evidence.

Making a decision about whether to have a test or which test is appropriate may require a second or third opinion. Women expect a test to reassure them, but instead it provokes more anxiety if the results are not clear or further testing is necessary. It is better to prevent complications with optimal nutrition and a healthy lifestyle, as emphasized throughout this book, thus decreasing your need for these investigations.

10
How to Prepare for a Multiple Birth

 Nutrition and exercise are the most significant factors in preparing your body for the demands of a multiple pregnancy and birth and for ensuring the health of your babies. Rest and relaxation are also important for health. Both movement and relaxation aid the distribution of nutrients within your body's systems and relieve physical discomfort as well as mental stress.

I never got to more than two classes. By the time the hospital would take me in a series, the doctor had changed my due date.

Exercise

Ideally, you have been exercising regularly long before your pregnancy. If not, you may be confused about what kinds of exercise to do and when to begin. During the early months you can learn correct posture to prevent backache with the benefit of sharing emotional changes in an ongoing support group such as a prenatal exercise class. I have been training instructors to teach such classes for more than twenty years and they are becoming more available nationwide. Most multiples come early, so it is a good idea to get into the earliest classes you can (and to learn how you can carry yours longer). Special classes for expectant parents of multiples are ideal if you can find them.

Private childbirth educators, physical therapists, midwives, doulas, clinics, and hospitals may offer early or ongoing classes. Sessions may be exclusively lecture and discussion or preferably balanced with exercises, relaxation, and comfort measures. The district or state chapter of the American Physical Therapy Association (1-800-999-APTA) should also be able to recommend an obstetric physical therapist. Some YWCAs and yoga studios offer classes in prenatal movement and exercise. The qual-

I knew I was having twins by the fourth month. That didn't stop me from doing anything. I felt great doing regular exercise and had an easy pregnancy. In the eighth month I learned that the twins were going to be triplets.

My doctor felt that it was my regular exercise sessions at the spa that helped me to carry my babies to term.

I swim sixty laps every day. Of course, I don't know if I'll keep it up to the very end — carrying quintuplets. But right now I feel fine.

Whenever my back began to ache I would go on all fours on the floor. It was paradise. I spent most of my labor in this position as well.

My therapist recommended a wide belt worn over the sacroiliac joints behind and under the abdomen in front. This gave me a lot of relief.

ifications and ability of instructors vary, of course, but if you are asked to do something that hurts, your body is telling you that it is wrong. Your instructor should have specialized training in prenatal and postpartum exercise, and ideally you can find a class for pregnant women. (Regular exercise classes may be too vigorous for expectant mothers of multiples. Besides, it is more appropriate and interesting to be in a group of peers.)

In addition to calisthenics and stretching, low-impact aerobic activity can be enjoyed recreationally. (Aerobic just means "oxygen burning," which is why it is important to keep breathing. If you are out of breath, you are into anaerobic metabolism.) Such activity is important to improve two vital body systems, blood circulation and respiration. The earlier you start gentle aerobic exercise, the better you will feel, particularly as you may find that even walking is difficult toward the end. Dancing, swimming, walking, and cycling are examples of this kind of easy exercise suitable in early pregnancy. Health clubs, Y's, and some hotels and motels offer access to a pool.

Swimming is ideal for expectant mothers, especially with multiples, because you float about nine-tenths of your body weight thanks to the buoyancy of water, which makes movement easier without stress on joints or the pelvic floor muscles. The Cochrane Review found that water gymnastics "appear to reduce back pain in pregnancy" as do specially shaped pillows, physical therapy, and acupuncture.

Listen to your body if you plan to continue with a sport or exercise program through your pregnancy. Jogging, for example, with the extra weight of twins or more, puts far too much strain on the pelvic floor. There is no point pushing yourself to run a mile while you suffer "falling-out" feelings in your undercarriage. However, with bed rest still a "standard of care," too many women are going to have a major challenge persuading their doctors even to let them get out of bed!

Carrying twins means making a double effort to stay in shape. Strong abdominal muscles are needed to protect your back as you move about through pregnancy. The pelvic floor muscles, which support your uterus from below, also must be in optimal condition to maintain urinary control. (There are more than 150 operations for urinary incontinence!) A complete description of the structure and function of these two vulnerable muscle groups can be found in my book *Essential Exercises for the Childbearing Year*, 4th edition, revised.

In their first guidelines for Exercising During Pregnancy and Postpartum, the ACOG considered multiple pregnancy to be a contraindication to exercise. This was removed in the 1994 update. (Their guidelines are aimed at cardiovascular workouts and consideration of abdominal and pelvic floor muscles is conspicuous by its absence.) The standard non-aerobic prenatal exercise program at my former clinic, the Maternal and Child Health Center in Cambridge, Massachusetts, is safe and necessary for any woman expecting multiples. I do not advocate unaccustomed vigorous exercise in pregnancy for anyone. Instead I emphasize body awareness — with particular attention to the essential muscles affected by childbearing.

Moderation is the key to any program. You cannot force your body to move quicker than its own pace. Do what you can comfortably and smoothly achieve while breathing normally *through your nose* and carrying on a conversation.

Warning: Double-leg raising and full sit-ups with outstretched legs are still being taught in many places to both males and females and are potentially harmful for everyone, especially pregnant women, with stretched muscles and softened ligaments. These strenuous trunk and leg motions put a dangerous strain on the lower back while they supposedly strengthen the abdominal muscles. Paradoxically, such exercises do not improve your abdominal strength because they are performed by substitute muscles (hip flexors).

Research by Swedish physiologist Per Tesch, reported in the 2003 book *Astrofit* by William Evans, adviser to NASA, found that the phase of returning to starting position of muscle activity was more effective in

Some of my friends used to wet their pants when they coughed, so I just thought it was normal in pregnancy.

I gave up jogging at three months, as the pressure on my bladder was too uncomfortable.

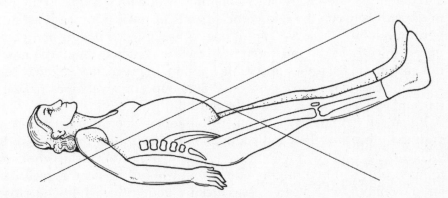

Raising both legs together can strain the lower back.

building muscle strength. (Have you not felt it more of a challenge to hike back down the hill than up?) The recommendation is to shorten the muscle for a count of two but lengthen for a count of six.

All exertion should be performed on *outward* breath. You can curl up as you breathe out, then inhale, and uncurl taking twice as long, while you exhale. Move slowly and rest frequently. Deep breathing and changes of position improve the circulation to compensate for the pressure from the large uterus that restricts the diaphragm above and reduces venous return from the legs and pelvis below.

A few exercises done properly and regularly will serve you best. Exercises must always be progressive to provide constant challenge and improvement — during pregnancy your increasing physical size will provide that progression. Changing the starting position or movement keeps your interest more than many repetitions. During pregnancy, as in life, everyone is different and needs to begin at the appropriate level for their condition.

The Abdominal Wall

It is quite prevalent for the center seam of the abdominal muscles to stretch widely at the midline (*diastasis recti*) when twins or more are inside. Check this seam before starting any exercises involving trunk-raising on your back. Also, check the gap frequently throughout the pregnancy, as the muscles can stretch apart as you grow larger.

Check the Center Seam

Lie down on your side and roll onto your back with bent knees. Press up and down the midline of your abdominal wall with a couple of fingers in the gap between the two vertical bands of muscles on each side of your navel. We all have a gap of one to two fingers: fingers and gaps vary. Now exhale and raise your head (which contracts these recti muscles so you can tell if they are parallel or not). In pregnancy you may see a bulging that looks like a sausage, a cantaloupe, or a watermelon! Postpartum, you feel for a gap after the third day.

If you can fit three or more fingers horizontally between the muscles, your seam has stretched and abdominal exercises must be modified. If your muscles pull apart with the weight of your head, it makes no sense to overload them by bringing your shoulders off the floor as well. Instead, continue with head raises, tucking your chin, while you cross your hands over the gap to help bring the muscles on each side toward

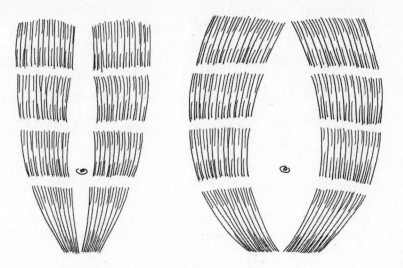

The muscles can stretch apart like a zipper parts.

the midline. After the babies are born you will need to continue this exercise until you can raise your head, then later your shoulders, and the space between the muscles is reduced to a width of one to two fingers. (More details can be found in my book *Essential Exercises for the Childbearing Year*.)

Appendix 4 summarizes the essential exercises to be done during pregnancy for as long as you can. These are the same exercises you will need to begin soon after the babies are born. The muscles you prepare are, logically, the ones you will restore — there is only one program to be learned. Mothers of twins often find it takes much longer than they expected to get their bodies back to normal. Getting the muscles into good condition prior to the birth makes this task much easier.

Curl-ups

You will notice from the illustrations that, apart from the all-over stretch, the knees are always bent. This helps to tilt the pelvis so you can more easily stabilize your lower back. For the same reason, the trunk is curled only halfway rather than to a full sit-up position. If you are not accustomed to doing abdominal muscle exercises, your front neck muscles may protest a little at the beginning. Remember to tuck your chin in first and then curl up.

Although the abdominal muscles are placed in front of the spine, they are nevertheless important muscles that support the spinal column. The various muscles of the abdominal corset work together in curl-ups. Straight curl-ups involve a forward movement of the trunk, and diagonal curl-ups bring one shoulder toward the opposite hip.

Begin curl-ups first with outstretched arms. Some women are able to come forward only a few inches. With time and practice, strength and distance will improve. Sometimes the upper back is stiff and cannot readily flex forward. You can check this by sitting with ankles crossed and seeing if your forehead reaches to the floor in front of you. After the outward physical signs of the pregnancy progress, which can happen as early as three to four months in a multiple pregnancy, just do what is comfortable. Muscles that have already started to stretch can be maintained in good condition, but additional strengthening cannot be expected.

Pregnant women who are in good shape, or begin early, perhaps can achieve one of the progressions of the curl-up exercises. It is harder to raise your head and shoulders off the floor with your arms folded across your chest (80 percent strength), and the 100 percent test is to clasp your hands behind or on top of your head. As your pregnancy progresses, the size of your abdomen will interfere, so revert to an easier arm position.

Raising the pelvis and lower back on hands and knees is a comfortable way to work your abdominal muscles against the force of gravity and takes the weight off your spine. Make sure your hands and knees are far enough apart to keep your upper back straight and avoid a "cat back."

Pelvic Tilting

When you do curl-ups, your pelvis is held stable while your trunk moves. With pelvic tilting the reverse occurs. You focus on your lower abdominal muscles. Your trunk stays on the floor while your pelvis is tilted back to align with your spine, pressing your waist toward the floor. Bending your knees makes this easier, so the first progression is to maintain the backward tilt of your pelvis while your heels slide slowly forward. Extend your legs only as far as you can while keeping your pelvis stable. When your abdominal muscles are strong enough to maintain the position of your pelvis while both legs are extended (heels in contact with the floor), you can progress to the next step, bicycling your legs in the air, in both directions.

Pelvic tilting can be done in a back-lying, all-fours, side-lying, kneeling, sitting, or standing position, or sitting on a gym ball. Pelvic tilting movements in all positions relieve stiffness and aching in the lower back — do them frequently.

Squatting

Squatting with your feet flat stretches out tightness in your lower back. While squatting, the pelvis is tilted back as far as it can go, so further active movement is not possible. This, along with the enlargement of the pelvic outlet, is one of the several reasons why a squatting position is chosen for birth in many societies. Dr. Sorger has assisted more than 3,000 births in the squatting position and the excellent outcomes were published in the journal *Birth*. If there are complications, such as the need for forceps, all the more reason to have the mother squatting so gravity helps. It is easier to squat with a partner (see illustration), on an incline, and in shallow water (the bath, a pool, a lake, or the ocean).

Posture

The position of the pelvis and its passengers is the keystone to good posture. As your pregnancy advances, your body weight moves forward, increasing the pull on your lower back. (High-heeled shoes tip the body and pelvis even further forward.) It becomes more difficult for your ab-

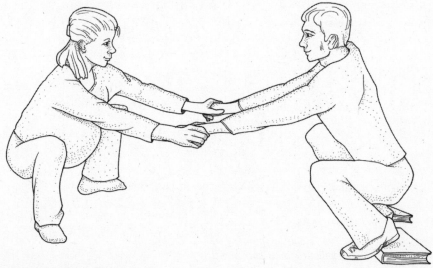

Squatting is easier with a partner.

Partner Exercises Strengthen Your Back and Improve Posture

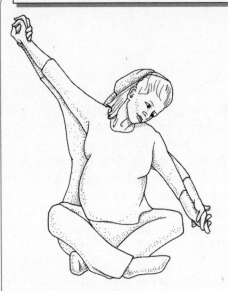

Bend from side to side while pressing against your partner.

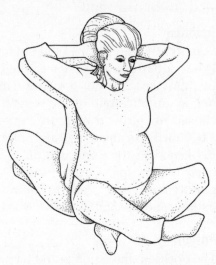

Press elbows together as you twist your upper back from side to side.

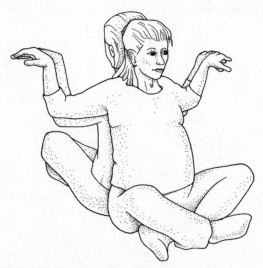

The "Hold-up" position with wrists touching challenges your back muscles.

dominal muscles to hold your bony basin in a good position. Your buttock muscles contribute by pulling your pelvis down from behind. A checklist is included to help you attain a comfortable and attractive stature.

The Pelvic Floor

Another muscle group that is particularly vulnerable during the childbearing year is the pelvic floor. Like a hammock slung within the pelvis, pelvic floor muscles must support the weight of your uterus and other organs such as the bladder and bowel. Because we mostly sit and stand, there is constant pressure from the load in pregnancy plus the force of gravity. Sudden increases in pressure such as a laugh, cough, or sneeze strain these muscles. If

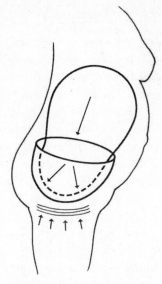

Multiples make a heavy load in the pelvis.

they are weak, urine leaks — one of the classic signs of pelvic floor dysfunction. Other symptoms include "falling-out" feelings, lack of sexual satisfaction for one or both partners, and inability to void completely. Smokers and people with chest problems who cough frequently have increased likelihood of pelvic floor problems, and these are aggravated by constipation and straining. Exercise, plenty of fluids, and high fiber will help prevent constipation.

The pelvic floor muscles run from your pubic bones in front to your coccyx behind and wrap around your three openings. These circular muscle fibers are known as sphincters and form a figure eight. The front half of the figure is shared by both vagina and urethra (the passage from the bladder). Exercises that strengthen the birth canal muscles also improve urinary control, making the muscles more supple for stretching during birth. Hormonal changes during pregnancy soften and prepare the tissues for such distention, which is achieved by the first baby so the second usually follows easily.

The pelvic floor is exercised automatically when you rise from a squat, so you either must do that several times a day or make time to do at least 50 contractions of these internal, invisible muscles a day. It is the same action as interrupting the urine flow. Contract the muscles only two or three times before resting as these muscles fatigue easily. The muscle contractions occur at the middle of the vagina and no bones move. The action of closing an eye is similar to that of contracting these sphincter muscles (although you must make a stronger effort with the pelvic floor). Just as you can close your eye very tightly, or make a very hard fist, in this manner you should do a strong, slow, uplifting pelvic floor contraction and hold it, progressing to 10 seconds. Sexual intercourse offers the best opportunities for practice and these muscles are important for the sexual response of both partners. Your legs are apart and your partner can provide feedback about the quality of your vaginal sphincter. Take care that the movement is an elevation, a drawing-up, then gradually relax. Do only the number of pelvic floor contractions that your partner can clearly feel and rest a minute or so before continuing. You can feel them yourself with your finger; also ask your midwife or doctor to evaluate the strength of these important muscles.

Many expectant mothers have little interest in sex during pregnancy, especially toward the end when their body seems to have grown out of bounds. For others, sexual enthusiasm increases in pregnancy, particularly in the middle months, which may bewilder some husbands who anticipate that pregnancy will be a low point in their marriage and sex life. Some men are very proud of the growing evidence of their contribution; others are concerned that the mother or babies will be hurt by sexual activity. Sensitive communication and good humor are assets.

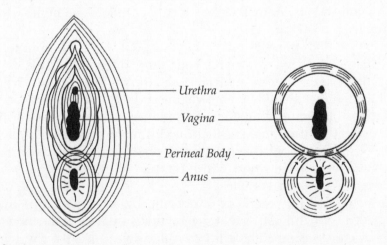

Urethra

Vagina

Perineal Body

Anus

The muscles that circle the birth canal also function in bladder control.

Any restriction that is placed on sexual activity for medical reasons should be thoroughly explained to both partners to avoid misunderstandings and resentment. Some physicians are very cautious in the case of twins because they fear that orgasm — from any means — may cause preterm labor. Preterm labor has never been proved to result from a couple's sexual activity; understanding this should spare couples from guilt.

Suggested Positions for Sexual Intercourse During Pregnancy

Lovemaking can be a challenge with a huge abdomen, but some of the following positions may be comfortable.

Man Kneeling

The woman lies on her back on the edge of the bed. Her feet are supported on one or more chairs at a distance so that the man is able to kneel between her legs. Pillows may be needed to bring the woman's pelvis to a higher level.

Side-lying, Approach from the Rear

The woman lies on her side with knees partially drawn up. The man lies on the same side, just behind her, with his chest a reasonable distance away to bring the genital organs into alignment. This position permits fondling and extra stimulation of the woman.

Right Angles

The woman lies or sits on the bed with her knees drawn up. The man lies on his side at a right angle so her legs can rest across his body.

Squatting

The woman squats with her knees bent or sits with legs extended. The man kneels and rests on his heels. (Some women have difficulty balancing in the squatting position or find that their legs go to sleep.)

Both Kneeling

The woman rests in a forward position with her shoulders on pillows and her knees bent. The man kneels behind or sits with outstretched legs.

Infection is no more a risk in pregnancy than at any other time as long as the babies are protected by intact membranes. Intercourse should never occur after the bag of waters has ruptured. Another contraindication is vaginal spotting of blood. This may occur after a head engages in the pelvis and the cervix sinks low into the vagina.

Although I spent the last few weeks in bed — too huge to move — sex was the last thing on my mind. Imagine trying to make love over a couple of active puppies.

Other Physical Considerations

The awkwardness and loss of balance that pregnant women experience are exaggerated in mothers expecting multiples. Daily discomforts can be minimized by wearing supportive footwear, bending your knees every time you reach down to the floor (that is, squatting), and rolling to one side to get up from the floor or out of bed. You should use care, and your arms, when getting out of the bathtub and maneuvering over other slippery surfaces.

Back-lying, while harmless for a brief episode of moderate exercise, is to be avoided in labor and for those on bed rest. The major blood vessels can be compressed between the uterus and backbone, which may cause dizziness and nausea in some women. Going on hands and knees offers a welcome change of position. The uterus is off the backbone and out of the pelvis, which relieves backache, too, particularly if you do some pelvic tilting in this position.

A Gymnastic Ball Serves Multiple Purposes

A gym ball is an essential piece of furniture and exercise equipment in my home. It makes a great footstool and a comfortable dynamic surface on which to sit when working at a desk or computer. I have been a distributor of these balls long before they became popular and available in toy and fitness stores. You will get hours of use out of gym balls and your kids with love them, too. There are many nice exercises you can do with these balls (see Further Reading).

If varicose veins run in your family, you may want to take some preventive measures. With twins, the blood volume and hormones are increased, which stresses your circulation. Veins require the pumping action of the surrounding muscles to push the blood back to the heart; therefore, exercise, walking, and frequent ankle movements with your feet elevated will help. Tight underwear, garters, knee-high

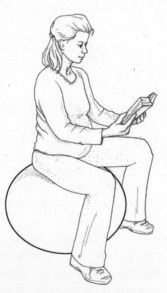

A gym ball makes a flexible seat.

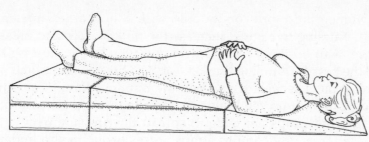

Take a break from gravity.

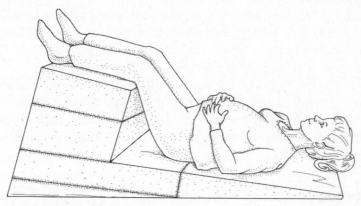

A flexible slant bed elevates your legs.

I found sandals to be the most comfortable footwear, and I could let out the straps as my feet got more swollen.

socks or stockings, and sitting with knees crossed can constrict your circulation. If your legs are swollen, you can raise the foot of your bed on 10-inch blocks to encourage the return of fluid to the heart at night, or during the day lie on an inclined air mattress, which will give your circulation some relief (from Aging in Reverse, www.ageeasy.com). Although exercise is important for the "venous pump," rest is also necessary so the kidneys have a chance to excrete the excess fluid.

Some mothers need support hose for leg swelling and the most effective type is custom-made by Jobst. It is important to put them on before getting out of bed.

Abdominal corsets help some backaches and pelvic pressure. It is preferable, however, to develop good muscles and to have any orthopedic problem diagnosed and treated. Spinal lesions and pelvic joint dysfunction respond to physical therapy.

The breasts contain no muscle tissue, so if allowed to hang by their own weight for prolonged periods of time, the tissues may stretch.

My husband used to massage my feet every night and I never got leg cramps.

Some women are more comfortable with a bra, others prefer to go without. Nursing twins will increase the milk supply and breast size; therefore, wait until after the birth if you plan to buy nursing bras to ensure the best fit. Nursing bras also absorb breast leaks; some women add breast pads as well. If you buy the trapdoor kind of nursing bra, you can walk around the house or go in the sun to air your nipples. Make sure the straps are wide to spread the pressure over a greater area, or you can buy comfort straps with silicone to slip under them (www.aswechange.com).

Stretch marks vary greatly with the individual and are less likely to occur if you take in enough vitamin C (for collagen repair). Many mothers of twins complain of intense itching of the abdominal wall. Oil massage has not been shown to prevent stretch marks but it is a nice treat. Coax your partner into giving you a regular all-over body massage with almond, coconut, or some other natural oil that is absorbed more effectively by the skin than mineral oil. Massage of the vaginal area with cocoa butter can enhance the circulation and increase the suppleness of the tissues for birth.

Relaxation

Simple rest at frequent intervals and enough sleep are essential in a multiple pregnancy, as your body is performing an amazing amount of work. Two or three times a day lie down or soak in a bath or put your feet up for *at least* 15 minutes. Perhaps you can line up a teenager or senior citizen to come in for a little while to mind any other children so you have some time to yourself. Many excellent vocal and nonvocal audiotapes and CDs for relaxation are available today, including my new *Inside Experiences: Guided Recall for Birth and the Time Before*.

Relaxation has both mental and physical rewards. Relaxed muscles allow better circulation, and when your body achieves a state of calm it helps quiet "the chattering monkey of the mind." Blend relaxation into daily living once you become aware of your own particular patterns of tension. Most people become tense in similar ways. As soon as anxiety develops, the classic body language shows flexion postures. The neck almost disappears as the shoulders are tensed and elevated. The arms and legs are usually bent and crossed, fingers are clenched, and the foot, if not tapping or wrapped around the other leg, points upward.

The solution is easy: extend the joints that are flexed. To allow the opposite group of muscles to contract, the tense ones must relax. (This is basic muscle physiology.) For example, stretching your fingers long relieves tightness in your hands. To relax your jaw, drag it downward actively. The jaw and hands are major tension areas because we use them so much.

At traffic lights, or on the phone, strongly pull *down* your shoulders, another typically tense area. Discomfort here begins in early pregnancy with the increased weight of the breasts and continues through into postpartum with all the mothering activities that require forward bending and lifting. Pause when you are writing or typing to stretch out your fingers. This way you can monitor your relaxation through the day to perform your tasks efficiently. Check for tense spots while sitting and standing. Mothers who learn simple relaxation skills find they cope much better with the postpartum period of disturbed sleep and incessant demands.

Stretch to Relax

The receptors in our joints relay messages directly to our conscious brain. Nerve endings in our muscles coordinate function and relay messages to the spinal cord and the primitive parts of the brain, but we are not directly aware of the messages they relay. Close your eyes and focus on your thigh muscle. It is difficult to determine how relaxed or tense it is. On the other hand, you know immediately if your knee is bent, straight, or halfway between. Joints, then, are more important than muscles in our awareness of relaxation.

Movement is an effective way to involve the mind, and yoga, which incorporates many basic stretches, is a good example. Yoga also builds strength and balance; its challenges and rewards lie in the confrontation of your own mental and physical limits. As you stretch into a posture and reach the edge of your tolerance, you learn that only by continuing to breathe, only by moving slowly toward the pain, only by freeing your body from the resistance of your mind is progress made. This letting-go is a useful preparation for childbirth and contrasts with the methods that emphasize distraction and control. The partner exercises in my book *Essential Exercises for the Childbearing Year* are a good way to help you learn surrender for labor and help strengthen your back muscles. Fathers enjoy these stretches, too.

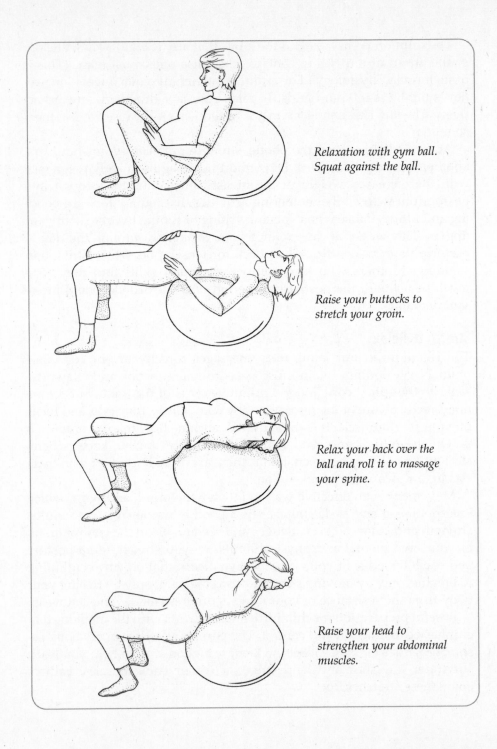

*Relaxation with gym ball.
Squat against the ball.*

*Raise your buttocks to
stretch your groin.*

*Relax your back over the
ball and roll it to massage
your spine.*

*Raise your head to
strengthen your abdominal
muscles.*

Relaxation can also be practiced passively, along the lines of transcendental meditation or its modification — the relaxation response, as described by Dr. Herbert Benson in his book of that name. Here one simply sits in a comfortable position. A state of relaxation is developed through concentrating on a repeated sound or mantra. Other techniques of meditation focus on one's breathing rhythm. Although it sounds easy, it is an art to observe rather than to control your breathing. As you learn to let go, you will notice your breathing becomes slower, more shallow, and you become aware of a pause between the outward and inward breaths. Finding these pauses or moments of nonactivity in your breathing cycle leads to deep relaxation — simply being. During labor you want to save energy. I strongly advise you to breathe normally and avoid artificial breathing patterns: see my book *Childbirth with Insight*.

Breathing awareness is an essential component of relaxation and exercise. Exercises in which stretches are maintained (rather than bounced) are done slowly, to enhance your awareness of your breathing. Start with an outward breath (there is always a reserve in the lungs) and the incoming amount of air will be spontaneously regulated.

Preparation for Childbirth

Couples who are expecting multiples need to be very well informed before the birth. Maintain your confidence in birth as a natural process, because the hospital staff, as well as family, friends, and neighbors, are probably anticipating complications.

The hospital you have chosen will send you details about classes, or your doctor may refer you elsewhere. Look for classes in the community taught by independent educators.

Childbirth classes generally encourage a couple to work together as partners. If the father of the baby (or a lesbian partner) is unable to attend, you will be encouraged to bring along a sister, roommate, parent, or friend. Whomever you wish to attend the birth should also attend the classes with you. It is important to check with both the doctor and the hospital so that any extra person (for example, a doula) besides your partner will be allowed to be present at the birth. Most hospitals in the United States now allow your other children as well as extra adults to attend the birth. Usually a crowd gathers for a multiple birth, people whom you have never even met; therefore, you have every right to have members of your chosen team present.

Important factors in selecting a class include the experience of the teacher, the size of the group, and the amount of discussion that is encouraged. Often much of the series is taken up with films, hospital tours, and lectures, leaving little time for group sharing and physical activities such as exercise and relaxation. The instructor may not have knowledge or experience about multiple birth. Special classes for parents expecting multiples are rare but check with your local multiples clubs. Amy Bustamante and Katheryn Hartigan, in Jacksonville, Florida, have modified the traditional childbirth class and inserted all the things that a mother expecting multiples needs to know — preterm labor, nutrition in a multiple pregnancy, NICU, nursing multiples, and the special needs of multiples once at home. They have also trained other mothers of multiples to help teach the classes. In addition to offering six weekend workshops on topics such as parenting and nursing multiples, they are offering Internet education (amybustamante@mybluelight.com or 904-334-5012).

In the United States more than half of twins and almost all triplets and higher-order multiples are delivered by Caesarean. Caesareans involve major surgery and prolong the postpartum recovery, especially for mothers having to care for two or more babies. Shop around for an obstetrician who is comfortable delivering multiples naturally. If you know for sure that you will have a Caesarean section, attend classes that prepare you for that and read Nancy Cohen's *Silent Knife: Caesarean Prevention and Vaginal Birth After Caesarean*.

However, you must also prepare for a vaginal birth by attending regular childbirth classes. Many mothers of multiples (especially supertwins) never consider the possibility once their Caesarean is planned, but some go into fast labor or deliver elsewhere. They are doubly stressed because of both lack of information and preparation during an emergency.

Childbirth education does not guarantee a painless labor, but studies have shown that prepared mothers need less medication and anesthesia. Remember that smaller babies are even more vulnerable to the effects of drugs.

There is so much fear around birth that we trust strangers in a medical institution more than we trust our own bodies. It is to them that we listen rather than to what is happening inside ourselves. The willingness with which a woman during labor, in her vulnerability, turns herself over to those who surround her has encouraged outsiders to "manage" the labor and birth. And the converse is true, of course. The alternative birth movement has done much to free women of these interventions, however well intentioned, so that they can extend both their minds and their bodies to stand on their two feet and give birth in their full power.

To balance the medicalization of birth, I include in the next chapter stories and photographs of women who birthed in water, or with midwives, or even at home. Today, it is easy to contact such women and chat on the Internet; and you can read inspiring stories of natural twin births on www.birthlove.com. Remember, it is the outcome that counts and less interference with Mother Nature almost always means better outcome.

11
Labor and Birth of Multiples

 Although complications can occur in multiple births, the mother's experience of labor was often easy until the Caesarean epidemic. (Caesareans are certainly quicker, but the recovery is longer — they will be discussed in the next chapter.)

The extra hormones in twin pregnancy soften the cervix prior to the onset of labor. Second and subsequent births are usually shorter and easier than the first, and naturally conceived twins are more commonly a subsequent pregnancy. Despite the growing trend to plan for surgery at the outset, in the absence of complications that would require surgery, you and your babies will do much better with vaginal birth.

Signs of Labor

Sometimes the membranes of one sac rupture and typically contractions follow within a few hours. At other times, the first sign is a mucus discharge, often bloodstained, from your cervix. If this is the only symptom of labor and you have not been advised otherwise, wait until contractions begin (probably within a day or two) before contacting your physician or midwife.

True labor contractions increase in both strength and frequency and may feel like menstrual cramps, gas, or pain in the lower back or groin. They usually build over time, but contractions can be very intense from the beginning in a rapid labor.

If contractions do not occur within a day or so after your membranes rupture and you are at term, Pitocin may be used to stimulate contractions. Most doctors prefer to deliver the baby within 24 hours after the membranes have broken, claiming that this precaution is to keep normal bacteria in the birth canal from invading the sterile uterine environment, where they may cause infection. For the same reason, it is important to avoid vaginal exams as well. Dr. Sorger recommends clinical observation of the labor or rectal exams instead. Vaginal exams should be considered only if a sterile speculum is used. Remaining at home means you are not exposed to the hospital germs, and you should take your temperature to check that you are not developing a fever (a sign of infection). You can also encourage labor to start, as described below for those who are overdue.

Deviations from the Due Date

Preterm Labor

As discussed in Chapter 7, preterm birth is the single most important problem affecting multiple pregnancy. Every expectant mother should be aware that the signs of preterm labor are the same as for term labor. However, they may be confused with other bodily sensations, especially if they occur well before the due date. Mothers often don't recognize these signs, which may be painless, and by the time they finally get to the hospital it is too late to stop the labor. (See Chapter 7 for a list of the signs of preterm labor.)

Preterm labor is much better prevented than treated, although prevention is not the result of any medical therapy or "magic pills." Excellent nutrition, sensible exercise, rest, relaxation, peace of mind, and emotional support all help to prevent preterm labor.

The medical treatment for preterm labor is hospital admission for bed rest and tocolytic drugs to diminish uterine activity. (See Chapter 19 for a complete discussion.)

Postmaturity

The expectation that twins will be preterm or at least "early" is so entrenched that little consideration is given to the possibility that they could be overdue. However, a 1990 review of the National Organization of Mothers of Twins Clubs' database of 4,445 sets of twins found that 13 percent were born after the ninth month. Even the medical literature has few guidelines on this point. The World Health Organization considers more than forty weeks postmature for twins. The technology today permits assessment of the babies' condition to determine whether labor should be started artificially.

Labor induced with Pitocin often lasts longer because the cervix may be unripe, and therefore more contractions are needed to stretch it open. In the year 2000, the rate of induction was 18 percent of all births — a 64 percent increase since 1989. Induced contractions are often experienced as stronger and more painful, although the monitor may not show increased intensity. Sometimes induction fails and may need to be tried again. You can also do nipple stimulation or make love to reach orgasm (both of which cause uterine contractions) or swallow an ounce of castor oil (which will activate your intestines) to get labor started.

The Course of Labor

Labor is divided into three stages, which always follow in the same sequence, although the nature and length of each stage vary greatly. The first and longest stage has two parts: latent and active. In the latent/early phase, contractions efface (thin out) the cervix and begin its dilation. (Effacement is measured in percentages and dilation or dilatation in centimeters.) With a multiple birth there is typically only one first stage: opening the cervix needs to be accomplished just once if the subsequent babies are born promptly. If there is a delay of hours, contractions may be needed to reopen the cervix. In the case of multiples, the cervix is generally a few centimeters dilated before labor begins; thus, the latent phase of the first stage can be short. Contractions become progressively stronger and last longer after the cervix is effaced and about 5 centimeters (halfway) dilated. This begins the active phase of the first stage.

When the cervix is fully dilated at 10 centimeters (also termed 5 fingers), the door is open for the babies to leave your uterus.

Each baby will have its own second stage, which is the journey down the birth canal through the mother's bony pelvis and vagina, ending with birth.

The third stage of labor follows with the arrival of the afterbirths, one or more placentas and membranes. These should be carefully examined to estimate the type of twinning (see Chapter 2) and sent to the lab for confirmation.

First Stage of Labor: Effacement and Dilation

In early labor, when contractions may be as infrequent as every half hour or so, it is best to carry on with your normal activities, which will keep

When I arrived at the hospital, the contractions were still light, and I had no urge to push even though I was completely dilated. Suddenly there was one strong contraction and a baby was there — in the labor bed, as planned. The second baby had been transverse but the doctor turned the baby to feet first and I pushed him out. I had twenty-four-hour rooming-in, which is something the hospital doesn't usually allow. This occurred only because I had a nurse friend stay with me during the night. Planning ahead of time paid off. I left the hospital twenty-eight hours after the births, and of course my two bundles went with me.

you upright and mobile. If this is your first pregnancy, it may take a while for labor to be established. This gives you time for carbohydrate loading, which the marathoners do before their physical challenge. Eat as many complex carbohydrates as you can, such as whole grain pasta, pancakes, and potatoes. These foods provide energy for the hours ahead in the hospital where you will most likely get nothing more than ice chips or water.

Lack of nourishment can cause many labors to become dysfunctional because the "engine has run out of fuel." Pregnant women usually feel hungry if they go without eating for even a couple of hours and to do so for a day or more, under the stress and physical effort of labor, leaves them ravenous and exhausted. When you are in active labor, you probably won't feel like eating, and at that point things move fast anyway. It is during slow, wearing labors that mothers need a constant intake of nutrients.

Laboring women are frequently denied food and drink, even water, in the rare event that general anesthesia may be needed. Food in the stomach can cause regurgitation into the lungs (the reason for fasting before surgery), but this rarely happens. Regional anesthesia (an epidural or a spinal) is used today for most Caesareans. General anesthesia, being more risky, is used only in extreme emergencies (when there is no time for a regional anesthetic to take effect) or if the mother has had a spinal fusion or refuses regional anesthesia, preferring to be "asleep." Should you need general anesthesia and you have eaten, the tube inserted in your throat before surgery takes care of the potential problem. The midwives at North Central Bronx Hospital in New York have encouraged their mostly high-risk mothers to eat and drink freely in labor for decades, and they have not seen one case of vomit being inhaled.

Stay at home as long as possible when labor begins. You have greater comfort and autonomy on your own turf. While some hospitals and birthing suites now have Jacuzzis, double beds, and rocking chairs and may even let you eat and drink, the security of your home is best. You should go to the hospital when you are in active labor, that is, when you can't talk during a contraction.

Medical records are usually sent ahead of time. The staff will take a history of your labor and do a physical exam, checking your blood pressure, urine, cervical dilation, and presentation of your babies.

The baby lying in the left half of the uterus is usually lower and presents first. When the head (or buttocks) sinks down into the pelvis, like an egg in an eggcup, the presenting part is said to be engaged. This, like dilation, may occur before the onset of labor because of the extra weight, pressure, and softening, together with an often smaller head in a multiple pregnancy.

Mothers of multiples, who are huge at term, have difficulty getting comfortable. Walk for as long as you can. Many pillows and frequent changes of position will help during labor. A large gymnastic ball, now called the "birth ball" in progressive maternity units, makes a comfortable mobile

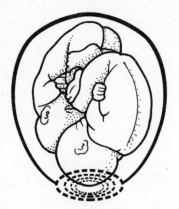

The cervix needs to dilate only once in a multiple birth.

seat. A Bodycushion® can be used for lying on your front, side, or propped up on your back. Lying flat on your back is undesirable for more than brief periods at the end of any pregnancy because the uterus may compress your major blood vessels against your backbone, which can lower your blood pressure, make you feel nauseous and faint, and reduce blood flow to the babies. The ACOG warns against exercise on the back but nowhere in its 700-page 2003 Compendium does it advise its members to avoid placing their patients in this very position during the vigorous exercise of labor!

Obstetric beds, typically found in birthing rooms, can be adapted to a variety of positions. However, mothers of multiples may have to go to the delivery room. (Dr. Sorger moves the birthing bed into the delivery room if hospital policy forces him to go there.) Hospitals prepare for potential complications with an intravenous drip, cross-matched blood, an anesthesiologist, and a pediatrician for each baby.

As soon as possible, look for a birth center or hospital that supports natural birth, with staff who will view you as "special needs" rather than "high risk." This is not an easy task and may require travel to other areas — but it's worth it for such an important event. Michel Odent, a renowned French obstetrician now living in London, points out that anxiety about possible complications makes it even more vital that mothers of multiples are supported in a low-key environment. Women journeyed from all corners of the globe to birth in water in his former clinic outside Paris.

One of my twins had her head engaged well before the birth. It is a family joke that she only had room to grow hair, because although they are identical, she had a head full of hair and her sister had almost none.

Can humanity survive obstetrics?
— Michel Odent, M.D.

The wallpaper and potted plants may be fancy, but are you allowed to give birth in any position that you choose? You need to be free to stand, walk, sit, rest on hands and knees, or squat. Many physicians will not allow a woman to get out of bed once the membranes have ruptured for fear that the cord will slip down and obstruct the blood flow. However, with the head (or buttocks) engaged snugly against the cervix, there is no room for the cord to prolapse.

The benefits of being upright for labor and birth have been well documented for so many years that it's a disgrace that so many women spend hours and hours flat on their backs — and they still do, in hospitals all over the world. Through three editions of this book, I have been complaining about this ignorance of physiology and disregard for comfort.

Gravity improves the downward force of contractions and increases their effectiveness. Less pain is reported by women who walk around freely, known in medical terms as "ambulation." There are fewer fetal heart abnormalities, less demand for pain medication, and less need to stimulate contractions with drugs.

Why are women invariably placed in bed to labor on their backs?

This is the time when a woman moves into her utmost power, her ultimate womanhood. Nature created us to give birth, as birds fly and fish swim. We can do this! Birth is what women *do*! A woman in her power will stand up for her rights on this momentous occasion, both in physical fact and emotional strength. Birth is as safe as life can be.

Alas, the culture undermines rather than reinforces her intent and ability.

The Increasing Medicalization of Birth

Among the top 25 inpatient procedures for the year 2001, eight were related to birth, a physiological process! Sadly, these obstetric interventions have not improved outcomes.

The Top 25 Inpatient Procedures in 2001

(Ranked by total payments of all third-party payers)

1 Manually-assisted delivery

2 Circumcision

6 Repair of other current obstetric laceration

9 Low cervical Caesarean section

10 Episiotomy

11 Artificial rupture of the membranes

15 Medical induction of labor

17 Fetal monitoring

MHE Source: Solucient (Evanston, IL), 2001

Medical Interventions

The intravenous tube (IV) unfortunately has become routine these days. This is "justified" on the grounds that it prevents dehydration because laboring women are usually not allowed to drink. A whole series of "in case" arguments are offered that include the possibility of hemorrhage and the need for blood, anesthesia, or drugs to stimulate the uterus or to relieve pain. Routine use of the IV implies that your body will not function without intervention; indeed, often the IV turns out to be the first step in a whole series of interventions. Once it is in place, it is easy to add drugs. You will feel more self-confident if you refuse an IV (unless there is a medical indication).

The electronic fetal monitor (EFM — using continuous ultrasound) is also routine despite evidence that it has achieved nothing but an increase in Caesarean sections. It was reported as the most commonly used obstetric procedure in 2000, used in 84 percent of labors, as well as ranked seventeenth in the list of the top 25 inpatient procedures in 2001. This means that 3.3 million women were confined to bed by this apparatus, which has failed to measure up to "evidence-based practice."

For twins, the EFM can print both fetal heart rates on the same tracing, with a third channel for contractions. Using two or more external monitors means strapping the mother to machines left and right. Also, the babies are exposed to ultrasound for varying amounts of time. The scalp electrode that is used for internal monitoring (electrocardiogram, or ECG) can be attached only to the head of the presenting baby. An external monitor has to be applied to pick up the second heartbeat. Internal monitoring, while more accurate, carries a greater risk — including infection, accidents, and hemorrhage because the electrode is inserted

My labor was progressing well until the doctor ordered Valium because he thought my blood pressure was getting a bit high. After that, everything seemed to come to a halt.

into the baby's scalp. Fetal scalp blood sampling is done to verify the monitor readings and to evaluate the baby's oxygen supply.

The IV and the EFM make it difficult, but not impossible, for you to move around. The belts can be removed for a while, and the IV bottle is usually on a mobile stand or it can be detached and carried by your partner or a nurse. A heparin lock (a small plastic tube) can be placed instead of the IV line to keep a vein open. Radiotelemetry allows the fetal heart rates to be recorded anywhere within the range of the nurses' station.

Sometimes, to speed up labor, the doctor will rupture the membranes if they have not already burst on their own. Artificial rupture of the membranes, however, creates a time deadline because of the risk of infection; and, furthermore, it is associated with cord prolapse, head compression, and bony misalignment.

In addition to the occurrence of false positive readings or faulty monitoring apparatus, EFM readings may be interpreted differently. Some couples, and most doctors, feel happier with constant surveillance by machinery. However, the information that the machines provide must be weighed against the intervention they entail. One has only to think of the women who delivered healthy undetected twins before all this obstetric wizardry! The babies' heart rates can be heard in traditional noninvasive ways, such as with a fetoscope. Rare accidents such as cord prolapse and abruption of the placenta can always be diagnosed by standard care.

Presentation

The presentation of the babies is determined usually by ultrasound. More babies mean less room, so they may stay in the same place for weeks. Multiples arrive singly, and any unusual presentations are handled as if only one baby were involved. As discussed in Chapter 7, about 40 percent of twins will both come headfirst (*vertex* presentation), like most singletons. This is the easiest way for everyone.

In approximately 60 percent of the other cases, one twin will be *breech*, most often Twin B. This second twin, however, can change position after the birth of the first, spontaneously or with help from the obstetrician. Internal version, a procedure during which the doctor manually turns the baby inside the uterus, can also be done if the twin is lying *transverse* (across the mother's pelvis) to bring that baby into a vertex position.

In a breech presentation, the arms need to be brought down, and the shoulders may need assistance through the pelvis. The head is the last part to be born. Buttocks may come out first or one or both feet, knees, or legs. Breech deliveries require more dexterity of the obstetrician, although if the mother assumes a squatting position, breech babies can be born spontaneously, especially after the passage has been opened by the first baby. Many twins are small for their dates, making breech delivery often easier than for a singleton.

Dr. Nial Ettinghausen in California assisted the births of many sets of twins and preferred the second twin to be breech, as "he could hold on to the legs better than the head"! Unfortunately, residents today are rarely trained in the skill of breech deliveries and are taught surgery instead. Predictably, few obstetricians will consider assisting a vaginal breech birth. Some will refuse a vaginal birth if the first twin is breech but will agree if the second twin is breech. Yet other doctors perform a combined vaginal-abdominal delivery. That is, the vertex twin is delivered vaginally, but the breech twin is delivered by Caesarean.

Ask your doctor what percentage of twin and breech deliveries she or he does vaginally. In 1938, quadruplets, all breech, were delivered vaginally in England. (Although their birth weights ranged from 1,445 to 1,815 grams, all but one died from breathing difficulties postpartum.) Dr. Derom in Belgium also delivered all breech quadruplets.

There is no medical consensus regarding delivery management for vertex and nonvertex presenting twin pairs. A study from Charleston, South Carolina, determined that breech birth of the second twin is the most cost-effective delivery. The cost of such a birth was under $6,000 compared with over $50,000 when the second twin was delivered by Caesarean. The length of stay was shorter for mothers. The infants had significantly lower rates of lung problems and neonatal infections (only 1 percent required the use of a ventilator); and they had a significantly shorter time in the hospital, most of them in the regular newborn nursery.

Comfort Measures

Back and upper thigh massage may comfort and relax you. Counter-pressure against your lower back and pelvis helps relieve the pain of contractions, which are usually felt in this area. Hot or cold packs feel good, too. Stand in the shower or soak in a Jacuzzi. Even if your membranes have ruptured, you should be allowed to take a shower. (Make sure you have help getting out of a slippery tub or taking a shower in case you get dizzy or feel faint.)

After Jason was born, I could feel Aaron inside wiggling around. The doctor was in a hurry to get him out but the baby didn't want to come. First an arm came down, and then a leg. The doctor finally pushed the arm back and pulled him out by both legs.

For labor, muster all your courage to surrender to the intense energy and power of the contractions. The stronger they are, the sooner your babies will be born! Breathe spontaneously at all times. Artificial breathing patterns have been the hallmark of childbirth preparation since the 1950s, despite the fact that mothers become exhausted and anxious when panting like small dogs during labor. The idea that this helps them feel "in control" denies the true nature of birth, which means no control — simply trust and surrender. Your body knows how to breathe right now and it will in labor too! Your breathing will be different, with moans, sighs, grunts, groans, and other expressive sounds. Artificial breathing techniques disturb this normal physiology and hyperventilation leads to dizziness, nausea, and feeling faint. (Too much oxygen constricts the blood vessels and impairs the release of oxygen from your red blood cells to your tissues. As a result there is less blood carrying less oxygen, which can affect your babies.) This risk is increased if your circulation is already reduced by regional anesthesia and by lying on your back. I discuss spontaneous breathing and "sounding" during labor in detail in my book *Childbirth with Insight* and demonstrated it personally in a video, *Channel for a New Life*, of my (noisy) last birth.

Medication and Anesthesia

Unless you have enjoyed supreme nutrition, your babies may be small or preterm, and they will be more affected by the adult dosages of medication and anesthesia. Doris Haire, President of the American Foundation for Maternal and Child Health (www. aimsusa.org), spent the year 2001 reading, analyzing, abstracting, and cross-checking the risks inherent in the use of approximately sixty drugs used in obstetrics. Virtually all these drugs cross the sieve-like placentas and the blood brain barrier, including oxytocin (Pitocin). Narcotics such as Demerol and sedatives such as Seconal depress the babies' respiration. Epidural anesthesia lowers blood pressure, makes extra demands on your heart, and slows down labor. Haire, in *Drugs in Labor and Birth*, points out that the package insert for the anesthetic Marcaine (used for epidurals) contains five pages of adverse effects. This insert also admits that there may be partial or complete loss of sphincter control and sexual satisfaction. Also, http://www.healing-arts.org lists extensive documentation of complications from epidurals (an incidence of approximately 23 percent according to Lewis Mehl-Madrona, M.D., Ph.D.; see Appendix 8).

Regional (epidural or spinal) anesthesia is safer than general anesthesia, and you stay awake. An epidural can be put in during the first stage of labor and continued through the birth and recovery phase. This differs from a spinal, which is a single shot given at the end to facilitate a delivery with instruments or for a Caesarean. Both types of anesthesia — particularly the spinal, which temporarily paralyzes the muscles — abolish your natural bearing-down reflex and thus interfere with your ability to push.

For regional anesthesia you will be asked to curl up on your side to open the spaces between the lower vertebrae of your spine. The area is cleansed with a cold antiseptic fluid. Next, you will feel a prick and soon after the anesthetic is injected, your legs tingle and go numb. For an epidural, an indwelling catheter remains so that the anesthetic solution can be topped up from time to time. This tube is taped securely along your back. Epidural anesthesia is effective for instrumental assistance. However, the use of epidurals themselves is associated with an increased need for instruments because contractions slow down and become less effective. This leads to further intervention — the need for Pitocin to stimulate the contractions. Stimulating labor with Pitocin has been linked to postpartum hemorrhage and jaundice in the newborn. Anesthesia causes delay in the delivery of the second twin and exposes this baby to its effects for a longer time. Babies born with epidurals often do not suck well at the beginning.

Second Stage of Labor: Descent and Delivery

The second stage of labor officially begins when the cervix is fully dilated. I would like to see it redefined as when the presenting baby descends onto the pelvic floor, stimulating the urge to push (unless you have been anesthetized). You will feel a reflex urge to push when the first baby is low enough on your pelvic floor to stimulate the stretch receptors in your muscles. These receptors communicate with your brain, which leads to the release of oxytocin (the natural form of Pitocin) to increase the power of your contractions.

Until this time, while the head or presenting part remains high, pushing will be too early and very tiring. There is often a physiological lull at the beginning of the second stage — enjoy the rest and wait until your body is ready for the "expulsive phase." During the second stage, nurses and doctors tend to cheer, instruct, and exhort. Ideally, you are experi-

I remember the nurses telling me that wasn't the way to push, but my doctor said to go ahead and do what felt right.

With my first delivery I did what I was told and strained for two and a half hours. The blood vessels in my eyes and cheeks were shot — I looked a mess the next day. With the twins, I just went with the urge when it came. It felt so good compared with the pain I had the last time.

encing your own inner direction that is more reliable. It makes no sense to push if your uterus is not pushing! Certainly a purple face and bulging eyes reassure the staff that the mother is indeed trying hard. Unfortunately, straining with the breath held is still taught and interferes with normal physiology. Such a forced expulsive effort is known as a *Valsalva maneuver*. When the glottis is shut tightly to hold the breath, a closed-pressure system is formed and the abdominal wall distends and moves outward.

The high pressure is transmitted throughout the entire body. This forced effort with the breath held tenses the pelvic floor, strains the midline of the abdomen, reduces blood flow to the babies, and causes fluctuations in respiration and circulation. Blood pressure is greatly increased at the onset of strain but within a few seconds it starts to fall because blood pools in vessels of the pelvis and legs due to high pressures in the chest. With reduced venous return, the heart has less blood to pump out to the lungs, uterus, and babies. The late Dr. Caldeyro-Barcia was one of the few researchers to look at the effects of forced and prolonged bearing-down efforts on the fetus. His studies led him to conclude that the Valsalva maneuver reduced oxygen to the babies and can increase the need for episiotomy by not allowing time for the pelvic floor to distend. He was President of the International Federation of Gynecologists and Obstetricians when he presented this research, which he undertook at my suggestion. Unfortunately, little has changed.

The body, however, has its own inherent wisdom, helped by a more sensitive threshold for oxygen deprivation in pregnancy, and the mother usually lets out a characteristic grunt. By pushing spontaneously — on *outward* breath — the pressure is released from above and the pelvic floor can relax and stretch.

Moaning and groaning — sounds of work with overtones of sexuality — are usually discouraged during childbirth because "air is escaping" and the "force is waning." However, this is the natural way that women respond. Misguided educators and maternity staff encourage long pushes with snatch breaths. Fortunately, women rarely sustain the strain for more than a few seconds. This is desirable, and regular breaths between bearing-down maintain normal physiology.

It is a prevalent but erroneous belief that to "push" you must have a "pocket of air" trapped inside by your held breath to "force down the diaphragm." On the contrary, the abdominal muscles contract on *out-*

ward breath — most effectively when exhaling air against some resistance. Examples of this include singing, blowing a trumpet, and inflating a balloon. During birth this is achieved by *partially* closing the glottis — which leads to the characteristic guttural sounds uttered by laboring women. Rest assured that your throat will be fine after your spontaneous sounds during pushing — the vocal cords become engorged with blood (hyperemia) to create the resistance and also to avoid later discomfort.

During physiological pushing, the breath is exhaled and the abdominal muscles move in toward the spine, shortening around the uterus. It is like squeezing a toothpaste tube. As the mother bears down on outward breath, her abdominals contract, and her pelvic floor reciprocally relaxes to open for the birth.

Instructions typically emphasize "doing" and "control," usually based on cultural ideas about elimination. The aspects of releasing, letting go, and giving can only happen — by definition they cannot be forced. You will *feel* and *know* what to do without being told. Those who seek the passion of childbirth must develop a sense of intelligent awareness — the link between body and mind. The first commitment is to learn total trust in your body. Birth, like orgasm, relaxation, and sleep, is spontaneous.

Episiotomy

Episiotomy, an incision to enlarge the vaginal outlet, may be indicated for fetal distress or a difficult presentation. Multiples are usually small and therefore episiotomies are unnecessary. Many obstetricians make this unkind cut "to prevent a tear," although episiotomy is a major cause of blood loss at birth, can extend into a tear, and must be sutured! Twenty-four percent of this modern form of genital mutilation extends into the anal sphincter and causes problems such as fecal incontinence.

A 2002 study from Australia published in *Birth* showed that, compared with midwives, obstetricians had five times the rate of episiotomies. Earlier Australian studies had shown that public patients were more likely to have an intact perineum than women with private health insurance.

A first-degree tear and often a second-degree tear do not need stitches, but larger tears do, just like episiotomies. For most women, a tear heals more comfortably than an episiotomy. Rates of this mostly un-

The nurse kept hissing at me to hold my breath. I told her (between contractions) that I had good reasons for wanting to avoid that. Then she said, "Well, at least you don't have to make so much noise." And I replied, "It is my birth and I'll make as much noise as I like!"

necessary intervention have been steadily dropping; and finally the ACOG has withdrawn its recommendation for routine episiotomy. Dr. Sorger's rate is 1.7 percent and correlates with the incidence of fetal distress.

Say NO! to cutting . . . both vaginas and penises.

The parents of twins may be so happy and excited to welcome the first baby that they momentarily forget that the other is still inside. On the other hand, it may be a challenge for the mother to bond with the first when more are to come. Putting the first baby immediately to your breast naturally stimulates contractions. It may not be immediately clear if the first infant has its own placenta and membranes. These may follow the first birth, or there may be one large placental mass or, less often, two separate placentas may be delivered after the second twin.

After the first twin arrives, the doctor or midwife will do a vaginal exam and press around your abdomen to determine if the position of the second twin has changed. You may be aware of increased movement with the extra room now available in the uterus. Between the delivery of the first and second twins, the cervix may close down a little if the second twin is not delivered right away. However, in most cases, contractions will dilate it again when the uterus is ready for the next expulsive phase.

Classic obstetric practice advises neither undue delay nor haste. The ACOG in its 1998 Educational Bulletin on multiple pregnancy stated that "the interval between delivery of each twin is not critical in determining the outcome of Twin B." Of course, vital signs continue to be monitored.

Third Stage of Labor:
Delivery of Placenta(s) and Membranes

Each cord is cut after it has ceased pulsing and has been identified so that each multiple can later be matched with the appropriate placenta. The cords are clamped — birth order is identified by the number of ties or clamps. Samples of cord blood are sent for laboratory analysis (and, we hope, zygosity testing). The placentas may be separate or fused and are usually delivered following the birth of both twins. About 60 percent of MZ twins have just one placenta. Arrival of the common placenta before the second twin is born is dangerous. If the placenta is not delivered spontaneously, it must be removed manually before the cervix closes.

Each placenta will be weighed and sections can be frozen for future DNA analysis if needed. Placentation greatly affects the growth and development of multiples; it is important to record this information accurately for the benefit of the individuals themselves as well as general research.

Some physicians like to see the placenta delivered within minutes, but in home births and in other countries, up to an hour is customary. Tugging on the cord to hasten removal of a placenta can cause hemorrhage. This third stage of labor, when hormones in mother and baby have peaked, is important for optimal bonding. Disturbances of this attachment period often occur because of haste to cut the cord or remove the baby for observation or washing.

Pitocin or another uterine stimulant is frequently administered during the third stage of labor to augment the contractions of the uterus. Nature arranged the uterine musculature in different layers, so that contractions naturally clamp off any bleeding vessels, preventing hemorrhage from the site of placental attachment. Thus it is extremely important that the uterus continues to contract after birth. Postpartum hemorrhage is more common after multiple birth, especially if there was interference in the labor or haste with the second baby or the placenta. Excellent nutrition builds a strong uterus that can contract adequately to stop bleeding from the large placental site. (Vaginal bleeding may be heavier and last longer after multiple birth owing to the larger area of uterus covered by the placenta.)

An episiotomy or tear is sutured after the placentas are delivered, but ideally you will deliver slowly and calmly with an intact perineum and will not need stitches.

Breast-feeding, which ideally commences as soon as possible after birth, stimulates your uterus to contract. Newborns at term have the ability to suck very soon, which stimulates an early milk supply and helps prevent engorgement of the breasts. Even if the babies just lick your nipples, this action will raise hormone levels, which helps lactation and your bonding. Babies can actually find the nipple themselves if placed skin to skin on your belly. This has been filmed in a remarkable video from Sweden, *Delivery Self-Attachment* (see Resources).

My babies were brought to me alternately for nursing in the hospital, but I think it is essential that both twins be brought in together. This way you don't prolong the fantasy that you gave birth to just one baby, which can delay the bonding with both.

Care of the Babies

After birth, mucus may be aspirated from an infant's nose and mouth with a bulb syringe. A catheter may be used if deep suctioning is necessary. (If an episiotomy was cut, there may have been inadequate squeezing of the baby's chest to help expel the mucus.) Oxygen will be administered to any baby with breathing difficulties. Heel prints, samples of cord blood, and wristband identification (A, B, C to indicate the order of birth) are done immediately after birth. Each baby should be put in different-colored wraps in the same crib and kept together.

In many states by law, silver nitrate drops or antibiotic ointment must be put in all newborns' eyes. This prevents eye complications that may arise if the mother has gonorrhea. The eye inflammation and blurred vision caused by these drops interferes with the babies' experience of bonding. Avoid or delay this procedure.

Although parents would prefer to have the babies remain warm and secure in their arms, hospitals usually place them in isolettes and take them to the central nursery "until their body temperature returns to normal." The cold air conditioning in the delivery rooms disturbs their temperature regulation, but babies can warm up quickly against your body. Thanks to increasing awareness of the importance of parental bonding with newborns, hospitals are becoming more flexible.

Apgar Scale

CATEGORY	SCORE		
	0	1	2
Appearance *(skin color)*	Blue, pale	Pink body, extremities blue	Completely pink
Heart Rate *(pulse)*	Absent	Below 100	Over 100
Respiration *(breathing effort)*	Absent	Irregular, slow	Strong cry
Muscle Tone *(activity)*	Limp, flaccid	Some flexion of extremities	Active, vigorous movement
Reflex Irritability *(grimace in response to stimulation of sole of foot)*	No response	Grimace	Cry, cough, or sneeze during suctioning

The nearer the total score is to 10, the better the baby's condition.

Newborn infants are assessed at one and five minutes after birth, according to the Apgar scale. Scores of 0, 1, or 2 are given for each category at each time interval. A perfect score of 10 is rarely given, as it takes a little while for the baby's circulation to adapt, even if the baby is a mature infant born spontaneously. Measurements are made of each infant's weight, length, and circumference of the head. A pediatrician will do a thorough evaluation of each baby's maturity and health. Assessment is made of posture, muscle and joint function, skin condition (some babies are born with fine hairs — lanugo — that disappear in postpartum life), creases in the palms and soles of the feet, development of the genitals, the areola around the nipple, and ear cartilage.

Parents are often unprepared for the appearance of a newborn baby. He or she typically has a disproportionately large head, molded irregularly. The body may be a little blue and covered with creamy white vernix that provided protection in the amniotic fluid. Large alert eyes are very impressive.

The parents of twins or other multiples become instant celebrities in the hospital. Staff and visitors are fascinated, and the mother receives flowers, gifts, and lots of help. The task of handling two babies seems formidable to the first-time mother, who may wonder if she can learn enough skills during a brief postpartum stay. Although you may start with just one twin at a time while the staff helps with the other, it is important to learn to handle two. Unless some assistance is arranged for your return home, you will suddenly have the job of both at once.

Because of the novelty of multiples, you can expect more attention and cooperation from the staff, especially with breast-feeding. If this is not forthcoming, ask for a lactation consultant or contact La Leche League. Some mothers have a problem making sure their babies are brought to them for night feedings, because it is often easier for the nursery staff to give a bottle and let the mother sleep. You will need as much practice as possible during your hospital stay, especially learning to put both babies to the breast together (which is a challenge in a narrow hospital bed). Breast-feeding helps your uterus return to its former size after being stretched for multiples. You may feel painful postpartum contractions in the early days, if this is your second or subsequent pregnancy, and these "after pains" are stronger when the babies nurse. The feeding of multiples is discussed in Chapter 13.

The most scary, but the most useful thing, was to learn to pick them both up together! When I finally had the courage and strength to do that, it was a great time-saver.

The Foreskin Has a Function:
Circumcision of Multiples = Multiple Mistakes

Soon after the mother has been cut (episiotomy or Caesarean), the knife is readied for the newborn boy's penis. You can see step-by step illustrations of one of the many procedures that create this disaster at http://www.CircumcisionQuotes.com/magcirc.html.

One hundred percent of baby boys oppose this mutilating surgery and so should you — their screams of betrayal and protest are ignored by those who are cutting. This abuse is typically done during the mother's postpartum stay (and in a room far away from where she can see and hear). Dr. Sorger refuses to do circumcisions and accept "blood money."

Circumcision remains the most frequent surgical procedure performed on males in the United States; the number of baby boys cut in the year 2000 was 1,214,312 for a total cost of $2.3 billion. The national rate is about 60 percent, although it varies widely. Medicaid currently funds over 25 percent of foreskin amputations, which costs United States taxpayers directly over $37 million annually, and indirectly far more.

Many midwives and doulas follow the example of "intactivist" and freebirth practitioner Jeannine Parvati Baker, who will not attend the birth of any parents planning this barbaric act. Europeans and Scandinavians look aghast when told that this is done in the United States. To them, circumcision is equivalent to one of the female genital mutilations performed in many regions of Africa and other parts of the world. There are laws in the United States against female genital mutilation, but inexplicably, not against male genital mutilation. No medical society in the world recommends circumcision, but it is pursued for profit by greedy physicians and by misinformed parents for a host of invalid reasons.

The tragic traumas (surgical, pharmaceutical, emotional, physical, and psychological) of Canadian twin David Reimer, who lost his penis after circumcision and was forced to undergo a sex change, is documented in *As Nature Made Him, The Boy Who Was Raised as a Girl*, by John Colapinto. At age 14, "she" learned the truth and returned to his real male self (surgically and hormonally). However, his life was in shreds, unlike that of his co-twin, who was left intact.

To "look like Dad" (which becomes "lack like Dad") is one of the common excuses given to deprive a baby boy of this protective and sexually significant part of his penis. However, one mother of identical twins, having witnessed the screams of terror and bloody agony as the first was circumcised, refused to allow the co-twin to be done. "But they won't look alike!" chastised her doctor. "Two wrongs don't make a right" was her reply.

Check the Resources for Web sites and other information to help you keep your son intact in the face of such abuse from the medical establishment. Be vigilant in hospitals where circumcisions are routine and all the babies in the nursery tend to be "done" — yours might be included. (There have been several lawsuits over inadvertent, as well as botched, circumcisions.) Preterm multiples often have the luck to escape, being too frail to undergo the operation (which has caused infection, hemorrhage, and even death in healthy term babies). Most of the world's males are intact as nature intended, and happily so! Your sons will thank you for being part of the majority, which they soon will be.

Natural Birth for Twins and Supertwins

Women must know and believe that natural birth for multiples is possible and they have the right to have it! The more women abdicate responsibility for their births to the medical profession and the more it is wrested from them by interventions, the worse the malpractice situation will be when their resentment surfaces later. Insurance companies unfortunately are increasingly dictating medical practice, to the detriment of the doctor-patient relationship. But taking responsibility means taking informed risks, and expectant mothers need to hear about good outcomes.

Professor Robert Derom, a Belgian obstetrician and longtime expert on multiple birth, delivered almost all of his triplets and quadruplets vaginally, including breech presentations. Because the overwhelming majority of obstetricians in the United States consider a *singleton* breech an indication for a Caesarean, it is important for American mothers to know how obstetric practices have differed in other times and places.

Dr. Louis Keith, who wrote the foreword to this book, assisted the vaginal delivery of two sets of triplets, at about 35 to 36 weeks, at the Cook County Hospital in Chicago during the first years of his residency. All infants did well. Interestingly, in a survey of the records of multiple births at the Chicago Maternity Center from 1901 to 1933, the perinatal

I recently immunized 2-month-old twins. The boy's reaction was the worst I have ever witnessed; he was so hysterical I thought he would throw up. His sister, who had not been circumcised, did not exhibit this "post traumatic stress disorder." At his 6-month check-up he cried less, but still much longer than his sister.

— Elizabeth Key,
Family Nurse-Practitioner

Nobody, but nobody, no matter how loving, no matter how well-intentioned, should have the power to steal precious parts of a body from a child before she or he even gets started in life.

I was extremely upset that I had had a Caesarean and it was my desire to have a nonintervention, natural birth this time. I felt the only way to get this was by having a home birth and was taken by the beauty and simplicity of it all. I knew I could never have that in a hospital.

mortality rate was about the same as today. All those multiples were born at home, delivered by midwives, nurses, and medical students to a population consisting mainly of immigrants living under adverse socioeconomic conditions.

Women must deliver where they feel safe. Remember that before the advent of hospital obstetrics, all multiples were born at home (of course, with some bad outcomes just as in the hospital). Others since have been born in small community hospitals or recently in birth centers. Midwives in the United States, while increasing in numbers, attended only 8 percent of the births in the year 2000 and very few involving multiples, but always *some*.

All the high-tech screening, intervention, and enormous expense that surround the delivery of supertwins today have *not* significantly improved outcomes *obstetrically*, although tinier and tinier babies are surviving because of developments in *pediatric* care.

The following anecdotes may inspire couples to shop around for a physician or midwife who will consider vaginal delivery, vertical or squatting positions, and nourishment during labor. Women and their partners who seek home births are generally highly informed and assume much responsibility for planning the event. The mothers whose cases I cite here all enjoyed excellent nutrition and prenatal care, gained adequate weight, and gave birth close to or even beyond their due date. In addition, they had good support and a resolute belief in their innate ability to birth normally.

Vaginal Birth After Caesarean (VBAC)

Many obstetricians are reluctant to consider a vaginal birth after a previous Caesarean. Their fear is that the scar will rupture, particularly in a multiple pregnancy where there is more stretching of the uterus. However, the transverse lower incision used today is stronger than the vertical or classical uterine incision done in the past. (The incision that is visible on the abdominal wall is not necessarily congruent to the one in the uterus.) As long ago as 1962, Dr. Alan Guttmacher described four VBACs of twins and stated that the indications for a subsequent vaginal delivery were the same as for a singleton — the absence of any conditions in the current pregnancy that constituted criteria for a Caesarean.

A good while ago (1988), Dr. Bruce Flamm demonstrated the safety of VBACs. Not one case of rupture occurred in more than 5,000 VBACs, and the study included 89 women whose scar was of unknown type. If the scar were to rupture, which is extremely rare, immediate surgery would deliver the baby. More typically, a slight opening of the scar (dehiscence) happens; but this occurs in only 2 percent of singleton and 4 percent of twin births.

According to Blickstein, VBACs are successful for twins at least 50 percent of the time. Instrumental deliveries (involving forceps or vacuum), especially for the second twin, require manual dexterity and experience from the physician. He points out that clinicians who are less experienced in twin delivery are more likely to report an adverse outcome following vaginal delivery or opt for a combined delivery when encountering minor difficulties delivering the second twin.

In summary, many clinicians who follow the cliché "no high-risk pregnancy should end with a high-risk delivery" may deliver twins by Caesarean section for many subtle reasons instead of clear-cut, evidence-based indications. Thus, the decision for a Caesarean in twin delivery, intentionally or not, is based on qualitative variables that are not quantified and on quantitative variables that suggest no advantage for a Caesarean in the majority of cases.

The rate of VBAC for singletons has been falling and varies widely by state: from 10 percent of births following a prior Caesarean in Louisiana to 42 percent in Vermont. Some obstetricians pay lip service to "allowing" women to go into labor after a previous Caesarean. The disheartening phrase "trial of labor after Caesarean" conveys a lack of confidence in the birth process. Too few doctors encourage their patients to plan a VBAC and too many readily agree to an anxious, poorly informed woman's request for another Caesarean.

If you want a VBAC, search for an obstetrician who genuinely supports VBACs for mothers of twins and can give evidence of success, but bear in mind that his or her hands may be tied by professional guidelines. In July 1999, the ACOG updated their standards of practice bulletin on VBAC, replacing their previous recommendations that a surgeon be "readily available" when a woman with a prior Caesarean was in labor. The new guidelines recommend that a physician be "immediately available throughout active labor and capable of monitoring labor and performing an immediate Caesarean." The practice bulletin, by stating that a contraindication to VBAC would be "inability to perform emergency Caesarean delivery because of unavailable surgeon, anesthesia, sufficient staff, or facility," has intimidated facilities and physicians. Many are now refusing to allow VBAC because they are unable or unwilling to meet the guidelines. Failure to adhere to ACOG guidelines can lead to malpractice litigation. (Of course, larger hospitals have medical staff and residents around the clock.)

Below you can read inspiring stories of mothers of multiples who set up VBACs. Mothers of multiples are increasingly candidates for VBAC, because they tend to be older and have borne more children, and because Caesarean rates are continuing to rise.

Amy Bustamante is a mother of triplets born by Caesarean at thirty-one weeks, who two years later had a HBAC* of a surviving twin at home in water. (She can be contacted at http://twins-n-more.tripod.com or amybustamante@mybluelight.com.) She writes,

> I wish I had had my three at home. We learn from our mistakes . . . for those of you wanting to experience a vaginal delivery after a Caesarean, my best advice is to take care of yourself, seek out help from those who have done it, be a good consumer with your care provider, and most of all have faith in yourself and birth.

Marcia Weaver was three days shy of 36 weeks when she went into labor with twins after a Caesarean eleven years earlier that had been done because her son was in breech presentation and the doctor scared her out of an internal version or a vaginal delivery. (She can be contacted at weaverdm@juno.com.)

> It was a very different labor for me than that of my singletons. Because Matthew, the one to be born first, was slanted a bit and didn't have room to get a straight shot down the birth canal, I stayed at 8 cm dilated for over 5 hours. I had gotten to the hospital around midnight and at 7 A.M. my doctor started manipulating Matthew and at 7:27 A.M. he was born. As soon as he was delivered, Hannah flipped to breech position and she was delivered at 7:37 A.M. feet first. Matthew weighed 5 pounds, 10 ounces and Hannah weighed 5 pounds, 7 ounces. They were perfect in every way with no complications. Again we were thankful to God for our double blessing and to our doctor for letting us try the natural delivery. They went home the next day with me.

Her obstetrician, Anita Showalter, D.O., a board certified OB/GYN, was a patient and mother before entering medical school. She trained

---

*Home Birth After Caesarean

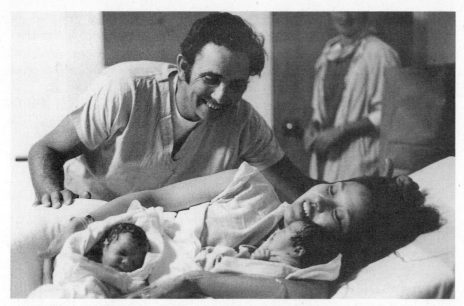

Natural childbirth brings joy to these new parents of twins.

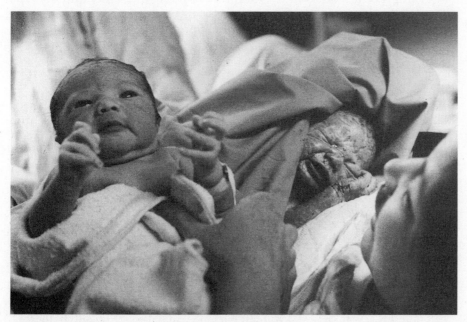

Healthy twins can be cuddled right after birth. The baby on the left has already been washed. The baby on the right is still coated with the protective vernix.

specifically to provide birthing alternatives and sensitive gynecologic care for women. Dr. Showalter routinely treats her patients with osteopathic manipulation, which she believes contributes to her very low Caesarean rate — about 3 percent primary (first-time), about 6 percent overall.

Doula Terri Moore describes a VBAC she attended for a mother who at thirty-nine weeks and two days gave birth to a total of 15 pounds, 9 ounces of gorgeous little girls:

> During pushing contractions, the mother — "D" — would talk to the babies, saying with each contraction, "Come on baby!" She was so determined and positive! She pushed out her first baby in only an hour and a half and while pushing through another baby. As soon as the head was born, D yelled triumphantly, "Yes!" Baby A arrived in a posterior position, looking up at Mom! She went right into D's arms and for the first time, was the baby on top, lying on D's belly, with Baby B underneath! Baby B was transverse, but was turned to a head down position by two obstetricians and delivered 45 minutes later.

Several recent studies in the literature support the safety and benefits of VBAC for mothers of twins. The references are in Further Reading if you need to convince your doctor, but perhaps it is better to find a physician who is already familiar with the evidence and has adapted his or her practice accordingly.

Hospital Waterbirth of Twins

British midwife Jane Evans, in a 1997 *Midwifery Matters* article ("Can a Twin Birth Be a Positive Experience?"), describes several natural hospital births in the United Kingdom of twins, including one in water. I admire her commitment to her clients' desires for no intervention and her disapproval of unwarranted attempts to medicalize the pregnancies and seize control of the birth process by physicians. You can read the details on-line at http://www.radmid.demon.co.uk/twins.htm.

Home Births of Twins

Andrea in New Zealand describes how she improved the presentation of her first twin:

> Your book was so positive about birthing vaginally. My second twin presented transverse from 28 weeks and just loved it that way. I stu-

pidly let someone perform an internal cephalic version on me after my first baby was born; thankfully they couldn't reach Amelia as she was too high up and I spent the next hour gently turning her myself with my contractions. I kept pressure on her bottom and gently pushed her up and over with the contractions, in between I just held my hand over her bottom and kept up the pressure so she wouldn't slip back. She was born face up weighing 8 pounds, 8 ounces, and it was great. I don't think I would have been so proactive if it weren't for the inspiration in your book.

Beverly, expecting twins, pregnant for the third time, decided she couldn't trust her midwives after they basically admitted that she would have a Caesarean. When they asked her, "How committed are you to a vaginal birth?" Beverly decided to look elsewhere for a midwife to attend her at home. She chose one in another state who advised her to follow the Brewer diet (see Resources). After her thirty-fifth week, she paid for the midwife to fly in. Her twin girls were born two weeks later, a half-hour apart, with her daughter sitting next to the midwife cheering her on. She concludes:

> The birth was everything I could have wanted but I don't recommend home birth for everyone. It takes a lot of commitment to the babies and not to your job, or other kids, or other commitments in life and that is a hard sacrifice to make sometimes. Also, not every twin pregnancy is set up so perfectly as mine. Having one amnion and one chorion would mean too much risk for a home birth (and my midwife told me she didn't do them).

A woman in Kansas delivered dizygotic twins at home, with transient complications. Although it was her second pregnancy, the first baby took four hours to push out. The second twin's cord prolapsed, so the mother took the knee-chest position and was given oxygen while the midwife pushed the cord back up. During the discussion about hospital transfer, when the mother was left alone, her instinct to birth the baby reemerged and ten minutes later she delivered a very alert and relaxed, completely pink little girl. The first twin weighed $5\,^1/_2$ pounds and the second 6 pounds, and they were born at forty weeks, one day after their due date. The mother, only five feet tall, had eaten well in pregnancy and had gained about 50 pounds. She taught aerobics until six weeks before the birth and nursed the twins for three years.

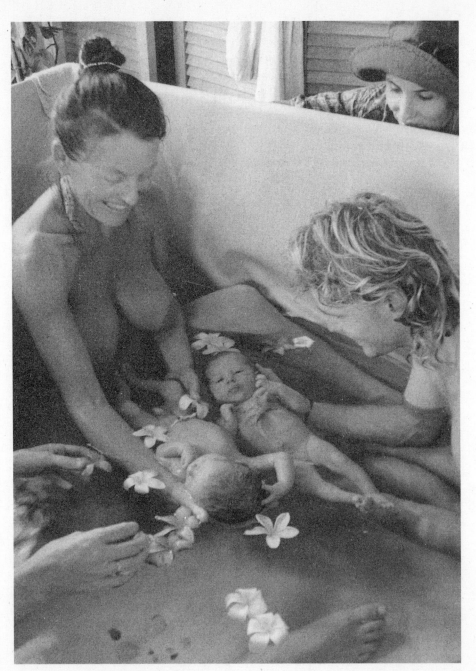

An ideal welcome into the world.

Freeda Cathcart's first child was born by emergency Caesarean and her second was born at home. She describes her third pregnancy with twins.

I knew my body could give birth vaginally but I wasn't sure how having twins was going to be different. I decided that the best way to proceed was to be prepared for both a home and hospital birth. During the pregnancy I concentrated on doing what I was able to do. I ate nutritiously. I regularly walked or swam for exercise. I took morning and afternoon naps. I knew that it was important to reduce as much stress in my life as possible and concentrate on enjoyable activities. Mothers who are in the best shape physically, mentally, and spiritually are better capable of handling the challenges that living brings.

It was very important for me to be able to trust the person who would be attending the birth. My previous experiences with the obstetrical professionals were not pleasant or reassuring. I felt that they weren't being upfront or supportive about allowing me to make decisions regarding my own care. I wanted to tune in and trust my own instincts. If I felt I needed a second opinion or medical care I knew my birth attendant would understand and support me. I did not have the same confidence in the obstetrical professionals to respect my intuition.

Labor started when my water broke and when my attendant arrived I was almost fully dilated. She determined that my babies were both in good positions to be born vaginally. In fact one baby was already starting to descend. I remember being a bit shocked that we were actually going to give birth at home.

I hadn't wanted to get attached to where the birth was going to happen because there were so many unknowns. I was more than willing to go to the hospital for the health of my children.

We were lucky to have prepared for a home birth because a mere two and a half hours after my water started to leak the first baby was born. He had a very short cord that needed to be cut before I could hold him in my arms. We were able to bond while I rested for about twenty minutes before fluid from the other sac signaled the beginning of the next birth. This baby started to show signs of distress. I knew it was very important to birth him right away and it didn't take long. He was white and somewhat limp so we covered him and started rubbing him right away. I don't think I've ever prayed harder

Our twins were born at home. We buried the placenta in the garden and planted two chrysanthemums above in memory.

in my life. I was so happy when right before our eyes the baby pinked up and then started to cry.

We were so distracted by the babies that we forgot about the placenta. I was still sitting on the birthing stool when the placenta went splat on the floor. That seemed to remind everyone that there was still work to be done. I walked over to the bed to drink an herbal mixture that helped to contract my uterus. I felt tired and elated — so amazed to have given birth to two babies, and so grateful they were both fine.

While I went to take a shower, the birth attendants changed the bed sheets and brought me some food to eat in bed. After they checked to make sure the babies were fine, they left. My husband and I were alone with our two new bundles of joy to cuddle and love.

Smells, sounds and feelings can influence the mother's ability to open up to birth healthfully. I am a survivor of child molestation. I believe it was crucial for me to be able to trust my birth attendants and to be in a setting that was familiar and comfortable for me to be able to open up and birth healthfully.

Jeannine Parvati Baker, author of several books, including *Conscious Conception* and *Prenatal Yoga*, delivered her twins at home. It was her second pregnancy, and she had experienced some bleeding in early labor and went to the hospital. After the bleeding stopped, she checked herself out, went home, and delivered the babies within a few hours with the obstetrician (who had followed her home from the hospital). The second baby was breech and she describes the experience: "I had the least pain of all my births with my breech baby. It even felt to me as if this was the right way to birth rather than vertex!"

Sheila Kitzinger, noted British childbirth educator and author, birthed her twin daughters at home. There has always been a tradition of home birth in England, endorsed by the medical profession, which dwindled as birth moved into the hospitals. Birth at home is currently being revived again there, as in Holland.

Alison Curtis in Florida writes her story:

I am wild, woman!!! I am what they fear the most — a menstruating, ovulating, copulating, orgasming, conceiving, gestating, birthing, lactating MOTHER. And all the while I have the gall to enjoy it. But I feel I have been punished and merely tolerated for my enjoyment of and success in my most creative and valuable process.

Those women who dared to say they wanted things to be different for them during birth had asked me enough questions that I dared to become their advisor, and told them that they, too, could have strong healthy children in powerful, empowering, undrugged births.

I became a Bradley Method® childbirth instructor at a birthing center with Jacuzzi tubs, double beds and two midwives.* However, when I became pregnant for the third time, they told me that if I wanted to birth there, I would have to limit my weight gain to twenty pounds and if I didn't, I would have to have my baby in the hospital. Firstly, I'm a big girl and also those restrictions went against everything I knew to be right.

I was blessed to have my old midwife to fall back upon. I wanted no ultrasound with this baby and she used a fetoscope, without acting like I was crazy.† I was measuring about 4 weeks further along than I thought I was, but we laughed and figured it was my baby fat.

Several happy strong pregnant months went by. My dear husband was able to relax when he heard I would have two certified nurse midwives in the house. (We all have our requirements.)

My due date was October 10. On September 17, while getting ready to go to a birthday party, there was a very quiet, internal pop . . . and a whole lot of water . . .

My contractions started out slowly and in a couple of hours I was in full-blown labor. I stayed in the shower and let the water wash over me. I was alone and contracting, it felt so strong and wonderful. I could NOT lie down; I had to labor upright. In the meantime, our helpers were assembling an inflatable birth pool. It was odd, but wonderful: our whole family, grandma, grandpa, aunts and uncles, cousins and one great aunt, moved the entire birthday party, from its original location an hour away and set up at our house, helping to take care of our children and support my husband while I labored.

I stepped into the birth pool and let go of tension I did not know I was holding. Contractions were strong. In the room were two midwives and an assistant, my husband, my older son, my sister-in-law and my brother, my mother-in-law and one of my best friends, and they were all so quiet and respectful. The energy in the room was

*Childbirth education program that is highly committed to natural birth; see Resources.

†A tapered wooden device to amplify sound.

A relaxed, loving atmosphere was just what I needed to have such a positive and wonderful birth.

I knew I wanted to have my babies at home. We had three midwives coming to the birth, plus a friend who was a nurse, and we live five minutes from the hospital. I decided that if something so tragic or awful happened that we couldn't make it to the hospital, then we would be better off at home anyway.

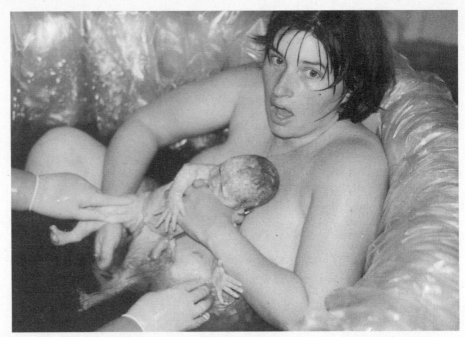

An unexpected twin on the way at this home waterbirth.

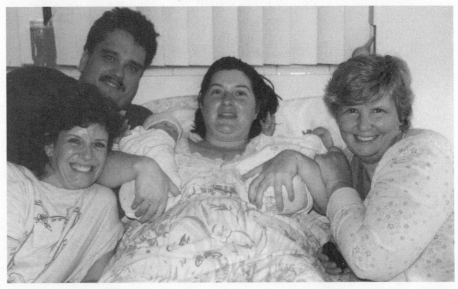

Alison cuddles her girls, surrounded by her husband and two midwives.

thick, strong and positive. One midwife encouraged me quietly to welcome my contractions, and in response to her soothing exhortations I did.

I felt my breath catch as I draped myself over the side of the pool. I began to push. It felt strangely different from my former births. When I pushed, it felt so heavy, like a strong man was leaning over me with his hands on my iliac crests, pushing with me. The baby was quickly born in the water. But it wasn't what I expected! I thought I was having a huge baby boy, but instead, I held a tiny vernix-covered pink little girl.

The midwives proceeded to cut Erin's cord. I was confused because I usually hold my babies much longer before their cord is cut. They wrapped Erin and handed her to her father . . . then my belly moved with a big waving motion . . . what an active placenta!

Have you figured it out yet?

Elizabeth was born head down, pink and perfect, 13 minutes after her co-twin Erin! They weighed 6 pounds, 8 ounces and 6 pounds, 4 ounces.

How wonderful do you think I felt?! I was a bad girl, I gained "too much" weight, I didn't take their tests, I didn't let them use ultrasound, I didn't let them do more exams than I felt necessary, I gave birth at home . . . I felt and feel POWERFUL.

I nursed twins. You don't know how the word *efficient* feels until you nurse twins, no wasted milk dripping on the other side.

I had never considered being a Bradley teacher, but that birth changed me and I must speak out to every woman and teach them how to say "NO!" louder and stronger and sooner than I did.

Nancy Sutherland, founder of Parents Centres in New Zealand, delivered two sets of twins. The first experience in the hospital led her to insist on a home delivery for the second set. After much searching, she found a midwife and also a physician to provide back-up care if required. She delivered a breech baby and a vertex baby without complications. (One of those twins is Diony Young, a renowned childbirth activist, author, and editor of the journal *Birth*.) Nancy made sure she found attendants who were old enough to have had a lot of experience and also to have worked with the Maori women so that they would appreciate and respect natural birth.

Dr. Ettinghausen delivered more than 20 sets of twins at home without mishap. Family practitioners, such as Dr. Greg White in Chicago, have attended home births for decades. His book *Emergency Childbirth*, written for firefighters and police, is an excellent guide in case twins arrive at home — planned or unplanned.

One Nevada mother delivered one of her twins — "by God and me" — in the car. The doctor had time just to roll up his sleeves to catch the other twin when the mother arrived at the hospital. In Arizona, a nine-year-old boy telephoned an emergency number when his mother went into rapid labor at home. While he followed the instructions of a dispatcher, both babies were born uneventfully.

Dr. Sorger delivered a second twin when the mother was transported from Connecticut to avoid a Caesarean! The first baby was born at home, but the mother refused to move to her local hospital after the midwife became concerned because the second twin had not descended. Instead, mother, midwife, and Twin A — against Dr. Sorger's advice — drove for several hours to Boston. Dr. Sorger met them at the hospital and ruptured the membranes. He quickly delivered Twin B who had some transient distress because of the shortest cord Dr. Sorger had ever seen — only about 6 inches!

Twins are routinely delivered at home at The Farm, a community in Tennessee. Its midwifery program has gained national and international attention for the excellent outcomes and low rates of intervention. Ina May Gaskin, chief midwife and author of *Spiritual Midwifery* and *Babies, Breastfeeding, and Bonding*, explains that the usual 7- or 8-pound weights in births at The Farm are due to the quality of nutrition and prenatal care. To date, fifteen sets of twins have been born at The Farm and only two have required transfer to the hospital. None has needed a Caesarean. Women seeking a natural birth are accepted at The Farm if they meet certain safety criteria.

The Maternity Center and its branches in El Paso, Texas, provided midwifery services for expectant mothers of twins at home or at the homelike center from its establishment in 1976 until it closed for financial reasons in 1987. The midwives had delivered more than one hundred sets of twins, with a very low rate of transfer to hospital. Many of the pregnant women were poor and high risk, and the staff at the center stressed nutrition, especially additional protein and iron.

Spontaneous Delivery of Triplets in the Hospital

Dr. Sorger assisted in the spontaneous delivery of triplets at thirty-five and a half weeks. The hospital insisted that the birth take place in the delivery room, but the staff wheeled the flexible birthing bed from the labor room so that the mother could remain in an upright position. She chose to be on her knees, embracing her husband, who in turn helped support her. With gravity assisting, each baby (all were headfirst) dropped out very easily. They all weighed between 5 and 6 pounds, and the time interval between the arrival of each triplet was about 20 minutes. The mother received no intravenous or anesthesia, and there was no tear or episiotomy.

Triplets Born at Home After a Previous Caesarean (Triplet HBAC)

This story began when Mary simply sought a natural birth after her first child was delivered by Caesarean. While the general policy held by the doctors in her small town was to allow a trial of labor for a subsequent birth, she felt that all she would have had was "hope with a very uncertain outcome."

Therefore, Mary looked for a midwife who would assist her at home. When it become apparent that "twins" were on the way, she felt it would be impossible to achieve the vaginal birth she wanted if she "plugged in to the medical establishment." Thus, she decided against an ultrasound, feeling that it would be only the beginning of a lot of medical interference. As the midwives would never have agreed to a home birth for triplets, Mary is glad that she did not have the ultrasound!

Carrying twins under the care of any of her local doctors would have meant a Caesarean at 38 weeks "to avoid uterine rupture from the uterus growing too large." Mary's midwife says:

> I agreed to help Mary and her husband do their prenatal care and see what things felt like when she got closer to term. I didn't feel right sending her off for a lot of obstetric technology she didn't want and a C-section she didn't need, so we started looking for ways to make it feel safe at home. They didn't want an ultrasound and I didn't take the possibility of more than two babies very seriously, although the father asked if I thought there could be more than two after reading *Having Twins*.

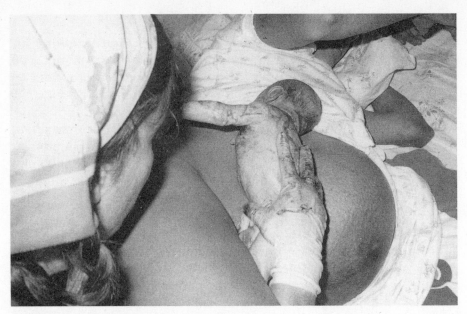

Home birth of triplets after a prior Caesarean.

Mary's husband was working in the home and available to help at the end of pregnancy. During the last few weeks, Mary rested in bed a lot of the time and was lucky to have a good friend staying with her. She helped feed Mary and provided the couple with invaluable emotional support. Eating every couple of hours, Mary took in about 200 grams of protein a day and gained nearly 70 pounds.

Two midwives took turns visiting Mary every other day to check her urine and blood pressure, which remained normal. *One week after the due date*, labor began. The first two babies were born, headfirst and uneventfully, nine minutes apart. At this point the family doctor, who had been listening to the heart rates and checking Mary's belly, said that she felt a head. The midwife reached in and felt a foot way up high, but the baby was facing Mary's front so the midwife turned her around to face the back. This breech baby was delivered ten minutes after the second. Next, with three umbilical cords dangling from her vagina, Mary pushed out the one single placenta and two fused placentas. No episiotomy was necessary, and there was only a slight tear after delivering the breech baby. The first-born was a boy of 6 1/2 pounds. The second-born was a girl who weighed 6 pounds, 14 ounces, and the third, the largest, was a girl weighing 7 pounds. The total weight of the three babies was over 20 pounds! All three babies nursed within the first hour and were entirely breast-fed for five months.

Mary had a little trouble urinating at first, as the size and stretch reflex of her bladder were diminished from months of pressure. This cleared up within a few hours after birth. For a week or so, her balance was shaky when walking because her skin and muscles were so loose that "her belly swung back and forth" when she moved! But she has three wonderful, healthy children, born without any medical intervention and for a total financial outlay of only $1,000 (although the midwives did not even ask for that much).

As midwifery services were not covered in her state by health insurance, the family practice doctor billed the insurance company. However, because there were no complications or special equipment, the insurance paid only for a single birth! This is deplorable, when no hospital birth of a singleton could be had for as little as $1,000 at that time. Perversely, inverse insurance reimbursement is yet another way to penalize natural birth. In this "triple high-risk" pregnancy — triplet, vaginal birth after previous Caesarean, home birth — the mother's competence and self-reliance should have been rewarded. She saved herself, the insurance company, and society at large hundreds of thousands of dollars in costs. In fact, Mary had a friend in her town who also had triplets but under the "care" of an obstetrician who restricted her weight gain and put her on bed rest. The babies were preterm and low birth weight, spending weeks in NICU and costing a fortune paid for by health insurance.

I believe all women should be supported in their birth choices. It is better to plan intelligently with committed caregivers than to do as one mother of twins did: she tricked a doctor into responding to her "single" delivery in a motel room because she didn't want a hospital birth!

Childbearing in Utopia (the Placebo Effect)

It would be an interesting experiment if government authorities and researchers would take a population of expectant mothers of twins and provide them with the best possible prenatal environment. In this fantasy, the women and their families would live all together in pleasant surroundings for sharing and moral support. They would be provided with the freshest, natural food of a wide variety, a pool for swimming, and classes in appropriate exercise, relaxation, meditation, and education for birth. There would be a daily massage. Midwives and doulas would take care of the women in consultation with obstetricians, so that these expectant mothers would have the support of other women, experienced in birth, through the entire labor and delivery. I know that the problems of multiples would occur less frequently in this utopia!

Steps have been made in this direction in Sweden and France, where mothers of multiples may quit work at twenty weeks on 90 percent of their pay. Both these countries have highly organized prenatal care for pregnant mothers of twins. Yet the preterm labor rate changed little. However, in France, the very preterm labor incidence was reduced with substantial savings in medical costs.

12
Caesarean Delivery of Multiples

Before looking at the use and overuse of Caesarean delivery, I will explain some nonsurgical alternatives such as instrumental delivery (forceps or vacuum extraction) and external version (turning a baby). Vaginal birth after Caesarean (VBAC) and home birth after Caesarean (HBAC) were covered in the previous chapter.

There is little evidence pointing to the best mode or type of delivery for women with a multiple pregnancy and certainly no evidence to suggest that Caesarean section should be the path to follow for mothers of twins. One limited trial found that for a second twin presenting other than as a vertex, a Caesarean was *"unlikely to be beneficial."* Rydhstrom found it was not possible in any of the Swedish twin studies of perinatal deaths, morbidity, and cerebral palsy to identify mode of delivery as a factor significantly altering the outcome. Twins delivered by Caesarean for placental abruption have a higher perinatal mortality than those delivered vaginally. In the 1990 study on triplets and higher-order births in the United Kingdom, the proportion of first-born babies needing resuscitation was lower after vaginal birth than after a Caesarean, despite the higher proportion of low-birth-weight babies that were vaginally delivered. Nevertheless, that path is well entrenched and, like the trend of increasing Caesareans worldwide, hard to reverse despite the evidence.

Many parents are not given adequate discussion and choices about the methods of birth or the types of anesthesia. The greater the intended intervention, the more they need information and explanations.

In multiple pregnancy, the two greatest contributors to mortality and morbidity are preterm birth and low birth weight — *prenatal* issues.

I did not want a Cesarean unless the babies were in danger. A sonogram revealed that they were both head down; my doctor still wanted to do a C-section, but I finally got my way.

 ## Alternatives to a Caesarean Delivery

Instrumental Delivery

In cases of headfirst babies who do not descend normally, Dr. Sorger would use forceps or vacuum extraction with the mother in the squatting position. Forceps are metal tongs that are placed on each side of the baby's head to pull him or her through the birth canal. In vacuum extraction, a suction cup is affixed to the baby's head.

The squatting position avoids problems with the mother's circulation that can occur if she lies on her back (supine hypotension) — especially with her legs in stirrups, termed the "stranded beetle" position by midwives. Squatting also takes advantage of the benefits of gravity and improved drive angle for the uterus, requiring less effort from the doctor to pull out the baby.

Instrumental delivery decreased to 7 percent in the United States in the year 2000, and Caesareans increased (23 percent).

External Version

Dr. Sorger has also externally turned several breech twins to a headfirst position — successes that have been published in two journals. With this technique, the mother lies inclined with her head lower to slide the babies out of her pelvis toward her heart. With gentle manual pressure, Dr. Sorger coaxes a breech or transverse baby to a headfirst position. Sometimes the midwife or the partner helps with another pair of hands. External version is usually done in the doctor's office, but if it fails the doctor can try again in the hospital using Terbutaline to relax the uterus. Talking the baby through this procedure is very important for a successful outcome.

Always include your babies in any discussions or procedures related to their welfare.

 ## The Caesarean Epidemic

In recent years, obstetricians have chosen Caesareans to avoid delivering difficult presentations vaginally, supposedly to make delivery less traumatic for very high- and low-birth-weight babies. This perpetuates the critical lack of experience with breech and vaginal multiple births and, of course, physicians are more likely to continue to do Caesareans when

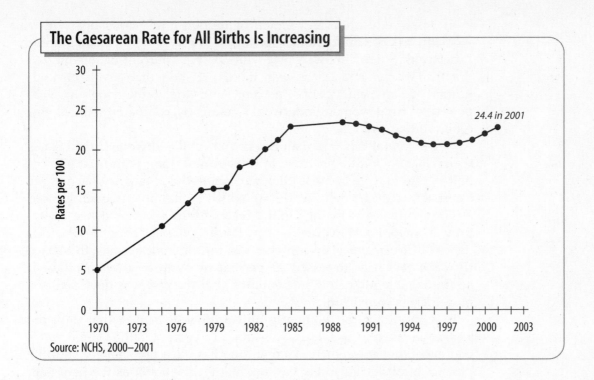

The Caesarean Rate for All Births Is Increasing

_24.4 in 2001_

Rates per 100

Source: NCHS, 2000–2001

challenged by such cases. Preterm babies do not always do better with Caesareans; it depends on how sick the mother is, too.

Almost one-quarter of pregnant women in the United States today undergo major abdominal surgery to bring their babies into the world, and an expectant mother of twins runs an extremely high risk of Caesarean delivery. In addition, in half of all multiple pregnancies one baby is breech, giving the typical obstetrician another "reason" to opt for a C-section. Mothers of supertwins are almost always scheduled for a Caesarean. In many states, courts have ordered Caeareans in individual cases, overriding the mothers' wishes.

The rate of Caesareans in the United States by the end of the year 2000 was a high 23 percent and it had increased during the prior four years. There was a 4 percent increase for first-time mothers, which "may be related to demographics and physician practice patterns," according to the NCHS. The demographics confirm this; for example, 15 percent of births in Hawaii involve a Caesarean but the incidence rises to 39 percent in Puerto Rico — islands at about the same latitude.

In Brazil, education and region of residence are associated with a woman's risk of undergoing a Caesarean. The 1996 Brazil Demographic and Health Survey showed that while only 13 percent of uneducated Brazilian women had a Caesarean, those with more than a secondary education had an incidence of 81 percent. According to the same survey, 20 percent of rural women underwent Caesareans, compared with 42 percent of urban women.

Understandable fear of malpractice suits in the litigious United States society has fueled the increase in Caesareans, along with trust in technology that may yield misleading data about the pregnancy, such as the external fetal heart monitor (EFM), which is the most frequently used obstetric apparatus in the United States (despite no evidence of improved outcome). However, in many South American countries the incidence of Caesareans is even higher and for different reasons. In Mexico City, the rate has surpassed 95 percent in some private hospitals! It began its meteoric rise in that country after the *peso* was devalued and obstetricians were losing money.

It is important for women in all countries to realize that until the 1970s, the rate for Caesareans was around 5 percent in the United States and even lower elsewhere. Women's bodies have not changed, but the practice of obstetrics surely has, and not for the better as the persistent high perinatal mortality rates show. Also alarming is the "weekend deficit" in the occurrence of birth interventions. The index refers to the ratio of the average number of births per day of the week to the average number of births per day of the year, with the base set at 100. The Sunday index for vaginal births in the year 2000 was 78, but 64 for primary Caesareans and 41 for repeat Caesareans. Clearly, doctors avoid doing deliveries and Caesareans on a Sunday! Necessary Caesareans would show an even distribution.

Indications for Caesareans

Surgery may be called for in emergencies such as fetal distress, prolapsed cord, placental abruption (preterm detachment of the placenta), or special problems known in advance such as placenta previa (in which the placenta blocks the cervical opening), active herpes infection, or transverse presentation of the first baby despite attempts at external version. Caesareans done because of the age or size of the babies are rarely justified and just add to the burden of care, financial and otherwise. Maternal conditions resulting from poor nutrition should be prevented as explained in Chapters 7 and 8.

The most common medical "reason" for a Caesarean today is a previous Caesarean. Other excuses include preterm or abnormal labor (a loose term that encompasses "uterine inertia" or "obstetrician distress," especially if an "overstretched" uterus is expected to "fail to progress"). A study in Israel found that the Caesarean rate for ART/IVF pregnancies was almost twice as high, and the only factor they noted was a nonprogressive labor during the first stage.*

Pelvic disproportion, another overdiagnosed indication for Caesareans in singleton births, rarely occurs with twins because the babies are usually smaller. However, there may be maternal indications, such as herpes, diabetes, and eclampsia. These last two are best prevented with excellent nutrition.

Many obstetricians consider a multiple pregnancy *per se* an indication for a Caesarean birth! On the other hand, numerous articles have appeared in the recent medical literature to persuade obstetricians to reconsider vaginal delivery for twins. However, Caearean delivery remains widespread for multiple births. In Aberdeen, Scotland, the rate of Caesareans for multiples, 29 percent, is not much more than the U.S. rate for *singletons*. The obstetricians in Aberdeen are clearly skilled in alternatives.

Risks of Caesareans

Risks for Babies

One quintuplet died after a Caesarean at a European hospital in 1977, and this loss cautioned the obstetricians involved. The highest-birthweight baby was the only one who did not survive, and they concluded that nature had arranged for a certain baby to engage in the pelvis and be born first — if born vaginally. However, with surgical delivery this unlucky baby was born last.

Delivery of twins by Caesarean entails risks for the babies. Respiratory distress and lower Apgar scores may result without the squeezing of the chest and lungs and other stimulation that occurs during the jour-

---

*Fetal surveillance, such as the EFM, confines a woman to bed and on her back, which gives rise to the kind of disturbances it measures!

ney through the pelvis. Either baby can suffer trauma during a Cae-sarean, especially if a breech baby is wedged in the pelvis. Parents are often unprepared for the amount of physical manipulation doctors may have to do — it is not always a simple matter of making a cut and scoop-ing out the babies.

The surgeon can accidentally nick the baby while making the incision, although this error is rare. I have two friends who were born by Cae-sarean and half a century later still carry the scar.

Riese of the Louisville Twin Study reported in 1988 that Caesareans did not offer any advantages or disadvantages for infants. The only dif-ference observed between Caesarean and non-Caesarean co-twins was that the preterm Caesarean-delivered infant was more active during sleep than the vaginally delivered co-twin, and this activity was related to temperament at 9, 18, and 24 months of age.

Risks for Mothers

Morbidity (nonfatal complications) is eight to ten times higher after a Caesarean and includes such problems as hemorrhage (blood loss is twice as much than with vaginal birth), transfusions, infection, reactions to anesthesia, decreased bowel function, and fever. Respiratory compli-cations that sometimes lead to pneumonia can develop if general anes-thesia was used.

The risk of death is less than one in 10,000 after a vaginal birth but rises to less than one in 2,500 after a Caesarean.

Mothers stay longer in the hospital after a Caesarean. Recovery from major surgery is an added burden to the mother who must return home to care for two or more babies. Although no muscles are cut and the in-cision is usually made just above the pubic hair (bikini cut), the trauma makes it more painful for your very stretched abdominal muscles to re-turn to their original length and strength, especially during the impor-tant early days.

Interview your doctor carefully about her or his usual practices. Hop-ing for the best is not enough; unnecessary Caesareans have to be ac-tively prevented. You will remember your birth experience forever; so will your babies. You want them to enter the world spontaneously. Be prepared to change physicians or hospitals and to write letters to hospi-tals, the Board of Health, politicians, and others to achieve the quality of birth you desire and deserve. Check the Internet for women who were successful in birthing naturally.

Combined Vaginal-Abdominal Delivery

Caesarean section for the second twin, after the first twin has been born vaginally, should be done only as the last resort. In rare cases, the second twin may remain too high in the abdomen to be born vaginally or the cervix may close following the first birth.

Dr. Sorger has never done a combined vaginal-abdominal delivery for any of his own mothers, but he assisted surgically in two such deliveries when he was called to help. He believes that this surgery can be avoided by prompt delivery of the second and by the obstetrician's skill and confidence in breech delivery.

Rydhstrom in Sweden observed that the increasing rates (from 0.3 percent in 1973 to 7 percent in 1984) of combined delivery are due to declining obstetrical skills and experience. In the most recent and largest study I found of 323 vertex-vertex pairs (both head down), the rate of combined delivery was 17 percent. The researchers did admit that "operator experience" could be a factor! Residents today simply are not skilled in breech delivery, if they are taught it at all. You must search for a doctor who has experience with breech presentation. More women should demand that all physicians who assume the title "obstetrician" have these manual skills.

According to The Cochrane Review, a Caesarean for the birth of a second twin in a non-headfirst presentation is associated with *increased* maternal fever and morbidity (nonfatal complications) and with *no identified improvement in neonatal outcome*. The review recommends that this policy not be adopted except within the context of further controlled trials.

Procedures for Caesarean Section

Thanks to the tireless efforts of consumers and childbirth education groups such as the International Caesarean Awareness Network (ICAN), partners are now allowed to be present during the surgery, which enhances parental attachment to the babies. In the event of complications, the mother needs the support and presence of her partner even more.

An IV is always given prior to surgery, and a blood pressure cuff is wrapped around one upper arm, because blood pressure tends to fall when regional anesthesia is used. A catheter will be inserted into your bladder. You will get an antacid for your stomach and a lead to a heart monitor. Your abdomen will be washed with an antiseptic and some of your pubic hair will be shaved.

My abdominal skin was extremely sensitive. I nearly screamed from the pain as I moved in the bed. I know other Cesarean mothers of multiples who had the same weird experience.

When my husband was allowed into the OR, there I was spread-eagled on the table, completely naked, with Betadine wash all over my belly. It looked to him like I'd been crucified. We didn't like all the people in the room either. To them it was just business, for him it was his wife and babies.

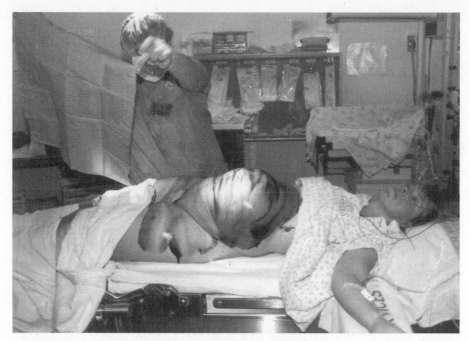

The mother is prepped with Betadine prior to Caesarean surgery.

A Caesarean is usually performed under regional anesthesia — a spinal or epidural — so that the mother is awake and can share the event with her partner. The other alternative is a general anesthetic, if there is a need for speed or the mother wishes to be "asleep." General anesthesia is used if there is some problem with the mother's backbone, such as a spinal fusion, that prevents regional anesthesia. Prior to the anesthetic gas, sodium pentothal or a similar drug is given through the IV to put you to sleep. Then a tube is placed in your throat (which is why it may be sore the next day) for the anesthetic gas. To diminish the effects of the anesthesia on the babies, the anesthesia is given as late as possible. In such cases, the presence of the father and the taking of photographs will help compensate for the mother's "absence."

Oxygen is often given to you during the delivery. Removing the babies takes only minutes. Although you will not feel pain, you will be aware of pressure and tugging sensations, especially if the babies are firmly lodged in your pelvis and take some effort to get out. If the lower twin lies transverse, a vertical (classical) incision may be made in the uterus. After the delivery, closing the uterus and abdomen can take up

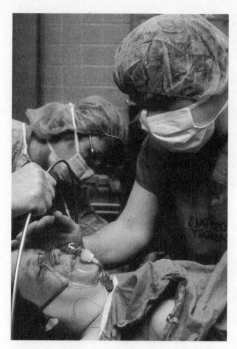

The mask is placed over the mother's nose.

to an hour. Make sure your doctor does a double layer of sutures in your uterus, because in recent times it has become quicker to do just a single layer, but this makes a future rupture more likely.

Skin sutures or staples may be used and removed up to eight days later. Dissolvable stitches are more comfortable but require more skill. Dr. Sorger never uses staples! Pitocin is added to the IV after the surgery to stimulate your uterus to contract and prevent hemorrhage.

With regional anesthesia you can fondle and nurse your babies, if they are in good condition, before the anesthesia has worn off. To ease the pain following surgery, transcutaneous electrical nerve stimulation (TENS) can be demonstrated, usually by a physical therapist. It involves a small battery-operated unit with strip electrodes that are placed on each side of your incision. Electrical currents applied to the skin travel faster to the brain than the slower sensations of pain; the effect is like scratching an itch. The increased comfort from TENS means less or no need for pain-killing narcotics, which pass into the breast milk.

For those who want narcotics, morphine can be given through the epidural catheter or through the spinal needle before it is removed. This medication gives pain relief for up to 24 hours after the surgery.

Nursing after a Caesarean is the best thing you can do, but a baby may be a little slower getting started after anesthesia. The suckling stimulates your uterus to contract so that it recovers faster, and nursing a Caesarean-delivered or preterm baby always raises a mother's self-esteem. Some women are told, even by nurses, that they can't breast-feed after a Caesarean. This is nonsense. On the contrary, you feel that even though the birth did not turn out as desired, you can fulfill this important biological function, satisfy mutual emotional needs, and boost your self-esteem.

My husband felt very left out that he was not allowed to be present, although everyone else in the hospital seemed to be.

I was not prepared for the acute pain from the incision, nor the heavy bleeding and deadening fatigue.

After the birth of my twins, it was obvious that my abdominal wall was too weak to support my spine. I felt dizzy and nauseated if I tried to stand or walk even a few steps without a binder. My doctor said no exercises for six weeks, so all I could do was wear a girdle. I know I would have gotten around much better if I had exercised.

I was very dissatisfied with the hospital treatment I received after my CS. They refused to give me any pain medication, so I never got to sleep. Once the twins arrive, the staff don't seem to care about Mother anymore. I could have used a lot more support and help trying to care for both babies after the surgery.

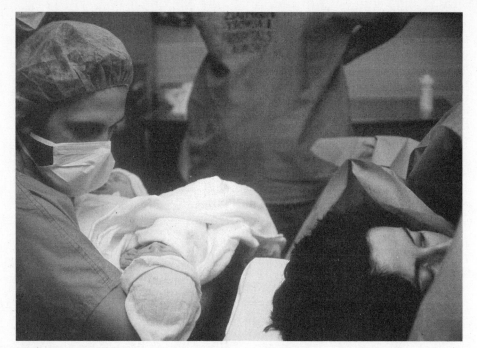

The father holds the babies while the mother is closed up.

Rooming-in is one positive way to use the extra time a post-Caesarean mother spends in the hospital. An electric bed is a necessity, not a luxury, especially for a mother of multiples. Caesarean mothers also appreciate sharing a room with another woman who has had a C-section rather than a vaginal birth.

Sibling visitation is even more necessary after the longer recuperation required by surgery and is permitted by most hospitals today.

For more information about Caesareans, see Further Reading or contact ICAN (www.ican-online.org).

Improving the Caesarean Experience

Michel Odent supervised the births of 72 sets of twins among 15,000 births while he was chief of the state hospital in Pithiviers, France. He did only six Caesareans (two of them for the second twin only), making a rate of 8.5 percent (much lower than the typical Caesarean rate for singletons).

Two more obstetricians, whom I personally know, Ronald Cole in

Texas and Bob Oliver in North Carolina, make a special effort to provide an optimal Caesarean birth experience. They protect the baby's eyes from the glare of the surgical lights and Dr. Cole plays calm music. Acknowledging that babies are highly aware, these obstetricians, or the father, explain to the baby what is happening. Dr. Oliver emphasizes how important it is to greet each baby, validating the fear and pain of being born Caesarean and to offer thanks for coming into the world.

If you know you will be having a Caesarean, you can begin right away to prepare your babies for this type of birth experience. Dr. Oliver recommends:

> Parents, especially the mother, need to describe exactly what may happen, that the babies will be surprised and maybe scared on hearing the sounds of the operating room, on feeling their mother being afraid, her body changing with effects of anesthesia. It is very important to tell the truth and not to sugar-coat what is going to happen, because babies know!

However, I must emphasize the importance of preparing for a vaginal birth. Despite plans for surgery, babies — especially multiple — can arrive quickly the normal way.*

New York psychiatrist Rima Laibow was amazed one day when her young son suddenly asked her why, when he was born, the people looking down at him had "half-faces" (wearing masks)! *Different Doorway* by Jane English explores memories of Caesareans and the effect of nonlabor birth on the developing personality.

Recovery after Caesareans

Deep breathing, "huffing" (a deep, rapid, forced outward breath quite different from a cough), and abdominal tightening, plus "bridge and twist" (page 483), are important to prevent the formation of gas. In the absence of normal intestinal movement (*peristalsis*, which temporarily ceases after the surgery), gas accumulates. This can be painful, especially around the third day. Begin deep breathing and abdominal isometrics, which substitute for the lack of peristalsis, in the recovery room.

Rehabilitation after Caesarean birth, especially for mothers of multiples, with their more distended abdominal muscles, is essential. Start

---

*There are several accounts in *Finding Our Way*, published by the Triplets, Quads & Quints Association of Canada, of women who found themselves in dire panic during an unexpected vaginal birth. They had never entertained the idea of that possibility, let alone prepared for it.

immediately and insist on seeing a physical therapist who can set up and supervise an exercise program before you go home. Those first few days are very important while muscles more easily rebound back to their former length. Although you may feel ill, depressed, and in pain, pulling your body back together is the first step. You have to take care of yourself before you can start caring for your new multiples and other children. (See Chapter 10 and the chart of exercises on page 483.) Detailed information on clearing the chest after general anesthesia or if you had a cold can be found in the chapter on Caesareans in my book *Essential Exercises for the Childbearing Year*.

13
The Feeding of Multiple Infants

Breast-Feeding

Breast-feeding is the simplest, cheapest, and most convenient way to feed babies, especially multiples. It requires no purchase, storage, refrigeration, preparation, or cleanup. Luckily we have two breasts to provide this always-available superb nutrition at the right temperature! Unbelievably, many obstetricians and perinatologists never even mention breast-feeding to mothers expecting multiples.

It is often easier to nurse multiples than a singleton, because the additional demand increases milk production. (Breast size has nothing to do with the ability to nurse, because sucking builds up the supply.)

Nursing is emotionally and physiologically satisfying for both you and your babies while providing them with the ideal food. The American Academy of Pediatrics and World Health Organization advocate breast-feeding as the most desirable method, yet it is not always well-supported by busy medical staff.

Your milk changes continuously to adapt to the infants' needs (and continues to adapt for the next couple of years). The money saved, up to $8,000 per baby per year, by not buying formula and all the related equipment can be used for household help, a diaper service, or appliances.

Nursing offers a special time to cuddle and bond with babies — only *you* can do it. This is the liberating aspect of breast-feeding; mothers who bottle-feed may find that they are serving refreshments while others enjoy giving bottles.

Doubters would say to me, "I guess you're not breast-feeding" when they saw I had twins. "Why not?" I would reply. "It's the most natural thing in the world — two babies, two breasts."

You have to take care of yourself, too, to nurse successfully. You need household help to achieve these goals.

I was told I would be too tired to breast-feed and not to bother.

I had a difficult time losing weight after my first pregnancy as I bottle-fed. So I was determined to breast-feed this time.

I regret that I never breast-fed my twins, but my doctor discouraged me.

I felt so privileged to be their sole source of food. I was essential to their survival.

Nursing twins is not the same experience as nursing a singleton, but for each baby it is just as important. And when you look down at those four little eyes and see two mouths break into milky smiles, it's worth it all!

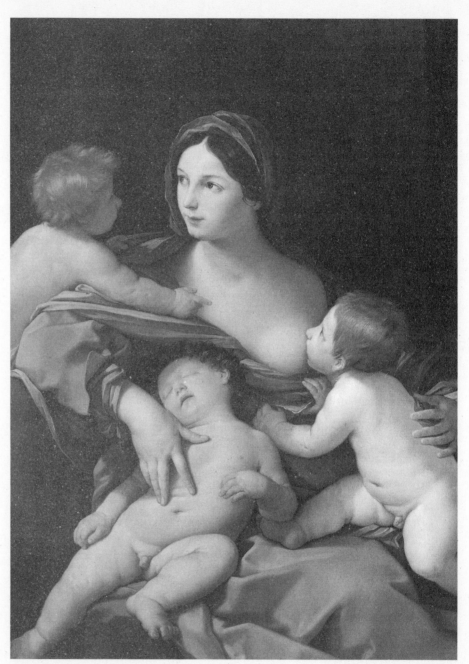

Guido Reni's famous depiction of triplets, "Charity."

Health Benefits for Breast-fed Babies

Some of the many benefits of breast milk include less indigestion and colic, enhanced immunity, fewer allergies, and better development of the palate and facial structures.

The University Medical Center in Jacksonville, Florida, listed some of the health benefits of breast-feeding versus formula.

- Breast-fed infants are three to four times *less likely* to have diarrheal diseases. Each year diarrheal disease kills more than 500 infants/children and 200,000 are hospitalized for this condition. Treatment costs range from $4 million to $10 million. Babies who consumed cow's milk were fourteen times more likely to die from diarrhea-related complications and four times more likely to die of pneumonia than were breast-fed babies.

- Breast-fed children have a 60 percent decreased risk of ear infections. By age three, one-third of all children in the United States have one or more physician visits for this problem, which costs more than $1 billion annually.

- Breast-feeding decreases the risk of respiratory infections by 80 percent.

- Breast-feeding provides a fourfold decrease in risk and severity of meningitis.

- Diabetes mellitus (Type 1) triggered by inappropriate bovine proteins (see the section on cow's milk formula) affects 120,000 children annually. Breast-feeding reduces the risk of Type 1 diabetes, especially if *only* breast milk is given during the first few months.

A 2002 update of a Cochrane Review found that professional support for breast-feeding produced a significant reduction in the risk of contracting gastrointestinal infections and eczema. In two trials with children suffering from diarrheal illness, the extra support was highly effective in increasing short-term, exclusive breast-feeding rates and reducing recurrences of diarrhea.

Infants who are breast-fed have lower rates of sudden infant death syndrome (SIDS). A baby who is suffering an allergic reaction to cow's milk protein is at greater risk from mucus in the lungs. This makes breathing difficult and for some infants deadly, especially in the pres-

The needs of the babies should be top priority, not what suits mother's needs, limitations, or lifestyle. Women have breasts so we can nurse our babies, and this must be emphasized.

ence of toxic gases that are emitted by some mattresses. Infants who died of SIDS showed responses similar to bronchial wall inflammation in asthma. In 1960 (and several times since) the British medical journal *Lancet* has reported that "Hypersensitivity to milk is implicated as a cause of sudden death in infancy."

Pumping and Freezing Breast Milk

If any of your multiples are in the NICU, they need your breast milk and if they cannot suck yet, you must pump.

Breast pumps can be bought or rented from hospital supply houses, pharmacies, medical equipment shops, lacatation consultants, and La Leche League groups, as well as some doulas and childbirth educators. Insurance often covers the cost of breast pumps, especially when ordered by your pediatrician. Before selecting any breast-feeding paraphernalia, consult the *Breastfeeding Product Guide* and the *Breastfeeding Product Guide Supplement* by Kittie Frantz (http://www.geddesproduction.com).

Hospital-grade breast pumps are necessary to initiate and maintain full breast milk production until your babies can take over. Pumping takes about the same time as nursing — eight to twelve sessions within 24 hours. It takes 10 to 20 minutes to empty the breasts. You pump less as the babies nurse more, until they are entirely breast-feeding.

You can express your milk and store it in the refrigerator for bottle-feeding, which liberates you from always having to be present for your babies to eat. The stored bottles can be used for preterm infants, outings, or when you need a rest or have to work. Remember to bring home a supply from the hospital.

Some containers are specially made for this purpose. Mother's Own Milk bags with the twisty tie tops that prop open are easy to fill and take up less space in the freezer. You can store them in a container according to date (the bags are *not* for expressing for premies because of the plastic that interferes with immunoglobulins in the milk). Mother's Milk-mate is another brand. Freeze small quantities to avoid waste.

Always have a drink at your side — a water bottle with a plastic straw so you can drink along with your babies, or a thermos of herbal tea or juice or both. A cooler is handy to have beside you with nutritious snacks and the sandwiches that your husband made for your lunch before he left for work, and maybe some of last night's left-over apple pie that was brought by a neighbor!

Antibodies in colostrum (the fluid made by your breasts before the

Breast-feeding is known to protect an infant against gastrointestinal pathogens, and epidemiological studies indicate that compared to breast-fed infants, formula-fed infants are at a greater risk of dying from sudden infant death syndrome.

— *Journal of Immunology and Medical Microbiology*, 1999

One nurse told me that the amount I had expressed was very inadequate for three babies. That made me depressed and I feel I would have continued longer if I had received more advice and support.

milk comes in, around day three) are very important for preterm infants. Providing breast milk for them is a boost to a mother's morale after the shock and disappointment of a preterm birth.

Nutrition for Nursing

Although stores of fat laid down in pregnancy provide energy for breast-feeding, lactation is a nutritional challenge that needs your continuing commitment. Around 400 extra calories *per baby* are required in addition to the daily requirements for twin pregnancy (a total daily intake of about 3,000 calories). You must continue to eat nutritious, well-balanced meals, drink plenty of fluids, and get adequate rest and relaxation. The essential fatty acids (EFAs, see Chapter 8) are very important too, as each baby will take 11 grams of EFAs daily from your breast milk.

Supply and Demand

Kittie Frantz, a pediatric nurse-practitioner in West Los Angeles and creator of many books and videos about breast-feeding, reminds us that the first year is about "trust versus mistrust" and that it was *God* who set up the breast-feeding system!

> It's the babies' job to drive the milk supply. This means even women with triplets and quads do fine. Four babies nursing = four times the milk. Among my clients, none used pumps but all had organized those around them to do cooking, cleaning, laundry and other chores.

Breast-feeding multiples works well because the supply of milk keeps up with the demand. Of course, it takes some practice in the beginning to position two babies at the same time who sometimes want different amounts of milk and who may suck differently. Some mothers prefer nursing and giving full attention to one baby at a time. Yet others feed simultaneously or alternate feeding separately and together.

Multiples may not coincide in their growth spurts and time spent nursing. A baby who sucks weakly can benefit from the let-down reflex stimulated by the co-twin nursing on the other breast. Alternate breasts so the smaller baby can have the benefit of the greater supply. This will help maintain a good supply in both breasts and gives each baby left and right visual stimulation and the chance to listen to your heartbeat, a familiar sound from the past. Alternating babies and breasts also keeps

When I was able to have more physical contact with the babies, I became more responsive and less depressed. But my depression did not really go away until I was able to nurse them all.

I was told I couldn't feed them together because then a baby-sitter will have to feed them together if I go out.

I find that I need to plan ahead for snacks so that I keep my food and water intake high. I'm back at work two days a week and I pump on those days. I have a direct relationship between the amount I eat and the amount I drink and the amount of milk that I'm able to pump. On days when I do not eat and drink as I should, I only pump about 24 ounces. However, on my best days, I pump 30 ounces. It's amazing!

I used to make lunch at breakfast time so that I never missed a meal.

I always kept a bottle of juice on the kitchen table, and every time I walked by I would pour myself a glass.

For the first six weeks, all you are really doing is feeding. I watched a mother who bottle-fed her twins and figured that she got only one extra hour off. Nursing twins means more frequent feeding at shorter intervals, but the convenience outweighs that extra hour.

My twins nursed quite differently. One sucked more vigorously. The other never needed burping.

At first I kept charts on everything, as you're supposed to. I soon dropped all of that. I just nursed my triplets when they wanted to be fed and I never had any problems. Maybe I overfed one and underfed another — but it worked out just fine.

your breasts the same size. If for any reason the milk supply in one breast is diminished, the baby who sucks more strongly can be placed on the other breast to increase milk production.

You may find it helpful to keep a record of each baby's feeding and bowel movements, or, on the other hand, you may be comfortable nursing your babies intuitively. As long as your babies have at least six wet diapers a day, they are getting enough. You will see and feel them gaining weight, usually about 4 ounces a week.

Dirty diapers vary with each baby: sometimes three or more a day, sometimes nothing for three days! It is important that the stool, if delayed, is soft and easy to pass, which is typical with breast-fed babies. (The definition of constipation is "hard stool.")

Babies soon become very efficient at sucking and can drain the breast in five minutes or so, although they often like to linger at the nipple, sinking deep into an alpha wave level of consciousness, their lips quivering with what Wilhelm Reich called oral orgasm. Mothers may experience orgasm too — nature designed nursing to be pleasurable to ensure survival of the species.*

You can be assured that your babies are feeding well if:

• there are six to eight soaking wet cloth diapers or five to six wet disposable diapers per baby in twenty-four hours during the first six weeks;

• each baby is having two to five bowel movements in twenty-four hours during the first six weeks;

• they are feeding at least 8 to 12 times a day for a duration of ten to forty minutes. Duration and number of feeding times per day will vary with each baby.

Breast milk can be stored at room temperature for about ten hours; in a refrigerator for about eight days; in the freezer compartment with a separate door for three to four months; and in a separate deep freeze for six months.

---

*However, cultural distortions of bodily pleasure, in the name of duty and the fear of incest, led to the absurd case of Denise Perrigo. Interviewed by TV personality Geraldo in 1993, she had reported pleasurable feelings during breast-feeding which led to her arrest. Despite more than one judge throwing out the case, she struggled with Social Services over the removal of her nursing child for almost a year!

Nursing Two Together

It may be easier to nurse one at a time at the beginning but when you can do two at once, the sooner you will halve the time spent feeding. If someone helps you at the outset to get two babies into position, you will be more inclined to nurse them simultaneously.

This time-saver of double-suckling increases your levels of prolactin, a hormone that facilitates milk production and the maternal emotions that accompany breast-feeding, as well as the "love hormone" oxytocin. The other breast is often letting down at the same time; thus, it is more comfortable to have them both emptied together. (Mothers of singletons have to use breast pads when the other breast leaks.)

Two babies are often hungry at the same time and ideally you feed them together. Otherwise you first nurse the one who screams louder at the fuller breast! Simultaneous feeding takes less time than demand feeding but may require waking one twin when the other awakens. The problem is that the sleeping baby may not be hungry but is encouraged to eat.

Many mothers prefer simultaneous feeding so that they can extend the time between feeding, but some prefer to let a baby sleep. You can see what works better for you and the babies, who might have quite different eating patterns. You can always nurse a baby separately for one-on-one bonding when opportunities arise.

Offer only one breast per baby, so that the foremilk and hindmilk, with the higher fat content, are both received.

Triplets are fed "on the circuit," that is, rotated on the breasts, preferably two at a time. Quads are nursed two by two and consume the same amount of time as nursing triplets.

Fathers are extremely important in providing encouragement as well as bringing the babies to you and helping with positioning, changing, and drinks.

Nursing on Demand or Schedule?

Demand feeding is regulated entirely by the infants: you feed them when they want to be fed. This is clearly the best situation from their point of view. According to the Cochrane Review, and contrary to the tradition of the "four-hour schedule," more frequent or on-demand breast-feeding is associated with fewer complications and longer duration of breast-feeding. Restricted breast-feeding was associated with increased incidence of sore nipples, engorgement, and the need to give some formula.

Breast-feeding is the only way you can hold and feed two babies simultaneously!

I enjoyed feeding the babies with one on each side of me. This way I could feed one and entertain the other. Lying on a couch or bed also enabled me to elevate my tired legs.

It's important to alternate the first baby at mealtimes, as the baby fed last usually gets more time and attention.

I am fortunate that my husband is so supportive. For the first twelve weeks, he got up with me for every nighttime feeding. He would diaper the babies, fix me a snack, and record the feeding. As hard as it was for both of us, we have somewhat fond memories of that time because we had so much opportunity to talk to each other!

My husband was very supportive. We both strongly agreed that breast milk was meant for human babies. I fed both babies at the same time since this saved time and neither twin had to wait. Seeing both satisfied simultaneously is such a pleasure.

Breast-feeding, which means a lot of close contact with each twin, is really helpful for learning to bond with each baby as an individual.

Engorgement is the major reason for discontinuing breast-feeding. Prevention is paramount. If it happens you must massage your breasts, perhaps use warm compresses, and express the milk.

No one else can provide this marvelous service to your infants except a wet-nurse. You will learn to recognize your babies' body language before they are howling. A hungry baby may turn its head (rooting), bring fingers to the face, and make sucking sounds to let you know that the milk bar is needed. Crying is a late "feeding cue."

Occasionally the babies' conditions place them on different schedules. For example, a weaker twin may need feeding every three hours while the stronger twin can wait four hours. Put a colored paper clip on your bra strap if you need to remember which breast was emptied last. Similarly you can color code your multiples' schedules to track who was fed what and when.

Positioning Multiples

There are various ways to hold babies together. Experiment with a variety of positions using pillows or special supports for nursing two together such as the NurseMate pillow, photo next page (see Resources).

The football hold is popular: the legs of each baby are directed backward under your arms while you cradle a head in each hand. This comfortable position leaves your hands free once the babies can stay attached on their own.

The babies' preferences may relate to their former life in utero. One mother reported that her son would not breast-feed if he was "under" his sister. The weight of his sister, when the mother used the cradle hold position, was something that he would not tolerate. When she switched to the football hold, which allowed each baby to be apart, he settled right down and breast-feeding went extremely well.

Another option is to position the babies so that their bodies are longitudinal, lying on each side of you on their fronts, or both lying parallel toward one side or the other. Pillows can be placed under the babies to support their heads and bodies or under your elbows. When you want to be discreet or don't have the space, put one baby on the left in the traditional position and the other on the right in the football hold. The babies' bodies can also be crossed on your lap and held in your arms.

Mothers who nurse while lying down find it very relaxing. Breast-feeding in this position is most useful for night feedings because you re-

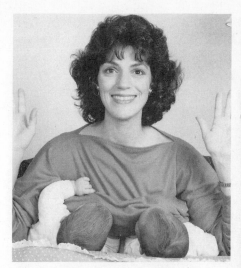

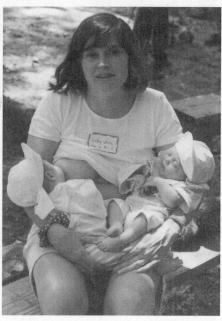

Nursing two babies at once is easier than giving bottles. The cushion ties at the back and has a zippered, removable cover. With the football hold, the mother's hands are free to burp a baby, help dress siblings, or read stories.

The cradle "V" position.

Infafeeders were a godsend for those hectic feeding times when I was alone.

The books say you are not supposed to prop their bottles, but coping on my own, propping makes a big difference.

main in bed with little disruption. If you attempt to sleep through the night in the early weeks, you may wake with engorged breasts. On the other hand, sleep deprivation can diminish the supply of breast milk, so allowing someone else to do the feeding at night can be a way to let you catch up.

Devices that prop a bottle should be used with care, as propped bottles can cause choking, ear infections, and dried milk around the neck. Of course, you have only two hands and the props come in handy, as long as you pay close attention during such occasions.

Troubleshooting

Night nursing is very important to establish and build a good milk supply. If the babies are small, they may take less at night but nurse more often. Mothers often get off to a poor start with breast-feeding because hospital staff and home-helpers feed the babies during the night rather than wake up the mother. This causes breasts to become engorged; and if the babies are satisfied with formula and have no interest in sucking,

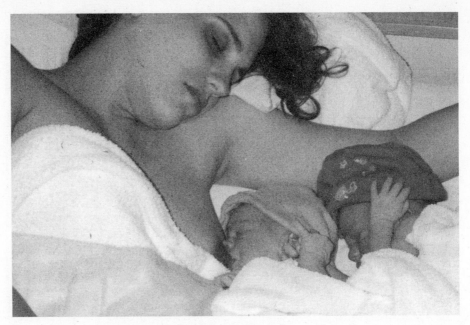

Learn to nurse lying down. One of the twins is dozing, too.

then mother's milk will have to be expressed. An engorged breast is difficult for the baby because the nipple cannot protrude adequately due to the tension of the tissues.

Milk supply is typically low at the end of the day as a result of the mother's fatigue and perhaps inadequate fluid intake. This is the time to have someone come in to tidy the house and start preparing the meal while you put your feet up and refuel.

Women who produce insufficient milk simply need to increase their fluid intake, improve their nutrition, and nurse more often. Brewer's yeast, nonalcoholic beer, and wheat germ can help, too.

Of course, breast-feeding is difficult for a mother of multiples who is single or working or poor. It is also a challenge for mothers who commute to the NICU with sick newborns and who often have other children at home as well. But these socioeconomic or logistical problems have nothing to do with the breasts' potential to produce the best food for your babies.

It is a good idea to air your nipples occasionally — sunlight is best. Vitamin E oil or lanolin helps to prevent dry skin and cracked nipples (which must have a chance to heal because nursing is too painful when cracks are present).

Tips for Nursing Challenges*

1. Herbs. Fenugreek and fennel can be found in capsules. A herbal tea recommended by Rosemary Gladstar in *Herbal Healing for Women* to enhance milk production contains milk thistle, nettle, raspberry leaf, fenugreek, and hops. These herbs can also be bought on the Internet.

2. Demand-feeding, even if it doesn't feel as if there is much milk, is important. Pay no attention to how often the babies feed.

3. Drinking too much water can be counterproductive. About 3 litres a day works well for twins.

4. Colic or reflux is different from hunger. Breast milk soothes a burning gullet and provides comfort to deal with the pain. An antacid and anti-reflux remedy can reduce the reflux until the stomach sphincter is stronger.

5. Ignore uninformed advice, however well-intended. It can exacerbate your own doubts and worries.

6. Pure lanolin and plastic breast shields help cracked, bleeding nipples within a couple of days. Air your nipples often, and in sunlight.

7. Positioning and latching techniques are critical when getting a baby both on and off the breast. (You may need to open the actual jaws with your fingers.)

8. Homeopathic remedies include *Galega Officinalis, Ricinus Communis*, and also *China*, which helps prevent exhaustion in breastfeeding.

9. Take one day at a time. It may be six weeks before breastfeeding is fully established. By this age the babies will feed less frequently, gain weight steadily, and the milk supply will be reliable.

Further advice on caring for the breasts may be found in *Nursing Your Baby* by Karen Pryor, Sheila Kitzinger's *Breastfeeding Your Baby*, and *The Womanly Art of Breastfeeding* by La Leche League.

Lactation Consultants

Despite the well-documented advantages of breast-feeding, mothers, and particularly those with multiples, require plenty of support and encouragement in the United States. In addition to ignorant remarks, jokes, and even disapproval about nursing multiples, mothers often hear con-

---

*Thanks to Connor Middelmann.

Even though I had two successful nursing experiences under my belt, nursing twins was very difficult. Even with the help of a lactation consultant, I got very sore at 3 weeks and AGAIN at 6 weeks. Unlike my older children, my twins ate every 2–3 hours in the night for 8 weeks. I'm delighted to report that (also unlike my older children who took much longer) my twins are now sleeping 10–12 hours through the night!

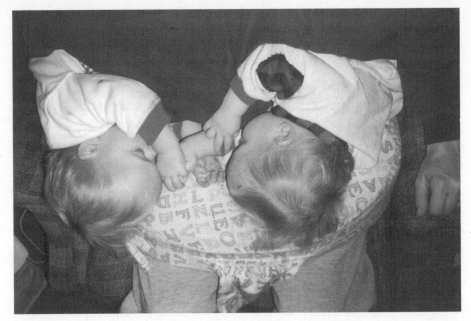

Double comfort.

flicting advice and may abandon breast-feeding at the first difficulty. Furthermore, there may be pressure to supplement with formula. Moral support is very important. *Before* you may need help, make contact with your local leader from La Leche League or with a lactation consultant.

A study showed that a lactation consultant needed to offer support to nine women in order for only one to breast-feed exclusively for just two months. Mothers who have breast-fed one baby may still need help because it can take several weeks to establish breast-feeding. Even if you nurse for just a short time it is better than not at all, but the ideal is three years.

"Many women in their 40's use IVF and reduce down to twins as their only chance of an instant family," observes a lactation consultant in Los Angeles. "They are very successful at breast-feeding if the 'fear mongers' can be kept away!" She advises against "baby nurses" often recommended by well-meaning people who believe that the mother needs this person who just "does" the babies. (These "nurses," who cost several hundred dollars a day, more than a real nurse makes in a hospital, are starting to emerge in well-to-do areas in the United States.) Often the mother is told that she can't produce enough milk without a breast

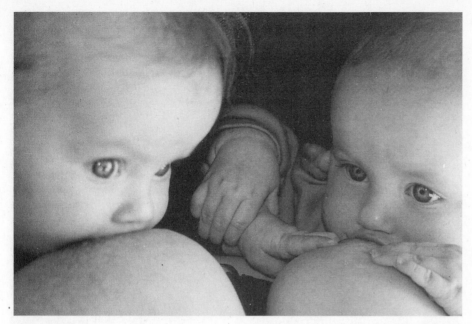

Bountiful bliss!

I called a breast-feeding counselor in tears because I felt I couldn't continue anymore. The nurse had put my babies on a strict 3–4 hour schedule and she made me pump to keep up my milk. I was always engorged and leaking and so frustrated.

pump; yet we all know mothers managed very well in the good old days! The "baby nurse" puts the babies on a schedule and offers to bottle-feed them at night so the mother can rest. As well-intentioned as this may be, it's a recipe for breast-feeding failure. Such an "expert" can disempower the mother, who feels she can do nothing right. Instead you need someone *you* can tell what to do and have it done! Someone who will help with meals, laundry, errands, whom you can ask to change one baby while you finish nursing the other. This helper should bring the babies to you at night for nursing and then change them. Some doulas offer these services as well as labor support so there is continuity of your relationship (see www.dona.com). To locate a certified lactation consultant you can contact the International Lactation Consultant Association — ilca@erols.com.

Once you find a lactation consultant in your area, call before the birth and tell her you are having multiples. Take her phone number along with you to the hospital. Lactation consultants may visit you there if you need specialized help at that time or at home. Although many hospitals do employ excellent lactation consultants, they may have time constraints and be unable to spend the amount of time a mother of multiples may need.

How else does one comfort a pre-verbal toddler, let alone two of them who are both sick or crying at once, without nursing?

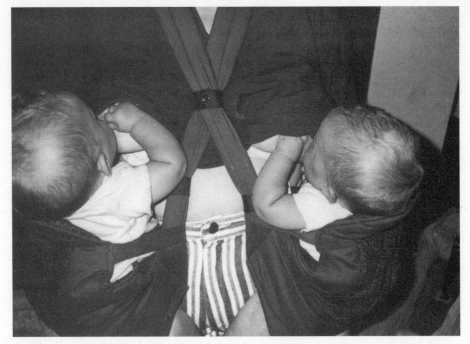

Two front carriers make a Mom mobile. The babies are upright and her hands are free.

Relactation

Amazingly, women who adopted an infant years after they gave birth, and even some women who have never been pregnant, with great persistence have produced some milk. Thus, if your milk was suppressed by medication and you now want to breast-feed, or if your babies were in the NICU and pumping was difficult, have faith. With enough motivation and support, especially from your partner, doctor, La Leche League, and other mothers who have succeeded — you can do it.

Relactation is initiated together with a feeding tube device, which can also help babies switch to the breast from the bottle. It is a plastic bag with a tube for the baby to suck. This bag can be filled with donor breast milk (preferably) or formula. The baby sucks on both your breast and the Lact-Aid tube, stimulating your milk production. As your supply builds up, you can gradually reduce the Lact-Aid fluid until it is not needed, which usually takes a couple of months. The process is faster and easier with twins because they provide double stimulation.

Weaning

One of the benefits of nursing as long as you can, up to two or three years, is that it is a wonderful comfort when the babies are sick or upset. Nature created a clever design: a baby cannot cry and suck at the same time. (Likewise if you are bitten, clamp the nose shut — to breathe the baby will have to open his or her mouth!) Also, breast milk continues to enhance their immune systems.

Your babies may wean themselves at different times, especially if they are DZ.

A 1986 survey of Mothers of Twins Clubs in the United States found that three-quarters of the mothers breast-fed their twins. But it was as high as 83 percent in the farm states of Iowa, Wisconsin, and Indiana. A 1985 Parents of Multiple Births Association survey in Canada found that half of the mothers who breast-fed did so for four or more months and 14 percent breast-fed for more than eleven months. These studies have not been repeated but I fear that with the double-income needs today fewer mothers are nursing.

Breast-feeding Substitutes

Substitutes for breast-feeding include: (1) breast milk expressed into a bottle, (2) complementary bottles of breast milk or formula to "top off" breast-feeding, and (3) supplementary bottles of breast milk or formula to replace breast-feeding.

Many articles for mothers of twins rationalize the bottle-feeding of twins to help mothers be guilt free with the decision. It would be more helpful to provide the information women need to have a successful breast-feeding experience.

Complemented Breast-feeding

The judicious use of formula or donor milk, in times of illness or extreme fatigue, can help prolong breast-feeding. If you complement breast-feeding with a bottle of breast milk or formula (up to a couple of ounces), nurse first. In the beginning, it is better to spoon-feed the substitute than to confuse the baby by switching between breast and bottle. (Babies find it easier to suck on an artificial nipple and after may reject the breast. Other babies may not like an artificial nipple at all despite the availability of different kinds.)

I breast-fed until my Cesarean wound broke down. I couldn't seem to get rid of the infection for weeks.

I found that one of the great bonuses of nursing, especially when they were toddlers, was the way it would calm them both down.

I'm a walking, talking, breathing example of a woman who successfully nursed twins, worked full time, lost 87 pounds, and lived to tell about it. My eight-month-old identical boys have only recently started to wean from the breast. I can honestly say that breast-feeding was the most relaxing, natural experience I have ever had. I nursed both using the football hold mostly.

To ease weaning, introduce the concept of taking turns with everything including nursing. Do other activities than nurse when you sit down, and look for opportunities to nurse them separately.

My doctor said that if God had meant for me to nurse triplets, I would have been given three breasts. I'm really angry that I didn't try because I have met other mothers of triplets who really enjoyed it.

When the twins were 8 months old, I decided to substitute one nursing session with a bottle of my breast milk. I felt I had the best of both worlds . . . I had the convenience of nursing, but I also had the freedom to take a break when I need it.

I breast-fed my boys until they were 3 months old. I would pump extra milk and freeze it. Also, by 8 weeks, I was giving my boys one formula feeding each night. This helped out more than I thought it would because I could ease up on the time I spent pumping. My parents did this until the boys were about 6 months old.

Supplemented Feeding

A total feeding session with a substitute for breast-feeding is called a supplement. With higher-order multiples, supplementing may be necessary because of too many babies, too little time, or health and organizational challenges.

Some mothers combine breast-feeding with breast milk given in a bottle, which allows partners and helpers to assist. This means all the babies are nourished with breast milk, if not always at the breast. Physical contact with the mother is reduced — but it is increased with the father. Mothers who supplement with bottles and wish to keep breast-feeding must do so at least eight times per 24 hours to maintain milk production.

Alternating breast and bottle may seem the perfect solution but it actually combines the disadvantages of both feeding methods.
 — **Karen Kerkhoff Gromada and Mary C. Hurlburt**

Cow's Milk Formula

Many babies have gas or colic, are fussy, and spit up if the nursing *mother* is consuming dairy products or if using a milk-based formula.

Problems with lactose and proteins in cow's milk have been linked to juvenile diabetes and more than 45 other diseases, according to the late Frank Oski, Jr., M.D., Chief of Pediatrics at Johns Hopkins Medical Center. There are at least 30 antigenic (causing allergies) primary proteins in milk, and digestion may increase the number of possible antigens to more than one hundred. Infants develop symptoms of allergic rejection to cow's milk proteins before one month of age. Most of the infants tested have two or more symptoms. About 50 to 70 percent experience rashes or other skin symptoms, 50 to 60 percent suffer from gastrointestinal symptoms, and 20 to 30 percent have respiratory symptoms. The treatment is simple: avoid cow's milk.

The American Academy of Allergy, Asthma and Immunology reports that cow's milk is the most common food allergy among children.

Cow's milk contains much higher proportions of protein and salt than breast milk does and it can strain infant kidneys. Clinical studies have shown that infants consuming cow's milk lose small amounts of blood from their digestive tracts. For this reason, the American Academy of Pediatrics recommends that infants below one year of age *avoid* cow's milk.

"We now think that iron deficiency at that age can lead to brain damage," remarked Dr. Lewis Barnes, a University of Wisconsin pediatrician.

> If you consumed only dairy products, you would have to drink 50 cups of milk to reach your RDAs for iron. If you have any doubts about this, check the nutrition label on the side of a cereal box. You will see that the iron status of the cereal increases by 1 percent or less, with the addition of $1/2$ cup of cow's milk.

An Australian study of children who developed diabetes found that children given cow's milk formula in the first three months were 52 percent more likely to develop diabetes than those not fed milk. Breast-fed infants had a 34 percent lower incidence of diabetes than formula-fed infants. In Puerto Rico less than 5 percent of mothers breast-feed their children. Instead, formula from cow's milk is used by nearly all. Meanwhile, Type I diabetes incidence in Puerto Rico is roughly ten times the rate in Cuba, where breast-feeding is nearly universal. The presence of antibodies indicates that bovine insulin might be spurring an immune system reaction against the child's own pancreatic islet cells. (Insulin regulates sugar metabolism in the body.)

Say "No!" to dairy products for you and your family.

Additional childhood afflictions which have been linked to cow's milk include asthma, rhinitis, eczema, milk-induced inflammation of the lung, stomach, and intestines, migraine headaches, Crohn's disease, and rheumatoid arthritis. Dairy products have been implicated in neonatal tetany, tonsil enlargement, and diseases later in life such as congestive heart failure, ulcerative colitis, Hodgkin's disease, attention deficit hyperactivity disorder (ADHD), and other behavioral problems.

Oski was one of the early whistle-blowers with his book *Don't Drink Your Milk*. Today Robert Cohen's books and Web site (www.notmilk.com) keep abreast of the hazards.

In the National School Lunch Program, however, milk is the only beverage that must be offered to children!

This book give facts about what is best for your babies. Many readers find this is entirely contrary to the views espoused by their health care providers but they, like the public, are victims of misinformation, politics, and advertising. Much more evidence against milk has accumulated since the previous edition of this book in which I warned readers about dairy products. Today the Internet allows readers to learn the truth for

> We are the only species that drinks another species' milk. It's a weird thing. We have not evolved to be exposed to bovine insulin protein.

themselves from such Web sites such as www.notmilk.com and www.pcrm.org.

Soy Milk Formula

Many doctors and mothers have turned to soy milk to avoid the well-documented problems with cow's milk. About 25 percent of American bottle-fed babies drink soy-based formula, which the New Zealand and Australian governments have made available only by prescription.

Parents who feed their children soy-based formula should be aware that some scientists are concerned about the estrogen-like substances in soy products, which are so helpful for women around menopause. However, the American Academy of Pediatrics is currently satisfied that no untoward effects have been observed so far.

Preparation of Formula

It is much harder to give two bottles at the same time than to give both breasts to two babies.

Arduous work is involved in purchasing and preparing formula, particularly for multiples, and the bottles take up a lot of space in the refrigerator. Also, you have to take along much more paraphernalia than your two breasts when you go out! Sometimes each twin requires a separate formula. Keeping track of who has drunk what and how much requires (color-coded) charts, which is more work than just letting them latch on to your breasts.

Formula comes in a ready-to-use or concentrated form or powder at the prices listed in the chart. Concentrate must be mixed with distilled or boiled water and any remaining mixture needs to be refrigerated.

Usually a batch is made up for at least a day or two at a time, which is less effort if everything must be sterilized. Some pediatricians consider the heat of an electric dishwasher or microwave oven adequate for sterilization. Certainly mothers discover short cuts. Most use the terminal method of sterilization, where the filled bottles (about sixteen for twins) are put together in a large pot or a couple of sterilizers for about half an hour and then left to cool. Milk is often heavily contaminated with bacteria regardless of the container. For triplets, it takes an hour and a half to prepare eighteen to twenty-one bottles for a 24-hour period.

Disposable plastic liners for bottles cut down on the soaking and cleaning involved. Special soaking solutions remove the milk residue from bottles to make for easier cleaning. Nursing kits are quick and easy, but they are expensive, as are professional formula services, which sup-

Cost Per Year of Infant Feeding

FEEDING TYPE	AMOUNT	COST PER MONTH		COST PER YEAR	
		SINGLETON	TWIN	SINGLETON	TWIN
Breast-feeding	200–500 kcal/d	$25	$38	$300	$450
Ready to feed formula	900 ounces per month, approx. 30 ounces per day of six 5-ounce feedings per 24 hours	$99 to $333	$198 to $666	$1,188 to $3,996	$2,376 to $7,992
Concentrated formula		$99 to $234	$198 to $478	$1,188 to $2,800	$2,376 to $5,600
Powdered formula		$54 to $198	$108 to $396	$648 to $2,376	$1,296 to $4,752

(Calculated by the San Diego Country Breastfeeding Coalition in 2001.)

ply everything. Remember to ask if there is a discount for multiples.

If the mother is alone and feeding the babies together, she can position them on a sofa or her lap or place them in infant seats and sit between them. One baby may be fed by hand, while the mother keeps an eye on the bottle propped for the other. When the babies can sit independently, the mother can hold a bottle in each hand. If they are not hungry at the same time, one may be content to watch and wait. A bouncer (they come in singles, doubles, or triples, with an optional toy bar) or swing chair is useful at such times.

Encouraging a mother to fix formula only adds to her outlay of money, time, and effort. Instead we should ask: How can breast-feeding be facilitated in this situation? Support for expectant and new mothers of multiples — such as home help, child care, travel assistance, and nutritional subsidies provided by health insurance — could save a lot of expense and distress, as well as providing valuable benefits for the family.

Warning: Dental Care

If you bottle-feed your infants you must take precautions to minimize future tooth decay. First, no child should go to bed with a bottle of juice or milk. This soaks the teeth and results in "nursing bottle mouth" — a typical pattern of cavities seen at four or five years of age. Similarly, pacifiers dipped in sugar or honey are harmful, however tempting it may be to quiet the multiples. Tooth decay begins between eight and twenty-

I know you are supposed to do all that sterilizing, but as a single mother and a full-time student I would rather spend my time with the twins.

four months, long before the average child is first taken to a dentist. Start a daily cleaning routine when each child gets the first tooth. A film of bacteria, called plaque, covers teeth and should be removed twice a day to ensure healthy gums and teeth. Parents of multiples may feel that this is yet another burden in their busy schedule, but it takes only a couple of minutes to wipe the gums of each child vigorously with two-inch gauze squares. This will pay off with savings in dental bills.

Introducing Solid Food

Solid food does not always improve sleeping patterns and it means work and mess. Five or six months is the earliest to begin, but you can wait longer, especially if the babies were born preterm, as more than half of multiples are. Until the second half of the first year, most food particles pass undigested through a baby's system.

Wait until the babies have some teeth, are clearly interested in food (grabbing at your plate and utensils, making sucking noises, putting fingers in the mouth), and can bring the food with their tongue to the back of the mouth to swallow. This may happen at different times for your infants.

Breast-feeding, of course, may be continued along with solid food for as long as you wish. Nurse first to maintain your supply.

The babies may differ in their solid food requirements and food allergies. Multiples, even MZs, can have different tastes and appetites. If one twin is always hungrier and asks for snacks or juice, the mother may automatically supply the other twin as well. Apart from overfeeding, this can lead to a social setback, where one child never asks for anything because the spokesperson has made the request for both.

An iron-fortified rice cereal is usually advised by American pediatricians to begin with, but other countries introduce different foods first. After the babies accept one food, strained fruits and vegetables can be added, just one or two per week to watch for allergic reactions.

When the infants gain enough balance to sit, usually at about six months, they can be placed in highchairs or portable seats that attach to the table with seat belts. Keep the chairs away from the walls and place them on sheets of newspaper (easier to throw away) or a large plastic tablecloth or shower curtain, to reduce floor washing. Have a couple of wet washcloths close by at meal times. Bibs usually have a container flap at the bottom to catch falling morsels, but the mess can spread further. I

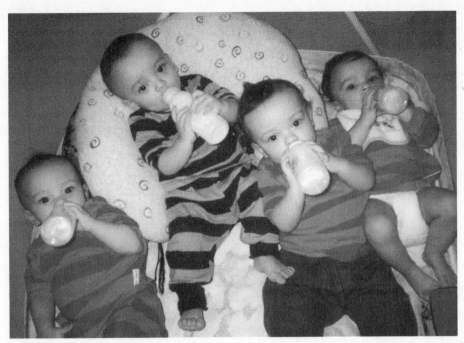

One day they will feed themselves!

sewed long "raincoats" of quick-drying nylon parka fabric that covered the neck to the feet, with long sleeves but open at the back. There was elastic in the wrists and neck, and just one quick Velcro closure at the back of the neck. This garment is quick to put on and remove and saves much laundry. Simply rinse it and let it dry over the sink. (Parents could use such a garment for themselves, too!)

Some babies will be happier dining side by side, or you can sit between them. The food doesn't fly as far if you all sit on the floor. One dish and one spoon are all that are required — for any number of multiples — until they want to feed themselves. One baby will be swallowing his or her mouthful and getting ready for more while another baby is being fed. They may play with a spoon or a toy while waiting their turn. With multiples you can be sure you won't be forcing solid food! Having to take turns inspires them to learn to eat independently.

Processed commercial baby food is the most expensive way to feed your infants. Sugar, salt, preservatives, and other chemicals are often added except in brands sold in health food stores, such as Earth's Best, which are certified organic and free from pesticides, herbicides, and in-

Introducing solid food to two babies at the same time is not always easy; and trying to persuade one that he will enjoy the vegetable puree of which he is deeply suspicious, while the other one yells for more, tests patience to the limits.
— Sally Salveson

I try to alternate where the twins sit at the table, which one is fed first or dressed first — wanting to be as fair as I can.

My babies were breast-fed prior to the meal, but they were still very hungry. Meals became a hassle as both babies demanded food yet were unable to do any self-feeding. I shoveled food into them as fast as I could using one spoon while alternating bites. Sometimes I used two spoons simultaneously! A suction cup toy on each highchair helped to distract them. An improvement was seen at eight months when they could gnaw on finger foods while I alternated spoonfuls.

I fed my twins in the bath so that the mess goes down the drain!

dustrial fertilizers. Foods can be ordered in bulk but it is easy and much more economical to prepare, in a baby grinder or blender, portions of food cooked for the rest of the family. Even easier, you can simply chew the food first and then give them a spoonful, partially digested, like the birds do! This is very convenient especially when dining out — ignore the stares of others!

When preparing food, remove the babies' portion before seasoning for the rest of the family. Vegan households should add vitamin B_{12} unless foods like tempeh are eaten. Cooking large quantities saves time. Small portions for the babies can be frozen in ice cube trays, plastic bags, or small food containers.

When the babies start to feed themselves, offer small portions in their bowls, which ideally are attached by suction to the table. If eating becomes a time for misbehavior, limit the mealtime. Removing one or more of the multiples may be necessary. Otherwise, ignore bad behavior unless it becomes unsafe. Remember to praise good behavior, something that parents easily forget, as they are preoccupied mostly with just keeping order.

Enjoy the early years when you can control their diet. It won't be long before the ubiquity of dietary junk outlets and the huge appeal of advertising and TV exert a much greater influence than you on their food choices.*

---

*Do read *Fast Food Nation* by Eric Schlosser, and *Fat Land* by Greg Critser.

14
Caring for Two or More

Taking Care of You, Too

During pregnancy your body had many months to adapt but after birth the changes take place in hours and days. The sudden loss of weight and fluid and hormonal adjustments may merge with an anticlimax that often follows an exciting and long-anticipated event. Your milk comes in around the third day after birth. All these changes on top of the arrival of two or more babies can make the most placid or experienced mother feel overwhelmed.

Many mothers of multiples find no time for rest, relaxation, or exercise. As a result, they postpone their postpartum recovery and give less and less time to their personal needs. You will benefit from rehabilitation started right after birth. Good physical condition will prevent discomfort and injury as you lift and care for your babies. It may be a long time before you sleep through the night, so you must learn relaxation skills and take rests at every opportunity (such as during breast-feeding).

Make it a priority to get out to La Leche League meetings (some are held specifically for nursing mothers of multiples) or mothers of multiples club meetings to share your concerns and feelings with others who are experiencing the same intense demands of parenting more than one baby at a time.

Postpartum Exercises

You should begin postpartum exercises the day after the birth. If you are recovering from surgery, do frequent deep breathing, abdominal tight-

Even in the hospital, the staff would ask me "How will you cope?" I would have appreciated answers more than questions!

We had to discuss how to balance our need for help with our need for privacy.

I wanted to feel that I could do it all myself, as I knew others had done. I resented the people who were helping me because I felt less competent.

When the boys were napping I would seize the free time for something spontaneous, something just for me. I knew I would never catch up with the housework, so weeding the garden or just reading a magazine would help my energy to return. I needed a break from the constancy of caring for the kids.

I wish I'd had some help. We sleep-walked through a fog of these early months and I'm sad we were not able to enjoy them.

After my quads were born, I could just pick up my abdomen, like a mountain of dough. It would just go, "blub, blub, blub" when I let go. I did frequent abdominal contractions, within a binder for support, and it was amazing how the muscles started returning to how they were before.

I was terrified of the twin skin thing the first time and now, even after five children (two sets of twins) in 4 ½ years, my abdomen is essentially back to normal!

All the new mothers of twins in our club are in awful shape. Postpartum exercise evenings are really popular because these women really need them.

Before my twins were born, I never realized how important my abdominal muscles were. I couldn't even stand up when I got off the delivery table. I was bent over at a forty-five-degree angle and my inside organs all went "slosh."

ening, and pelvic tilting with your knees bent. Pelvic floor contractions help to heal the tissues if you had an episiotomy or tear. Even if you had a Caesarean, it is important to do pelvic floor exercises to prevent incontinence and prolapse that often result from the weight of the babies on this muscular shelf during the months of pregnancy.

Your uterus will return to its normal size over the next six weeks, and breast-feeding stimulates the appropriate hormones to help. However, be prepared for quite painful contractions during the first few days if this was your second or subsequent pregnancy. After a Casesarean, which is major surgery, you may be very depleted from (sometimes heavy) bleeding, pain, and fatigue. Arranging for personal help in the hospital for the first days is a good idea.

The same exercise program is followed after the birth as before. Check your abdominal muscles and follow the instructions in Chapter 10. Progress the pelvic tilting and curl-ups as described. *First you shorten your abdominal muscles, then you strengthen them.* Do lots of isometrics — when you are on the phone or feeding a baby, remember to "pull your belly-button toward your backbone." *Hacking* — a quick light chopping movement with the outer border of your hand — helps to bring life back

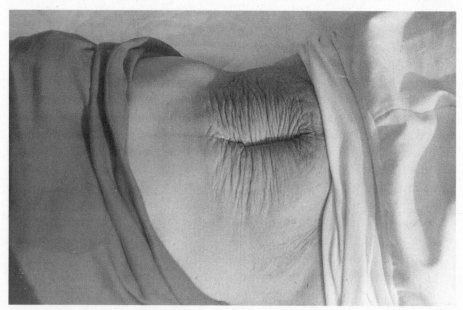

"Twinskin" will improve with abdominal shortening.

to the stretched belly. These techniques are demonstrated in my video *Baby Joy: Exercises and Activities for Parents and Newborns* (see Resources), which offers more than one hour of movement, massage, and water activities, as well as calisthenics that each parent can do with a baby. Also, you will learn how to carry a baby "by the base" to encourage head control and to spare your wrists and thumbs.

Sleeping

Prevention of Crib Death (Sudden Infant Death Syndrome — SIDS)

Crib death continues to be the most common cause of death among infants in the United States in their first year, with the risk peaking between age two and four months.

The American Academy of Pediatrics recently adopted a new policy regarding infant death occurring during sleep, and the cause of death is now identified as suffocation. The United States "Back to Sleep" campaign, which advises parents to SLEEP BABIES FACE UP, has resulted in a 38 percent relative decrease in the rate of crib death.

However, many babies still die, and many more get misshapen flattened heads from sleeping on their backs. Research published in the Journal of The American Medical Association in 2001 found that the use of a home monitor did not reduce the risk of crib death.

Denton Davis, M.D., in Colorado, reports on his web site http://www.criblife2000.com/ that:

> A breakthrough in understanding this syndrome occurred when Barry Richardson, a chemist and material preservation expert from England who has published more than 250 scientific papers, demonstrated in 1989 that fungal organisms commonly referred to as mold or mildew can produce a toxic gas from antimony. A compound of antimony was placed in baby mattress PVC as a fire retardant in the 1950s. Richardson warned that PVC mattresses containing antimony as well as phosphorus and arsenic should be considered dangerous, because fungal activity had the ability to convert these three elements into potentially toxic gases. He also advised parents that by turning a baby on his or her back the risk of exposure would be decreased. His next recommendation was for parents to isolate their babies from exposure to PVC and mildew by the use of a thick polyethylene cover.

When you are besieged on all sides with advice on how to cope with twins, it is easy to forget that what every baby needs, most of all, is a healthy mother. Extra rest and good nutrition are absolutely essential.

My abdominal muscles after the birth were unbelievable. I felt I could put my hand in and touch my backbone.

No matter how tired you are, do your postpartum exercises every day. They are really important to help you feel well and able to cope.

A New Zealand forensic scientist, Dr. Jim Sprott, had previously postulated (in 1986) that crib death was due to toxic "nerve" gases generated by fungal activity on chemicals present in the baby's crib. In New Zealand, the country that formerly had the world's highest crib death rate (2.1 deaths per 1,000 live births in 1994), the incidence has dropped to around half following nationwide publicity advising parents to wrap babies' mattresses in accordance with a specified protocol and to use bedding on top of the wrapped mattress which is not capable of this gas generation.

Since this publicity commenced in late 1994, an estimated 120,000 New Zealand babies have slept on mattresses wrapped in accordance with the protocol, and there has been no reported crib death among them. The crib death rate of the New Zealand European ethnic group has fallen by around 75 percent.

According to Dr. Sprott, who has a Ph.D. in chemistry, every step in the toxic gas theory for crib death has been proved.

The partial success of face-up sleeping in preventing crib death actually confirms the toxic gas theory. Since the gases are generated in infant bedding, a baby sleeping face up is less likely to inhale them. However, one reason why face-up sleeping is only partially preventive is that the gases can be readily absorbed through a baby's skin, especially if the skin carries traces of certain detergents.

The rising rate of crib death from one sibling to the next also confirms the toxic gas theory. If a mattress contains compounds of phosphorus, arsenic and/or antimony and certain household fungi have become established in the mattress during previous use, when the mattress is reused by another baby gas generation commences sooner and in greater volume. The crib death rate is very high among babies of solo parents, who, for economic reasons, are more likely to buy or use secondhand mattresses.

The high crib death rate among twins is not the result of being a multiple. Low birth weight and/or preterm birth increase the vulnerability of a baby to the toxic gases. Imminent risk to the surviving co-twin is posed if that twin continues to sleep on the same mattress/bedding as the twin who has died of crib death.

Mattress-wrapping must be carried out in accordance with a strict protocol. For full information contact Dr. Sprott by e-mail (sprott@ iconz.co.nz) or visit http://www.cotlife2000.co.nz/. On this website you will also find information about Dr. Sprott's book, *The Cot Death Cover-Up?*

Where Should the Babies Sleep?

You have many options: the babies can sleep in your bed, their own bed in your room, the same crib or separate cribs in another room, or in cribs in different rooms. Multiples prefer to sleep together, or with one or more siblings. A Twin and Multiple Birth Association (TAMBA) study in the United Kingdom found that 90 percent of parents chose to have their twins sleep together in the beginning, although half were sleeping apart by three months. Multiples who sleep apart from each other at home usually had done so in the hospital.

Co-sleeping reduces apneic (breath-holding) episodes that occur with babies who were born preterm. A recent Polish review found that co-bedding helps maintain temperature regulation, circadian rhythms, and feeding and sleeping patterns. Staff in many NICUs now realize that twins do better in the same isolette.

Parents usually place twins in the same crib on the solid rationale that they have already spent a long time side by side. Some parents start by putting them at opposite ends, only to find later that they are snuggled together, perhaps even sucking each other's thumbs! Other parents use one crib but divided in half with a padded board; the babies will let you know if they like that idea! There is also an L-shaped crib called Double Delight that fits in a corner.

When twins awaken, they often entertain each other, watching overhead mobiles or playing with each other's toes or fingers.

Playing recordings of heartbeats or classical or soothing music is easier than rocking the babies to sleep every night, which they can end up demanding. Sometimes a parent has to be present a few times without feeding or picking them up (which is difficult) until they learn to go back to sleep. The family bed avoids this task of "sleep training." If the sleeping patterns are chaotic, you may want to keep a chart to determine what is going on.

It is ideal when babies nap together. On difficult days, it may help to put them in the car for a drive, as the motion usually lulls them to sleep. Then the mother or father can just relax or read while parked until the babies awaken.

Co-Sleeping: Parents and Babies

From the babies' point of view, sleeping in their parents' bed provides continuity of the warmth and body contact they enjoyed before birth.

There is never any trouble getting the twins to bed. They always have each other for company.

If you don't have sleep, you can't go on.

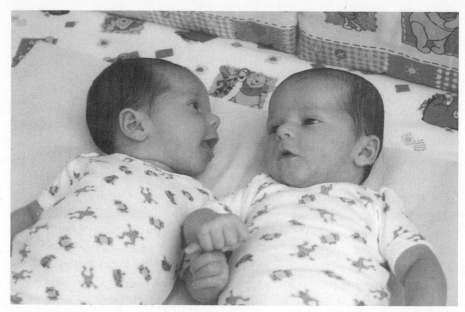

Twins shared the womb...

Co-bedding of and with twins means better settling and more sleep for everyone. Breast-feeding mothers often co-bed with their babies because they can be nursed to sleep. Jean Liedloff showed in *The Continuum Concept* how babies who feel secure in infancy become more trusting and independent later. The benefits of parents and babies sleeping together and other issues are discussed in *The Family Bed* by Tine Thevenin and *Sweet Dreams* by Paul Fleiss, M.D., and Frederick Hodges.

Newborns may take a few weeks to settle into a steady, quiet breathing rhythm. On the other hand, hearing a few snuffles from your babies beside you is very reassuring. Even with triplets and quadruplets, you can take turns between babies sleeping in pairs and those next to you. Mattresses on the floor are practical; some parents use bed rails at night.

Night Waking

The age at which an infant first starts to sleep through the night varies widely. Some twins both sleep through as early as eight weeks.

Parents understandably respond quickly to the twin who wakes up to avoid disturbing the other. A smart twin enjoys this reliable tactic to get Mother's attention! One child may want more nursing and cuddling time than the other. While you attend to the more demanding twin, your

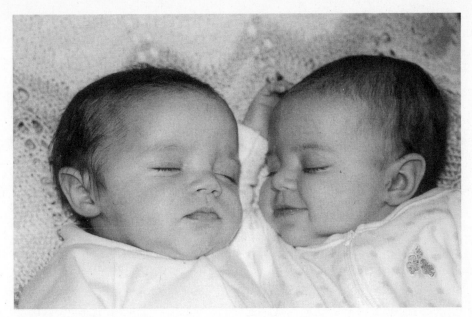

And they like to sleep together...

partner or helper can entertain or just hold the other baby and let him or her fall asleep.

Some mothers prefer to wake the babies and feed them both before the adults go to bed. Always clean up the changing area and refill your water bottle, so you are ready for next time.

Night Help

Your sleep needs must be taken care of to enable you to take care of the babies. Fathers help to bring the babies to you and to change them, but they have to go to work in the morning. Night help is thus even more important than day help, especially in the beginning. Routines with multiples for night sleeping and day naps are very necessary if you are to get any rest at all.

Bathing

The kitchen sink or laundry tub can be used for bathing babies. The height is better for adults and the surrounding sides are better for the babies than a bathtub. Some parents use bath seats attached by suction cups to the regular tub. *Always pay close attention to your babies, especially*

I used to bathe both babies each day. After all, you need only one tub of water and they seemed to sleep better.

I arranged for help with morning baths when my triplets were very young. I could then give each baby undivided attention during the bath and dressing.

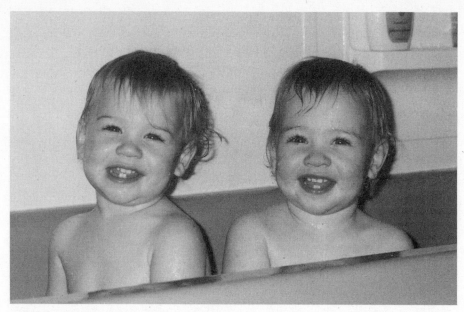

Which one did you wash already?

in a bath. Two can concoct much more mischief than one, especially by turning on hot water. Choose bath toys carefully for safety.

Many parents bathe just one baby a day and others bathe babies every couple of days. It is necessary only to wash a baby's diaper area and face regularly and to provide clean clothes. Rashes can be dried with warm air from a hairdryer.

Baths also calm restless infants. Bath time can be fun for babies and parents, especially in the water together. Support just the head as a baby floats on his or her back and wiggles with delight in the buoyant water. Babies can move in all directions in water just as they could in the uterus. The added challenge of gravity requires babies to redevelop these skills after birth; and that can take up to four months to roll from front to back, and up to six months to roll in the other direction.

Fathering/Co-Parenting Multiples

Fathers are sometimes more apprehensive in the beginning with multiples, but the admiration of others compensates. Dads who participate in the birth experience develop close bonds with the offspring sooner and today they are present even at Caesareans.

Ideally, your partner can take time off from work or go on flex-time. On the other hand, financial challenges may require that your partner take a second job, reducing assistance at home. The amount of support you anticipate from your partner is central to your coping with multiples. Partners feel lots of additional pressure after the babies arrive — to bring in more money, to help more at home, and to give loving support to the mother — despite getting no more than a few hours sleep at a time, perhaps for months.

Clubs for parents of multiples help fathers learn from other fathers about childcare and development in general, with special advice regarding twins. Multiples spend more time with fathers than do singletons. One study found that two-year-old twins considered the father the primary caretaker. First-time dads of twins are happy and proud of their complete family unit in which each adult "has a baby." During the night, Dad can be a great help bringing the babies so you can nurse without having to get out of bed, or he can give one baby a bottle too, bring you a drink, and change diapers.

Parents can exhibit wonderful teamwork as they constantly interchange multiples. For some it is intuitive, but others need to create an action plan. It's very important to make sure each parent takes turns with each baby.

Suggestions for fathers include the following:

- The more time you spend with your babies, the more confident you will be as a father. It will be easier to see them as individuals. Look after the multiples by yourself so your partner can have a break and so you understand what it is like to be alone with the whole crew.

- Be prepared for total maternal absorption in the babies for several months.

- Get together with other fathers in the same situation — join a club for parents of multiples.

- Check out the Web sites that deal with multiples (see Resources).

Grandparents

Grandparents, other relatives, and significant people can keep life as normal as possible for you and also any siblings, especially in the early months when you are so occupied with the new arrivals. Introduce your

The small size of our twins made my boyfriend nervous about handling them.

My husband used to escape out the door as soon as possible in the morning. Now the babies are such fun to watch, he doesn't want to leave for work!

I gained two children but lost my wife, and I didn't particularly like this zombie who looked like her but had no time for me or our marriage. It took me about three weeks to realize that if we were to keep our marriage intact, I'd better pitch in and be a partner. Once that brilliant thought was turned into action, I became a zombie too, but at least then we were a matched set again!

My husband took a while to get used to my neglect of him and the decrease in our domestic standards.

I could never have survived without my husband's help — especially at night. I just nursed the babies in bed and he did the fetching, cleaning, and changing.

My parents helped enormously. I know not all twin families have this option, but my mother and father had both babies overnight every Saturday. I would pump extra milk and freeze it. They picked them up around 5:00 P.M. and dropped them back around 9:00 A.M. This allowed my husband and me to get one full night of sleep a week.

Friends and neighbors gave more practical help than my family. They were always prepared to help cook or do the laundry, not just visit and coo over the babies.

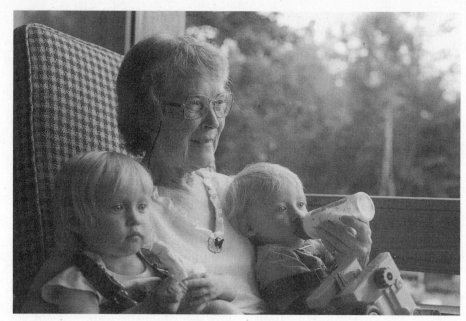

Grandparents help meet the needs of each twin.

parents to other grandparents of twins, provide them with literature, encourage them to treat the multiples as individuals — calling them by name, bringing separate gifts, and spending time with each one.

How Families and Friends Can Help

1. Provide night help.

2. Give baby clothes (at least 12-month size unless the babies were preterm) or equipment. A rocking chair, a video camera, and a cordless phone are welcome gifts for a family with multiples. They will receive more than enough stuffed animals and receiving blankets!

3. Donate a few weeks or months of diaper service.

4. Bring food such as a casserole or a whole meal.

5. Organize the neighborhood to cook a meal per day for the first three months, with assignments marked on a calendar.

6. Offer to bathe, feed, and baby-sit the multiples.

7. Offer to grocery shop and take one or more of the babies with you.

8. Help clean the house or arrange for someone else to do so.

9. Give a gift certificate to the mother for a massage, facial, exercise program, or pool or health club membership.

10. When the babies are older, invite one or more to stay overnight.

11. Invite other siblings out for treats.

12. Give the parents a weekend away.

 ## Increase Your Efficiency

Changing two or more wiggly babies can be wearing — keep a bowl of small toys near the changing area to occupy little hands and minds.

Get a large plastic trash container for used diapers. Store clean diapers and baby clothes on open shelves or in laundry baskets. Collect clutter in plastic crates until someone has time to put it where it belongs. Soak dishes in the sink until you have time to wash them or load the dishwasher.

Plan menus and make more than one meal at a time — for example, while you stir the oatmeal for breakfast, prepare the spaghetti sauce for lunch. Make double quantities of whatever you cook and freeze one. You can do all this and still keep an eye on your babies and talk on a cordless phone if you use a headset!

Twin consultant Pat Malmstrom recommends a simple chart with labeled clothespins — no need to find a pen — for tracking baths, feedings, and so on.

Patronize drive-through stores, cleaners, and banks. Even the 7-11 chain of convenience stores is testing drive-in services as I write this. Use on-line services for bill payment, ordering in bulk, and finding items for multiples.

 ## Baby-sitters

It is more difficult and expensive to find care for more than one baby and mothers of multiples predictably suffer from social isolation, more so if they have recently moved. People make irritating comments (such as "How do you manage two babies? One is almost too much for me," or "I've always wanted twins, you are so lucky!" or "My two are just eleven months apart, so I know just how you feel") which increase your feelings of isolation. You long to be with others who have experienced the intense demands of parenting more than one baby at the same time. Per-

---

The housework will always be there but your adorable babies will grow up so fast. You will never get it all done!

I prepare as much as possible early in the day, because by late afternoon my energy level is very low. The crockpot is a big help, as are two pressure cookers, and both keep the nutrients in the food.

Going out with twins often was a prolonged expedition. It was a great help to take along small snacks for me, too.

Two Yahoo groups are very helpful: Clothdiapertalk and BTL Diapering. I was paying more than $100 a month for the disposable diapers and their disposal.

haps you feel reticent about spending time with single-birth mothers since your challenging situation may seem to trivialize their concerns.

First, look for someone who is comfortable with twins or more, and whom you trust and believe could cope with the babies. You may need two baby-sitters to care for triplets or more. To help sitters, write down details of each baby's schedule and preferences.

Make arrangements with other parents of twins to take turns baby-sitting in order for each set of parents to have a break.

When one twin is sick, you may need a sitter to entertain the well infant, who may resent your diverted attention. It can be very demanding when both are sick, depending on what kind of medication* or therapy they require. If all have to see a doctor, you will need someone to help unless you can arrange a home visit.

Keep infants together if one has to be hospitalized, and it is ideal if you can stay with them, too. Otherwise the sick twin will have the double stress of a separation from mother plus co-twin. You will then need to explain what is happening, where the twin is staying, and how long it might be before they see each other again. It helps to talk like this even to infants — they understand on some level, which adults rarely appreciate.

Venturing Out and About

An Australian study found that 74 percent of mothers did not go out without the twins and 92 percent never went out alone without their partner. It is a challenge to go anywhere without another pair of arms to handle two or more babies who may all cry or want to eat at the same time.

In other countries, many mothers of multiples do not drive or do not have a car. This puts many activities out of reach, especially during inclement weather. Your mobility with two or more babies may be restricted by narrow elevators in apartment buildings and public transport.

Many mothers feel it is just too much trouble to go out in the early months despite their understandable frustration at being tied down. They would rather have people come to them. In retrospect, these same women will emphatically advise others to have a break from their babies as soon and as often as possible! It is important for your sanity, they ad-

---

*Useful herbal remedies are echinacea for colds (start at the first sign) and valerian, chamomile, or passion flower to help sleeping. See *Prescriptions for Nutritional Healing*.

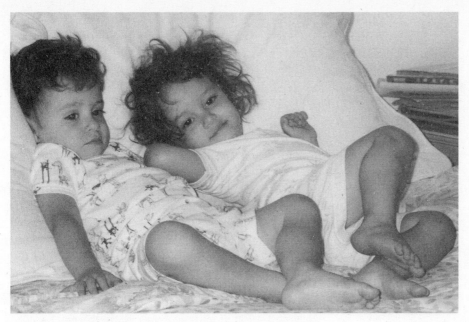

All mammals enjoy bodily contact, especially when watching TV.

I resented advice to get away from my babies. Bonding with twins takes much longer than with a singleton, and I needed all the time I could find to adequately mother each infant.

I like the attention at the mall. It makes me feel I am very special on days when I feel harried and frustrated.

vise, to get out even if just to the hairdresser or to have a quiet meal. Taking an hour away for a walk is a welcome respite.

However, parents need to take the babies out so they receive their share of fresh air and admiration. If there are older dependent siblings as well as the multiples, the best options are a minivan and drive-up windows, fortunately common in the United States. Parents of multiples should qualify to park in the handicapped spots. In Sweden there is a button with the icon of a pram on the buses and trams that alerts the driver to wait for the mother to load the strollers onto the movable ramp.

Be Prepared

Just as you want changing stations at each level or at each end of your house, you need to be "ready to go" with diapers and supplies. This means restocking the diaper bag after each trip and putting it in the car for next time. As well as packing more diapers and spare clothes than you think you will need; also pack stain spray, wipes, and a pomander of cloves and cinnamon to conceal odors. (Hang one inside your trash-can diaper pails, too.) Recycle plastic bags from the supermarket for the dirty diapers.

Many different designs of diaper bags can be carried or worn today. Backpacks and a waist pack for money and keys leave your hands free.

If you are giving bottles, take some extras in a lunch box with a cold pack just in case — errands often take longer and babies can be unpredictable.

Equipment

Your most important piece of equipment is that which makes you mobile! The right wheels help you feel more confident to get out on your own sooner and feel that finally life is returning to normal.

Babies prefer body contact and you can carry one or two babies on your body. Options include soft fabric carriers, backpacks with metal frames, and slings that can be worn in various ways. When the babies are small, two may fit in some styles of slings. Maxi Mom Double or Triple Carrier and Gemini Twin Carrier are designed especially for twins and triplets. These versatile carriers can be left on the babies while in their car seats. Maxi Mom offers twelve positions and comes with an instructional video.

Carrying anything on the back improves posture. When you transport your multiples in this way, you will feel less like a celebrity parade when you go out. This gives you a break from the curious public and helps any other siblings to feel included.

When loading the children into the car, put them all into the car first and then fasten each child into a seat. When disembarking, get your stroller out first and set it up in front of the car door. Release the seat belt and place each multiple one by one into the stroller and fasten again.

Strollers

Two or three newborns can fit in a stroller for transport and also for sleeping — inside or outside. In former times, it was considered important to let babies take their naps in a shady garden for the fresh air. Make sure you can easily lift the stroller into the car.

Check mothers of twins clubs, secondhand stores, and the Internet for used equipment. Thanks to the great increase in multiples and Web sites for them, it is easier now to find something used *when you need it*.

Side-by-side strollers are more difficult to handle and are too broad for some doors. Umbrella-type single strollers can be hooked together for twins. These are compact and portable, and they can be used singly when needed. Parents of quads have done well with a side-by-side twin

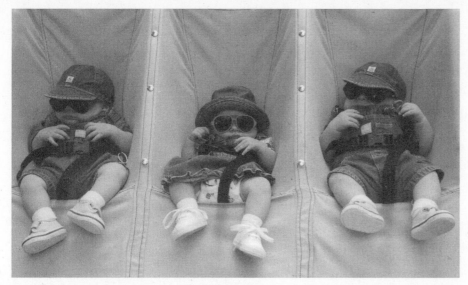

Movement helps them sleep and keeps you awake.

I found that a large single pram, with a twin at each end, was more convenient than a double pram. Separate back rests are a good idea so that one baby can sit up while the other sleeps.

We use "Sassy seats" for our ten-month-old twins. They are collapsible chairs that clamp onto the table and are held in place by the child's weight. They are cheaper and take up much less space than regular highchairs. Also our girls are very small and the chairs fit them better. They are easy to transport and have proved invaluable in restaurants since many seem to have only one highchair and we have two babies!

stroller (because two babies can fit in each seat through the toddler years). A booster seat can be attached to single strollers when the twins are toddlers.

To avoid pushing two prams or strollers, which requires another person, the ideal solution is a mobile transport specially designed for multiples. The top quality strollers like the Perego and the Runabout have excellent resale value. The Runabout has easy-to-clean molded plastic stadium seats (on an incline). Limousine strollers allow face-to-face interaction or the babies can sit in tandem. Rotate the seating arrangements as well as the toys that dangle on the rails. (More information is available in Chapter 16.)

Many parents abandon the stroller when the children loosen their seat belts and try to get out and run in different directions, but this is the time when the stroller is most useful to keep them secure. With encouragement, perseverance, and perhaps harnesses, you can continue to use this helpful equipment until they are age three or four.

Car Rides and Shopping

Beginning with the trip home from the hospital, babies should be secured in infant car seats, which is required by law almost everywhere.

Initially we put all the triplets in one carriage. Now two fit in the carriage and one of us takes the other in a backpack.

Nobody expects triplets, and people are always asking if I have twins, as the boy is a bit bigger than his sisters.

When people ask, "How do you tell them apart?" I reply, "I look at them!"

The first question people usually ask is "When did you find out you were having triplets?" Next they say, "How adorable. May I hold one?"

It didn't take long for the novelty of having quads to wear off as far as shopping is concerned. I am afraid I just push right on now to avoid time-wasting encounters with the public. People never think of quads; they always ask if I have two sets of twins.

Health care providers should routinely assume that the parents are invariably exhausted, often overwhelmed, and sometimes seriously in need of help.

As your children become more mobile, train them to accept restraints in cars (remain stationary until they buckle up). A comparison of the various types of car seats can be found at the Web sites listed in Resources.

In the supermarket, you can pull the stroller of multiples while you push the cart of groceries. Or you can put both babies in one shopping cart, lined first with a blanket, and push that cart while you fill another one with groceries. Small children can sit side by side with both legs in the space intended for one leg. Prop them up with blankets at each side if needed. Alternatively, one twin can sit strapped in an infant seat that is also buckled onto the cart while you carry the other one in a sling or back carrier. You can also put the second infant seat in the main area of the cart. If you have triplets, you can wear one on your body, or with quads, one on your front and one on the back. Some supermarkets now offer fancy carts designed for two children.

Bring some small toys to the store and tie them to the cart (or you will be busy picking them up). Once babies can stand, the carts can tip over, so pay close attention. Accidents are the leading cause of death for children. This is perhaps the time to take just one baby along and have a sitter for the rest.

If a mother use leashes for toddlers, her arms tend to be pulled in different directions! Another idea is to have a piece of colored rope with knots, or hand loops, so each child can hold on to the "tandem line."

Babies overcome people's social reserve, and you will receive comments that are naive or sarcastic as well as complimentary. Most mothers are pleased to be sociable with interested, polite people and enjoy the opportunity to feel special. Inevitably, there will be times when you resent intrusive comments.

On the other hand, you will meet accommodating strangers. One couple was getting out bottles to feed their babies in a restaurant when a couple nearby offered to feed and amuse the babies so that the parents could enjoy a peaceful meal together.

Doctor's Visits

A separate appointment should be made for each baby. The first slot of the day or after lunch is ideal. A companion is a help. Better still are home visits, more likely abroad than in the United States.

Twins Can Be a Hard Happiness

Experiencing Overload

A recent study done by Twins and Multiple Birth Association (TAMBA) in Ireland, which has the highest rate of twins in the British Isles (15 per 1,000), found that the problems faced by parents when they went home with the twins included:

- Financial strain

- Lack of government assistance (only 2 percent received any)

- Mothers not admitting that they were not coping for fear of losing the babies

- Feeling isolated in the house and finding the crying very stressful

- Demands of caring very great and not enough sleep

First-time parents are gaining skills under more difficult circumstances with multiples, although they can focus on the new arrivals without concern for any other children. Women who are already mothers can benefit, too, from guidance and support. In fact, they have had the experience of immersion in a dyadic relationship, just mother and baby, and these mothers may feel distressed because they cannot provide the exclusive attention to each multiple that they did to their singleton. This is true even of affluent families with plenty of help. Outsiders rarely comprehend the stress and distress that mothers experience relating to plural babies of the same age with the same needs.

Women who conceived with infertility treatment often develop an idealized vision of themselves as a future mother. Career women in particular may be hard on themselves when coping with multiples turns out to be much more challenging than they had anticipated. They are often the last to admit they need help because of their intense desire for pregnancy during an often years-long struggle. Now that they have their prize, they don't want to be put down for complaining.

Bringing home just one baby or dealing with an ongoing medical problem with one or both is a severe anticlimax. During pregnancy, parents typically construct an image of how their healthy robust newborns will look; and the greater the discrepancy with the reality, the more they need to grieve that lost image.

The hardest thing about twins is comforting both when both are fussy.

Twin Escalation Syndrome: That's when each one tries to outscream the other!

My best advice is to just do the best you can. No one can expect more from you. If your house is a wreck and you have sandwiches for supper, who cares?

It might be "twice as nice" when twins are older, but at first it sure is "double trouble."

Having twins was extremely stressful for the first three to four months. Between caring for the two of them I got no more than one hour of sleep at a time. I became impatient and violent and I often got confused about where I had left a baby. I came dangerously close to abusing all three of my children.

I was a preschool teacher so I was used to handling small children of the same age. But it is not something anyone learns in Parenting 101!

The ongoing fatigue and sleep deprivation, which continue for months and sometimes years, threaten a mother's mental health, unless she has good support, especially from her partner, and *plenty of home help*. Mothers who feel too tired or too busy or can't be bothered to go anywhere may be showing early signs of depression. Such mothers feel too burned out to be rational and acknowledge their own needs. A mother alone, without help, is sitting on a time bomb. The United Kingdom report *Three, Four or More* includes many stories of women who reached the breaking point before their doctors and local health services would take their plight seriously.

Marital Challenges

Expectant parents can picture the extra work of multiples and the effects on older children, but few anticipate the effects on the marital relationship. Rifts may begin in pregnancy with prenatal complications, bed rest, or anxiety about preterm delivery. After the birth, the father may have to work overtime for more income, one or more multiples may still be in the hospital, and there is no time for shared activities except baby care. These new and conflicting demands on your time can exceed your personal resources, emotionally and physically. The exhaustion and constant care of the multiples push sex aside for longer than after singleton birth. This is a phase in which the couple become parents first and foremost and spouses second.

Depression

Depression tends to come on a few weeks or months after the birth. Bringing multiples into the world is surrounded with so much attention and excitement that any "baby blues" in the beginning may hardly be noticed.

Fatigue from the job of feeding and changing multiples around the clock is the biggest contributor to postpartum depression, which if prolonged can affect the babies' development. Research by the Louisville Twin Study showed that the psychological dynamics between twins are basically the same as between any other siblings less than two years apart in age. Mothers with closely spaced children are at three times the risk for depression compared with mothers of single children. A La Trobe University Twin Study in Australia found depression to be five times more common in mothers of twins; 76 percent of mothers of twins reported being constantly exhausted compared with 8 percent of mothers of singletons.

Furthermore, mothers who experienced depression prenatally are more likely to experience it postnatally, especially if they were on bed rest. Twin consultant Pat Malmstrom calls the condition *twinshock*.

Caesarean delivery, with its medication, anesthesia, and separation from the newborns, is another contributing factor. Coping with multiples while recovering from major abdominal surgery and often commuting to be with one or more babies still in the NICU (or different hospitals) stretches any new mother's limits. False reassurance such as "you are coping marvelously" makes things even worse.

Parents of multiples are at higher risk for drug and alcohol abuse, family violence, and divorce. In Japan it was found that 10 percent of child abuse victims were multiples, ten times the rate in the general population. The abusers are mostly mothers in poor health and usually just one twin is the victim. Child abuse can be physical, verbal, or emotional, or it can simply be neglect. In the United States, child abuse is nine times more frequent in families with multiples — half the time it involves a sibling and neither of the twins. Parents Anonymous and other hotlines for times of crisis are listed in Resources.

Young people are bought up today to regard their possessions as controllable. They are sometimes affronted to discover that babies are by no means user-friendly; it is not possible to switch them off or turn the volume down, or trade them in for a different model. . . The neglect or ill-treatment of babies arouses such pity and anger it is hard to think straight about it. . . . At what point in the cycle of deprivation would it be most expedient for society to break in and concentrate more help and more resources — there is only one possible answer. At the beginning.
— Elaine Morgan, *The Descent of the Child*

We have seen that caring for two or more is too much for just two parents in the early days. The reality is that regular help is needed, starting at night in the beginning. Take the comments by new parents in this chapter very seriously, so that organizing assistance in advance becomes your top priority.

Depression was a major negative factor in my pregnancy. As a working professional, giving up my career to be on bed rest for twelve weeks and then to care for my sons was a forceful blow.

My twins were preterm and colicky. I thought I would go crazy trying to console them because they seemed to cry all the time they were awake. I would go into another room and punch pillows in frustration, screaming like they did. It made me feel better to release my, yes, resentment.

When I felt overwhelmed caring for triplets, I would stop and imagine how it would be with quads or quints. Finding things to laugh about proved a real safety valve . . . keep your sense of humor and know that "this too shall pass."

My self-esteem was critical for mothering my girls. The work was so much, so repetitive, that I kept motivated by realizing that I was coping with two babies whereas most mothers only look after one.

Many well-meaning people help with physical tasks. My husband did everything he could around the house. I had to learn to ask for emotional support. It helped so much to receive compliments and advice that was not judgmental.

15
As Multiples Grow

The first six months may seem easier when you look back to this time before the babies could crawl and throw food! During the next six to nine months they will learn to crawl and walk. While their development is fascinating to watch and you now get more sleep, multiples moving in multiple directions is your next challenge.

Twinproofing the House

Babies explore the world around them by putting everything in their mouths to taste. Breast-fed babies have strong immune systems, fortunately! Crawling multiples arouse concerns about safety. However, restraints and devices such as playpens, jump seats, and gates interfere with curiosity and development of body skills. Instead, create one big secure area for their play.

Children learn quickest if they are allowed to complete an activity; they then move on to something else. As Joseph Chilton Pearce points out, a child who is constantly stopped from taking out pots and pans, for example, will seek the experience again and again until the learning circuit in his or her brain is complete.

Remove what you can from the reach of your multiples and secure everything else. Bolt bookshelves and other furniture to the walls. Turn down the temperature of your hot water heater. Keep the telephone number of your local poison center handy. Educate your infants about "Mr. Yuk," a comic face on luminous green stickers for marking dangerous substances. Keep some ipecac in the house; it will induce vomiting if a baby has swallowed anything undesirable. (Always call the

The days are long, but the years are short.

I was so tired by the end of the day that the thought of entertaining friends was out of the question. Instead, we would invite people to brunch, which suited us much better. If we did invite guests to dinner, my husband would always get take-out Chinese food.

Most mothers of twins had better get used to not getting much sleep for a while. If you accept this, it doesn't bother you as much as if you fight it. Attitude is so important! My twins are two and a half and just started sleeping through the night.

My girls were climbing out of their cribs deliberately (not just falling out successfully) by age 15 months. I left the side down for them so they wouldn't get hurt since I was losing the battle of keeping them in, and before their second birthday, we bought twin beds.

They start out on their own every night but end up together by morning. They still sleep together in a queen bed although there have been rumblings from them that they want to have their own rooms.

poison center at your hospital first — some substances should not be regurgitated.)

 ## Bedtime

Sleeping arrangements may change as the babies become more active, and although they will sleep longer at night and start to give up one or more of the daytime naps, your sleep may still be interrupted.

Cribs can become hazardous: there are many accidents each year with babies who get stuck between the bars or between the mattress and the frame. The safest bed is a mattress on the floor.

As twins grow, each parent can read each child a different story and tuck in the child with his or her own cover and toy. Encourage relatives to take one multiple at a time for an overnight stay. (This may be useful to improve sleeping patterns.)

Later, there is the challenge of first getting them to cooperate in going to bed and then to go to sleep. It helps to have initiated good habits.

Make sure the room is empty of attractions that they can reach, especially in combination. You may want to install a barn or Dutch door, where the lower half can be locked to contain the multiples, but you can swing open the top half to check on them.

 ## Outings

Social occasions are very important for multiples, who spend so much time with each other. Unfortunately, inviting twins or triplets is daunting to parents of singletons; and as a result, multiples receive fewer invitations. People also assume that multiples have a built-in playmate and don't need the organized diversions of a single child, but separate outings and separate friends are especially necessary for multiples.

Interaction

First-time mothers of multiples sometimes want to have a singleton to enjoy the exclusivity of relating wholly to one infant. That same one-to-one interaction, the recognition of each baby mirrored by the mother, is also very important for an infant's identity and development. Parents must spend time alone with each child. This is also helpful for language development, which lags for multiples. Their mothers tend to speak less and in simpler sentences of direct requests and commands to the unit.

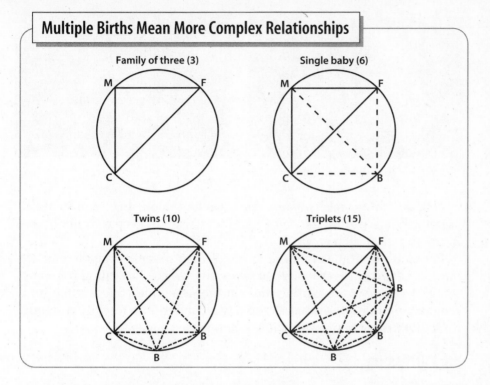

Multiple Births Mean More Complex Relationships

Family of three (3)

Single baby (6)

Twins (10)

Triplets (15)

Caring for two babies is not just doubling the workload — it is caring for three relationships. The extra one, two, three, or more family members exponentially affect the number of relationships within the family. When twins arrive, a family of three gains more than triple the relationships — for triplets it is five times as many and for quadruplets 21 times, as illustrated above. Quintuplets mean 28 new relationships, all becoming more complex as the babies individualize.

Opportunities for directing your attention to each individual include repeating the name during changing, feeding, carrying, and soothing, and routinely describing what you are doing and why.

The Importance of Play

Babies need to spend time on the floor learning to crawl, sit, and walk. Avoid walkers that can fall over. Parents may be dismayed by the mess from sand or paint spread around by the pair or group at play, but consider keeping a room just for them where they can explore, be fed, and be messy.

Make a foam mattress for a folding playpen and the twins can sleep as well as play when you are visiting.

We put up seventy-five feet of welded fencing with a locked door for $90. It's not the most attractive fencing, but it does the trick. It encloses a sandbox, swing set, children's pool, and other weather-resistant toys. We can easily remove the fencing when the triplets are older, but it's great for peace of mind now.

We found that a playpen was very confining for two babies, so we bought a Kiddy Korral, like a portable fence, which gave them a larger, safe area to play in.

I realized I couldn't wait for my days to be less hectic. I had to carve time out for myself. I had to make sure that I got out of the house, every day. These things don't just happen. I have to organize them, and until I did that, I was an emotional wreck.

I've learned to seize the moment, stop whatever I am doing, and give my full attention to the child who interrupts. When I do this, these snatches of quality time give me a chance to enjoy that one's uniqueness.

We both enjoy watching the babies play together. This must be one of the most special treats for parents of twins.

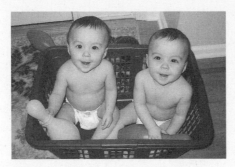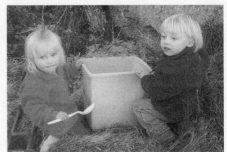

Twins always have a playmate.

A basket on wheels is handy for collecting items that accumulate all over the house during the day, or you may want to keep a clutter basket in the corner of each room.

Parenting multiples is more stressful than parenting singletons. It's hard to keep your cool when there are two voices screaming for something. If you try to discipline them at the same time, one is often grinning or giggling at the other. If you have to move both forcibly, it is more difficult to carry two crying kids than one (see pages 330–336).

Dressing

While infants do not care how they are dressed, new parents of multiples receive many identical sets of clothing as gifts. Understandably, most parents are proud of their multiples and enjoy dressing the babies alike in the early years. However, always dressing them identically (to create a unit) may suggest some ambivalence about having two babies or more. Psychologist Ricardo Ainslie makes the point that one does not outgrow one's twin, like a transitional object (security blanket, bedtime toy), and that identical dress can reinforce the transitional nature of the twin relationship. He found that 90 percent of parents dressed their twins alike, at least occasionally, as did 86 percent of DZ same-sex twins, and 70 percent of mixed-sex twins.

Identical clothing is usually associated with institutions that like to create anonymity and sameness, such as schools, hospitals, and prisons. It is also associated with "unit bonding" rather than attaching individually to the babies because the clothing allows the group to share a single, same image.

Ask yourself: Does it benefit me or my babies to emphasize their being part of a set?

Dizygotic twins may look very similar at an early age and some parents may want to treat them as if they were MZ. Such parents feel that unless the twins are dressed identically, their twinship will not be obvious. They may also have some ambivalence about relating to them individually. Multiples appearing as a team also draw attention to the parents and make them feel special. However, because individuals in Western cultures do not usually dress identically and parents usually do not dress siblings alike, this spectacle makes the other children in the family feel out of place. In fact, siblings may demand to be clothed like the multiples to share some of the attention! Some parents even create father-son, mother-daughter outfits to wear with mixed-sex twins.

Matching outfits are fine to commemorate special occasions or for photographs, but dress children differently for everyday activities.

Be sure to dress children differently in situations where you want to be sure other people can tell them apart.

Dressing twins alike is not without its problems, even for those parents who fancy the idea. If one half of a set of clothing is stained, torn, or lost, the entire combination is no longer complete. Matching sets invite more scrutiny. Twins themselves can be fussy, noticing the slightest blemish that can lead to conflict. A psychological imbalance may develop when one twin demands the perfect item and the other accepts damaged goods. It is less interesting to sew duplicate garments from the same fabric, although this economizes on patterns and leftover fabric.

On the plus side for different outfits, remnants are usually cheaper and insufficient in quantity to make two outfits. Sale items can rarely be found in duplicates. Secondhand clothing in sets is available only through multiples' organizations. Stores do not always have identical garments in the right size. Both DZ and MZ twins can differ in height and weight, and they grow out of their clothes at different ages. Furthermore, as they get older they may not always agree on the outfit of the day. Twin children become annoyed when they are mistaken for the other and welcome having different clothes and hairstyles.

Parents who plan to select different clothing frequently complain that it is easier to grab two or more of the same from rows of identical gar-

Treating twins as unique individuals does not depend so much on how they are dressed but rather on how closely the parents have bonded with each baby.

My twins choose their own clothes and sometimes will quite independently select the same outfit. I'm not going to start a fight just to get them to look different.

Dressing the twins in the same outfits has a great advantage in a crowd or at a busy playground — it is easier to spot them.

I think parents of twins have a difficult time in the beginning when they try to become attached to more than one baby. Dressing the babies alike can help the parents bond with the unit. Later, it becomes easier to discover each twin as an individual.

One day I was feeling ready to throw the twins at the wall. I couldn't stand their non-stop crying. Instead, I dressed them alike (which I never did) and took them out in the stroller. I needed the admiring looks and comments to help me feel I had taken on a big job and was doing OK.

In that first six months to a year of their lives, I saw more bare bottoms and open mouths than I did of any personality traits, so the idea of favorites was pretty ludicrous.

— Sheryl McInnes

I was so relieved to learn at our twins club meeting that I was not the only mother who felt more for one twin than the other. We all agreed that by expressing this we were able to make a conscious effort to get closer to the other child.

My husband and I take turns to take one of the twins out individually once a week.

I often feel furious when someone says, "Oh, how easy it must be because twins keep each other company." Parents push themselves to the limit to give their best to the huge demand for time and attention.

It is hard for parents of twins not to compare them and make comparisons with the "average" baby in the books as well as with friends' babies.

We encourage everyone to use the twins' names or to refer to "your brother" or "your sister" rather than "your twin."

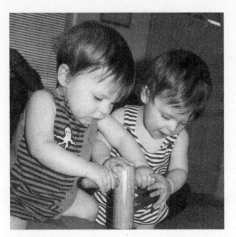

Two can figure things out more easily than one.

ments. One solution is to buy different colors. Of course, twins can wear identical outfits at different times or coordinate colors.

Dressing alike is great fun on occasion but should stop when the children take an interest in choosing their own clothes (and they will enjoy dressing alike sometimes). Not only does this clarify that establishing individuality at an early age is more important than twinship, but different dress enables teachers, classmates, babysitters, and relatives to identify each twin without confusion. It is important in an emergency to know their separate identities in order to ensure that both are safe.

 ## The Balancing Act

Some parents harbor guilt feelings from giving unequal attention to the babies, neglecting other family members, or showing preferences or disappointment. They may be overprotective toward a twin who was sick.

Eye contact is very important; in fact, the more visually responsive twin typically gets more attention. The other may need more input from you to respond. The primary caregiver needs to be aware that individual attention in the first few months influences the development of the babies' vocabulary later on.

Attention deficit hyperactivity disorder (ADHD) is more common in multiples, a condition that may be aggravated by the fact that parents constantly shift their attention to the different members of the set, so as not to favor one. On the other hand, intense one-on-one time may overstimulate a baby as parents compensate for their inability to give undivided attention to all.

Every mother does her best, though in hindsight, it may never measure up to her ideal. You deserve to be understood and supported while you parent your multiples as best you can. There is no such thing as the perfect mother! When auditing the time spent with each baby,

Karen Kerkhoff Gromada, author of *Mothering Multiples* and editor of the former periodical *DoubleTalk*, advises: "Think — if these children were a year apart, would I be so worried about treating them exactly the same at all times?" Instead, individually praise or reward each child for their own differing achievements.

 ## Toilet Learning

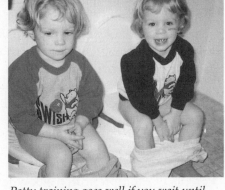

Potty training goes well if you wait until they are ready.

Children reach sufficient neurological development to control bowel and bladder function after at least 18 months. Before that time, lucky breaks may occur, or more often it is the parents who become trained. Multiples may be slower than singletons in learning control — they may be about two years of age before they are interested. Experiment just a few times in the beginning, starting with the one who seems ready. If they don't catch on, postpone it for another month or so.

A child will give some signs to indicate that he or she is ready. This often happens when you notice that fewer diapers need to be changed during the day or the child is dry after a nap or even overnight.

Some parents start with the bowel movements if the toddler has a dirty diaper at a regular time.

Obtain two potties or one potty and one toilet seat; sharing is not practical during this transition. Small plastic jars around the house are handy for boys. Baby Bjorn's "little potty" is deeply molded to support an infant in a sitting position, even as young as four to six weeks, and is used by mothers who wish to do less diapering.

There is a Web site for parents who are learning "elimination communication" (EC) based on the fact that African mothers, for example, who do not have the option of using diapers, can sense when their children need to eliminate. This is very important when the babies are carried on the mother's body! You can go to http://groups.yahoo.com/group/eliminationcommunication, or http://www.committed.to/ec, or consult the book *Diaper Free: The Gentle Wisdom of Natural Infant Hygiene* by Ingrid Bauer.

Treat each child as if that were the only one — that is to say she (the mother) will be trying to find the differences between each infant from the moment of birth.
— Donald Winnicott

I think a lot of parents are so zealous about how to treat the twins. They look so hard for problems that they often create the problems they find. When you grow a plant, you give it light and water, but you let it be a plant.

I always felt guilty because I couldn't give two children as much love and attention as one. My pediatrician made me feel a lot better when he said that public attention would make up for it.

Treat your children as the individuals they are. Give them what they need, whether their needs are the same or different.
— Pat Malmstrom

We heard our young twins name-calling, and one of them said, "I can't even call you ugly — you look just like me!"

It is important to accept and understand emotions if kids are going to learn safe and healthy ways to express them.

Parenting obliges you to set limits and enforce consequences.

Children, as great imitators, learn more quickly when they can observe adults or, in the case of multiples, each other. Multiples may not be ready at the same time but they have the advantage of peer approval and motivation. After one has led the way, the others are usually quick to follow. Your job is to praise success and help your children be comfortable around the bathroom and new equipment.

The Snug-To-Fit diaper, with Velcro closures, fits infants weighing 8 to 30 pounds and can double as training pants because a child can pull them up or down.

Sharing and Squabbling

Parents of multiples often ask whether discipline for all or neither is appropriate when a culprit will not confess or when one or more insists that the mischief involved teamwork. Punishing both is unfair and leads to bad feelings on the part of the other.

Punishment should never involve sending a child to bed or depriving the child of food (except treats). Reprimand the multiples individually in private. *How to Talk So Kids Will Listen and Listen So Kids Will Talk* explains that punishment only breeds resentment and loss of self-esteem. The authors suggest more creative alternatives to show children that behavior has consequences in life.

It is the parents' job to discipline their children. Each family will create its own rules in response to situations that arise with their multiples. Here are a few general tips:

- Lower your voice. Even animals put their tails between their legs if you whisper your disapproval! Children may temporarily enjoy an angry outburst from parents; it gives them a sense of power, but that may also lead to feeling out of control if limits are not set.

- Stop the stroller if they stand up and wait until they are seated. Stop the car until they buckle up, or sit quietly as if you have plenty of time to wait. They will soon get bored with causing delays.

- Discuss matters only when everyone is calm and playground voices have returned to normal. It helps to acknowledge the feelings: "I can see that you are frustrated because . . . BUT we use words not fists to . . ." You want them to learn how to communicate and resolve their differences.

- Identify problem *behavior* only. Assume that the child knows better and can modify his or her actions. Separate *feelings* (encourage their full expression) from *actions* (that must remain within the bounds of safety). Arguments will diminish when a parent owns his or her own feelings, for example: "I feel upset when I see you hitting your sister." As the children grow, stay out of their disputes, intervening only for safety; in such cases, take care of the victim and deal later with the aggressor. Children quickly learn that they can attract parental attention for bad behavior, often more easily than for good behavior. It is thus important to remember to praise the peaceful times and pleasant interactions. That is a challenge for parents of multiples who are so busy just keeping order.

In Great Britain, thanks to the pioneering efforts of pediatrician Elizabeth Bryan, there are clinics for multiples, where parents can take twins who, for example, are biting each other. Others can seek advice in chat rooms on the Internet and from parents in their local multiples clubs.

The ability of twins to amuse themselves is one of their great advantages from the parents' point of view. Of course, there are times when biting and fighting can overwhelm the most patient parent. One family found a taste of vinegar was the right medicine! A few minutes of time out — with a timer — is effective. Time out is usually given as a minute per year of age: five minutes for a five-year-old. Persistence is necessary if the child is kicking and screaming. One mother told how she would tie the door shut, because it helped her to "react to the behavior rather than reacting to the reaction to the punishment." Another good suggestion, when it is safe to do so, is to give *yourself* time out instead of the troublemakers.

Shouting and spanking show that the adult has lost control and is resorting to unfair stronger physical power.

Providing several duplicate toys, especially in the early years, makes life easier for the parents. If twins were squabbling over the red racing car, then peace can reign if you can produce another one. Even the same color may be demanded!

Twins learn to share and take turns earlier and more easily than singletons do; they already shared the womb. However, like all children, they learn to share their possessions gradually. Once a child has devel-

I used to feel that discipline was some kind of universal truth that parents are supposed to know and I never felt I knew it.

Some days my husband would come home and find me sitting in the playpen, alone, crying, while the babies crawled around the room. I'd explain, "This is the only place where they can't attack me."

Discipline is the name given to rules parents make to help their children stay out of trouble while the children learn how to keep themselves out of trouble.
— Judith O. Hooper

Children would rather be praised than punished but punished rather than ignored.

I used to say to my children when they misbehaved in public, in an audible voice so they knew the people around would hear, "You have just put me in the position of making sure you learn that this behavior does not work."

Our twins each have their own cake and invite their own friends and sit at opposite ends of the table.

I already had a set of twins so they found it quite normal when two more babies arrived!

We came up with the idea of letting each child choose a Saturday morning activity in turn.

oped a sense of ownership and understands the concept of "mine," the next level is learning how to share and exchange. It helps for each multiple to have his or her own clothes and toys labeled with his or her name, in a separate place. (Many twins are often able to distinguish their identical toys such as stuffed animals by smell.) Multiples need toys that promote cooperative play — jigsaws, Legos, seesaw, balls, games — as well as individual coloring books, pull toys, and building blocks. With the exception of hammers and other "weapons," encourage them to choose their own toys, pets, and hobbies.

Parents of multiples know that sharing one gift creates difficulties. Multiples are understandably disappointed when they receive one item for the set or identical gifts at Christmas or on birthdays. Visitors and caregivers should relate to each child individually, by name, spend some one-on-one time, and give separate gifts and cards. Similarly, multiples themselves prefer to give separate gifts and cards.

Birthdays

Some parents choose to celebrate birthdays on different days for each child, alternating the actual birthday each year. Other parents give back-to-back parties or celebrate one birthday a week later, so that each multiple will feel special. Sending out separate invitations and taking a photo of each twin with his or her separate cake is the way singletons celebrate. The solution of one father of twins was one large cake with two halves decorated differently with its own set of candles. Sometimes multiples have different birthdays if they were born around midnight. A birth on New Year's Eve may put twins' birthdays in different years.

Separation and Independence

Multiples may have infrequent opportunities to be alone and learn self-sufficiency. Rarely do they get a chance to benefit from solitude to develop greater self-awareness. Parents may feel that the babies need to be together or that it is onerous to organize separate outings. However, experience with adult twins who function poorly because of their co-dependence indicates that separations are important. If you start when they are young with short visits, then adjustments to preschool and kindergarten will be much easier. (See Chapter 18.)

One-on-one outings relieve the frustration parents feel about having to divide their time and attention. This enhances bonding and the enjoyment of each individual whether the outing is with a parent, sibling, or grandparent. The babies begin to experience being on their own and having their uniqueness reinforced.

As you organize life in your home, make sure the children from an early age learn to help. Encourage them to do what they can accomplish, such as putting dirty clothes in a hamper, hanging up towels, bringing dishes to the sink, putting shoes away, and feeding animals.

Taking Advantage of Discounts

Twins and triplets infrequently qualify for discounts or freebies because they are less novel these days. It is always worth asking, however, and checking with the clubs for multiples. Donations and discounts for quadruplets and more are discussed in the next chapter.

Returning to Work

In the United States, unpaid maternity leave of a mere 12 weeks is ridiculously inadequate. The job outside the home is the priority in that patriarchal system, and at stake is the welfare of the next generation. In Scandinavia and Europe, paid maternity or parental leave can be as long as 18 months! Portugal has one extra month of leave for twins and for breast-feeding mothers. When multiples arrive and no additional leave is granted, the babies miss out, having to share their mother for what is already a very short period of time.

Women with careers (apart from raising multiples) may be anxious to resume them again soon. Other mothers are not ready to do so, but financially they may have to return to work, particularly to hold on to their job.

A home-based business may work very well, but some mothers need to get out of the house. One mother of twins started a used toy and equipment business. I have helped families replace their outside incomes by working from home for a company that provides home metabolic testing and customized supplements (contact info@elizabethnoble.com).

Further help on raising multiples can be found in the many publications for parents of multiples and Web sites, as well as books such as *The Art of Parenting Twins* by Patricia Malmstrom and *The Joy of Raising Twins* by Pamela Novotny. *Mothering Twins* relates the personal stories of five mothers.

Three of everything: bottles; food; diapers; prams; car seats; wipes; shoes; toys. How can these costs be shared?

These are first children (and last!) so there are no seconds to pass on.

Why should our children be disadvantaged for all having the same birth date? Multiples means multiple everything — including cost.

Don't be discouraged by people who say, "You poor thing" or "I'm glad it's you and not me." Later, your ego will be boosted when they exclaim, "I don't know how you manage so well!"

Haircuts were the only thing I ever recall where I got two for the price of one. And the barber made me promise not to tell any other mothers of twins.

Sleepless nights worrying over money can last much longer than the sleepless nights with babies.

No one chooses to have a multiple family and although we love our children, the cost is frightening and childcare demands prevent my return to work.

16
Having Supertwins:
Triplets, Quads, and More

As we have seen, a vast increase in the birth rate of higher-order multiples began in the late 1970s as a result of fertility treatments. About three-quarters of supertwins result from assisted conceptions. Between 1971 and 1998 in the United States, there was an increase of about 80 percent for twins, 500 percent for triplets, and over 100 percent for quads compared to a 10 percent increase for births in general.

In the United Kingdom until 1992, only 22 percent of supertwins were the result of ART, but for the years 1999 and 2000, 65 percent resulted from IVF. These higher-order multiples accounted for 18 percent of low-birth-weight babies and 44 percent of very-low-birth-weight babies in the United Kingdom. Most of the infertility treatment in the United Kingdom takes place in the private sector; thus, those providing the services do not confront the costly consequences for the National Health Service for the bearing and raising of the multiples. In the United States, infertility specialists are not necessarily the doctors furnishing prenatal care and deliveries.

According to the U.S. Centers for Disease Control (CDC), one-third of the increase in triplet births can be attributed to a shift upward in maternal age, but the remaining two-thirds are due to increased use of ART. Although multiple birth survival rates have improved more rapidly than for singletons, the CDC also noted that, compared with infants born in single deliveries, triplets have twelve times the risk of dying within the first year of life.

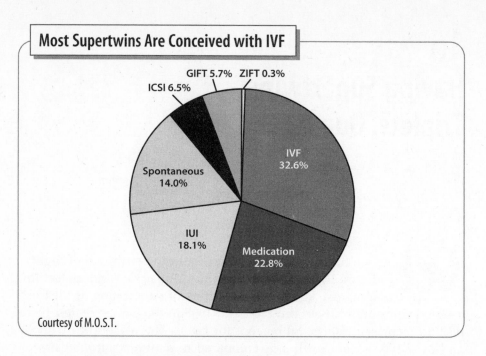

Most Supertwins Are Conceived with IVF

GIFT 5.7% ZIFT 0.3%
ICSI 6.5%
IVF 32.6%
Spontaneous 14.0%
IUI 18.1%
Medication 22.8%

Courtesy of M.O.S.T.

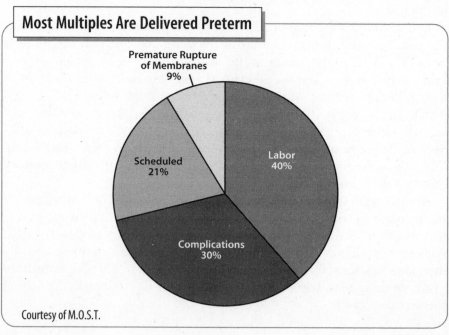

Most Multiples Are Delivered Preterm

Premature Rupture of Membranes 9%
Scheduled 21%
Labor 40%
Complications 30%

Courtesy of M.O.S.T.

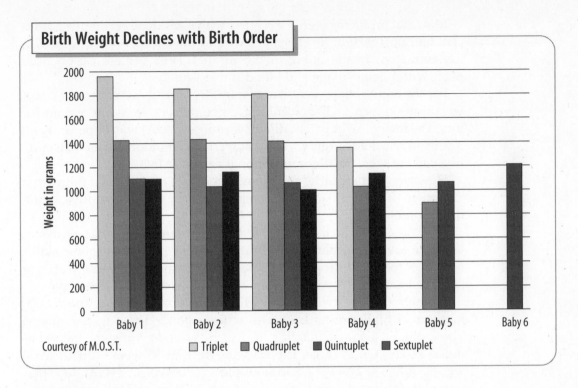

Birth Weight Declines with Birth Order

Weight in grams

Baby 1 Baby 2 Baby 3 Baby 4 Baby 5 Baby 6

Courtesy of M.O.S.T. ☐ Triplet ▨ Quadruplet ▨ Quintuplet ■ Sextuplet

Outcomes

A February 2001 study by Yudin et al. in Canada involving 150 sets of triplets, 14 sets of quads, and one set of quintuplets showed that little has changed for supertwins since the previous edition of this book. More than three-quarters of the conceptions resulted from ART, 85 percent required at least one hospital admission prior to delivery, and 98 percent of the mothers were placed on bed rest at home or in the hospital. Preterm labor occurred in 68 percent and preterm rupture of the membranes in 31 percent. Preeclampsia or pregnancy-induced hypertension was reported in 17 percent, 8 percent had anemia, and 4 percent had a cervical suture. Eighty-eight percent had a Caesarean; of those, 15 percent had the operation because of "maternal discomfort." However, in 17 percent of the triplet pregnancies, all babies were delivered vaginally. The average gestational age was thirty-one weeks. Stillbirth accounted for 31 percent of the deaths. With 89 percent of fetuses and 91 percent of live births surviving, the perinatal mortality rate was 108 per 1,000.

Maternal problems were associated with Caesarean section — 12 percent had postpartum fever, sepsis, wound infections, and endometritis (inflammation of the lining of the uterus). Four percent experienced postpartum hemorrhage and blood transfusions.

For the babies, 40 percent had respiratory distress syndrome and surfactant was given to 37 percent. Fifty-five percent were put on ventilators. The incidence of patent ductus arteriosis (PDA) was 11 percent and 3 percent required surgery.* The rest were given Indomethacin. Twenty-five percent were small for gestational age (SGA).

However, 90 percent of the infants were free of deficits at follow-up. The other 10 percent had either cerebral palsy or visual, cognitive, or auditory problems.

As always, maturity was the key factor. For infants born at 28 weeks or later the severe morbidity (cerebral palsy and deficits in motor skills) was 13 percent but dropped to 9 percent if born at thirty-one weeks or later. At less than 28 weeks gestation the incidence was 44 percent.

Mothers of Supertwins (M.O.S.T.) summarized the data from 1,000 mothers of higher-order multiples who responded to a questionnaire. The mothers' average weight gain was 51 pounds, but some gained as much as 110. On average, triplets were born at 33 weeks, quads at 31 weeks, quints at 29 weeks, and sextuplets at 30 weeks. Seventy-four percent of the mothers were hospitalized at least once, and the average time when that occurred was at 25 weeks. Half the admissions were for preterm labor.

Barbara Luke's study of babies born before they reached 30 weeks showed no substantial differences in birth weights, length of stay, or financial costs between twins and higher-order multiples. After 30 weeks, however, the average birth weight of both triplets and quads fell behind those of twins. Compared to twins she found:

- Average birth weights were 28 percent lower for triplets and 45 percent lower for quads.

- A newborn's time in the hospital was 86 percent higher for triplets and 279 percent higher for quads.

*PDA is an open communication remaining between the aorta and the main artery to the lung. This normally closes at birth to allow external breathing.

- Costs related to the birth averaged 287 percent higher for triplets and 418 percent higher for quads.

- Quads gained the least weight per two-week period.

Costs for hospitalization decreased, of course, the later they were born. Forty percent of the quads were born before 30 weeks and 80 percent of the mothers had used ART and were first-timers. The average weight gain for these mothers of quads was 1.24 pounds per week, not nearly enough for a full-term pregnancy.

Preterm rupture of the membranes (PROM) occurred in 40 percent of the cases with quads (compared with 19 percent for triplets and 17 percent for twins). In contrast, John Elliott, M.D., reported in 1994 that there had not been a single case of PROM in 15 sets of quadruplets that he delivered. Furthermore, there was not a single case in 71 supertwin pregnancies reviewed by Collins and Bleyl. As always, we must look at the women who do *not* have a certain complication and find out what they did for prevention.

Quadruplets were delivered vaginally at home until 1957, when the first Caesarean quadruplets were delivered in England. In 1938, a set of quadruplets, all breech, was delivered vaginally in England. (Although their birth weights ranged from 1,445 to 1,815 grams, all but one died from breathing difficulties postpartum.)

◉ Who Has Supertwins?

Influences on the natural occurrence of supertwins are similar to those for twins, as discussed in Chapter 3, but the high number of assisted conceptions confuses the data. For example, in Europe today the lowest rate of triplets occurs in Poland and the highest in the Netherlands.

There have been some exceptions to the general rules concerning the conception of multiples: Japan has the lowest twinning rate in the world but the highest rate of identical triplets and quadruplets reported outside Nigeria. In central India between 1960 and 1965, the frequency of triplets was as high as 1 in 880 births, but the rate declined in the 1980s to 1 in 1,700, which is still higher than the rate in Indian cities (1 in 4,000). There is much we do not yet understand about the conception of multiples.

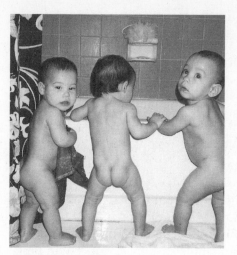

Triple the fun at bathtime.

Triplets

Older women are two to three times more likely to produce triplets. In 1975, the incidence in the United States was a mere 5.3 percent, but it rose by 1999 to 22.8 percent for women aged 30 to 39. In both 1999 and 2000, the rate was 144 per 100,000. Based on maternal age alone (excluding ART and OI), the rate should have been about 49 per 100,000. Triplets born at less than 28 weeks gestation have a higher mortality rate than comparable singletons, but triplets born at 28 to 36 weeks had comparable or better outcomes than singletons of similar gestation. The average age of triplets at birth is 32 weeks, but they do best between 34 and 36 weeks. Their average birth weight is 3 pounds, 12 ounces or 1.8 kilograms.

Zygosity

Triplets can be three "fraternals," which are called trizygotic (from three different eggs), or a "pair and a spare," which are monozygotic (two identical, from one egg) and one singleton. (Boklage suggests the possibility of the extra triplet being half of a MZ twin pair whose other member vanished in early pregnancy.) Among naturally conceived triplets, about half are DZ, one-quarter are MZ, and the other quarter are TZ but a lot more are TZ after ovulation induction.

Of the group studied in The Triplet Connection's survey, 6 percent were MZ, 28 percent were TZ, and 66 percent were singleton plus MZ. One boy and two girls were the most frequent combination. More triplets are born in April and May than in any other months. Weight gain and increasing maternal age were associated with a longer duration of pregnancy and higher infant birth weight.

Always keep in mind that many mothers have carried triplets uneventfully (and formerly unknowingly) to a good maturity and birth weight and delivered without medical intervention, even at home. Mary (see Chapter 11) went to 41 weeks and had her triplets at home after a prior Caesarean! These events were described in the chapter on labor and birth to reassure mothers of twins that if triplets can be born normally, surely twins can be, too!

 ## Prenatal Care

The diagnosis of triplets and higher-order multiples is rarely missed with the extensive use and increasing sophistication of ultrasound technology. Yet, occasionally one baby has overshadowed another and an extra appeared at birth!

Although some obstetricians may never deliver triplets, quads, or more, make sure you have a physician who at least has experience with the natural childbirth of twins. For quadruplets or more you will probably be referred to a perinatologist who practices in a high-risk hospital (Level III) with a neonatal intensive care unit (NICU). This avoids a transfer to another hospital if any of the babies require specialized nursery care.

Look for a doctor who is committed to a vaginal birth, because most triplets are delivered by Caesarean today, although this has not been shown to improve outcome. Remember that supertwins are smaller and thus fit easily through the pelvis.

If you visit the NICU during your pregnancy and take a Caesarean birth class, this will reinforce your commitment to eat well, rest often, and visualize the birth of healthy babies *naturally*. Recovering from major abdominal surgery is an ordeal in addition to the burden of taking care of three or more babies. I repeat, surgical delivery has *not* improved outcome.

Nutrition, Hydration, Weight Gain, and Education

The cardinal rules for a healthy pregnancy are even more important for the challenge of supertwins. *Nutrition is the single most important factor in outcome* and, fortunately, something over which you have complete control. Mothers expecting triplets need to eat for four and mothers of quads need to eat for five. Barbara Luke recommends 4,000 calories and 200 extra grams of protein per day for triplets. Mothers of triplets should gain at least 60–70 pounds. If you are carrying quadruplets, you need 4,500 calories and 225 grams of protein daily. Eating this much is certainly difficult, especially since there is less room inside your stomach because of crowding from your uterus. Decreased levels of activity mean less appetite too. Yet what you eat builds your babies!

> My doctor did an ultrasound and remarked: "They're stacked in there like cord wood, with no room to turn!"

Eat like a horse and drink like a
whale.
— Janet Bleyl,
The Triplet Connection

Pre-pregnancy weight is significant, and many mothers of higher
multiples are below normal weight at conception (which also plays a
role in conception difficulties that may have led to the hormonal treatments that resulted in a supertwin pregnancy). The evidence is quite
clear: mothers who had the larger, healthier babies and carried them
longer gained at least 50–75 pounds and had better nutrition than mothers who had smaller, less healthy babies. Responses (more than 10,000)
to a medical questionnaire sent by The Triplet Connection indicated
that, with rare exceptions, mothers of supertwins who gained less than
35 pounds delivered very preterm babies.

A newspaper article in 1997 reported the birth of quadruplets at Valley Hospital, New York. The mother, Annette Sherman, determined to
hold out longer than Bobbi McCaughey who gave birth to the Iowa septuplets, reduced her activity to avert early labor. Toward the end, she
walked only from the bed to the bathroom. *Her doctor encouraged her to
watch her weight, and she gained just 30 pounds* (italics mine). No wonder
the babies weighed between 3 and 4 pounds and had to spend at least a
month in the NICU.

This is one time in your life when you have the best possible reason
to gain weight. You will lose most of it quickly after the birth, especially
by breast-feeding.

One expectant mother of triplets was hospitalized for observation because she had achieved an (excellent) gain of 50 pounds by thirty weeks.
She was recommended to go on a restrictive diet, but she had educated
herself about good nutrition and threatened to sue!

A nurse working in a doctor's office in North Dakota was in the habit
of walking two miles each day when her triplets were detected. Her
doctor ordered bed rest from the sixth month, but she refused and kept
walking, even up to a mile a day at term. Her healthy 7-pound triplets
were born uneventfully and were the smartest kids in their class at age
six. Of course, she had the advantage of prior conditioning, but the
point I make is that you can have super success with supertwins.

It is up to the expectant parents of supertwins to be highly informed
and to educate others, even health care providers who generally know
little about nutrition and often eat poorly themselves.

Eating small amounts constantly makes the task of maintaining good
nutrition and good weight gain easier and also helps keep energy levels
consistent. Remind yourself every day how much your babies need food
to grow. Keep nibbling nutritious snacks and drinking smoothies,

whether hungry or not. Many mothers of multiples have said with remorse "If I'd known then what I know now, I'd have made myself eat more."

Adequate fluids are also essential, up to 20 glasses per day depending on individual factors such as climate and activity level, to maintain an adequate blood volume to prevent preterm labor.

Getting Off Your Feet

Rest is extremely important. The greater hormonal changes in the first trimester make you very tired, and in the last two trimesters the extra weight and pressure bring even more fatigue. However, lying flat with larger multiples can be uncomfortable, and mothers find it nearly impossible to stay in one position for long. Recliners, adjustable chairs, sofas with arm rests, or electric hospital beds may be better than a bed. An overhead pull bar is a great help,* and a firm wedge is needed to support your overextended belly when you lie on your side.

The topic of routine bed rest is covered in Chapter 19. It does not prolong pregnancy or improve outcome for singletons or twins. Itzkowic, as long ago as 1979, found that bed rest also was of no value in prolonging triplet pregnancies.

Being "put on bed rest" is a sentence that has been tried for almost a century with no proven benefit and continues to be prescribed out of fear and lack of alternatives. If it did any good, and the Cochrane Review showed that it can actually be harmful, the obstetric outcomes would not remain so consistently bad. The preterm labor rate and incidence of low-birth-weight babies have increased with each edition of my book! Only *pediatric* rescue has improved the outcome of those babies who are born too soon and too small.

Mothers with good outcomes do not spend weeks or months of their pregnancies in bed. In cases where a cerclage is in place, your cervix has been stitched closed and bed rest makes no sense. Of course, if a baby's foot is hanging out of your cervix or you are bleeding or have other acute symptoms, you will then need to be hospitalized.

Comfort Measures

Use cocoa butter, vitamin E, or any vegetable or nut oil for the itching and often painful stretching of abdominal skin. My favorite is cold-

With my first child, I felt these intermittent tightenings, but I didn't notice them with my triplets. With supertwins, contractions are contractions and more than four an hour is scary.

*Make sure you bend your knees and exhale when changing position.

pressed castor oil. Brushing the skin with a loofah helps remove dead layers of cells and makes it easier for your skin to get rid of waste products.

Regular massage helps mobilize the extra fluid and relieve muscle strain. All of us, expectant mothers of supertwins most of all, should enjoy a weekly massage. There are even practitioners who specialize in massage for pregnancy.

Aquatics

A swimming program should not only be routine for mothers of multiples but ideally should be covered by health insurance. In water, you will experience only one-tenth of your body weight. This relaxation is extremely beneficial for an "irritable uterus" and can diminish or stop preterm contractions. This pleasurable exercise demands very little effort, yet it reduces swelling and maintains healthy joints, muscles, and cardiovascular system. Hospitalized expectant mothers should seek a daily float with exercise in the physical therapy department, if hydrotherapy pools are available, even if the mother has to be transported in a wheelchair. Today many hospitals are installing large whirlpool baths in the labor suites, which you could ask to use. Even though you cannot swim in them, the pressure of the water reduces swelling and you can do stationary exercises.

Reducing Exertion

Ultrasound exams tend to be long and rigorous with three or more babies. Make sure that you lie on your side for ultrasound scans to avoid a drop in blood pressure that can occur if you lie a while flat on your back.

Heavy lifting and impact aerobics (running, jumping) make no sense if you are carrying supertwins. But a worse strain physically is a job requiring you to stand for eight or more hours a day. Ask your doctor to write a prescription for disability at 20 to 22 weeks. In France, the preterm labor rate has dropped to 4.5 percent now that expectant mothers can take leave from work at 24 weeks.

Preterm Labor

Janet Bleyl of The Triplet Connection has had contact with more than 19,000 families plus 2,000 more expectant parents each year. She found that very few had been able to detect (painless) preterm labor contractions and recommends home monitoring. She cautions that if doctors wait until the mother reports contractions, by then it may be too late. Some women will begin to have contractions from 18 weeks, and it is important to stop contractions before the cervix starts to dilate. Bleyl recommends home monitors made by Tokos Medical Corporation or HealthDyne Perinatal Services (see Resources). These organizations will also help you find a home monitoring nurse near you who can explain home monitoring in detail and advise you about health insurance coverage.

Although no benefits of monitoring contractions at home have been proven for twins, home uterine activity monitors (HUAM) have helped mothers expecting supertwins. Furthermore, home monitoring should give mothers freedom from strict bed rest, although they are often prescribed together.

Bleyl recommends that home monitoring be done twice a day beginning at 20 weeks and that biophysical profiles should start at 32 weeks and continue twice weekly after that, even if labor has been controlled. (See Chapter 19 for more details on home monitoring.) Many stillborns occur after 35 weeks, perhaps as a result of a placenta that can no longer function adequately from poor nutrition.

Caesarean Section for All Supertwins?

In these days of almost inevitable Caesarean sections for supertwins, we must remember the 1988 study by Thiery, Derom, and colleagues in Belgium. They reported an 81 percent vaginal delivery rate for 16 triplet and higher-order deliveries. Sixty-eight percent of the infants were born before the thirty-sixth week. The perinatal and neonatal mortality rates for infants weighing at least 1,000 grams (2 pounds, 3 ounces) and born after 28 weeks were 7 percent and 3 percent, respectively. Caesarean section resulted in *more* complications for the mother compared with those who delivered vaginally. The authors doubted that the outcome for the babies could have been markedly improved by performing more Caesareans and time has proved them right.

Some other countries have a lower Caesarean rate for supertwins than the United States does for singletons, but Caesarean rates are rising almost everywhere. A recent study in England and Wales reported a Caesarean rate of 80 percent for quads and 72 percent for triplets if the mothers had

Many people think vaginal delivery of multiples is too risky or downright negligent. I was very encouraged by the chapter on "Supertwins" and I went on to deliver my triplets vaginally at 34 weeks. My boys were healthy but did stay in NICU for a month, and Noble's info prepared me.

I found it hard to ask for help. I know it was silly, because I like to help people, but I felt so overwhelmed that asking for others to do things for me somehow made it feel worse. It's okay to say that things are not fine and that you are not coping and that you desperately need help. If you ever felt like a squeaking wheel needing grease, now is the time to speak up loud and clear.

The needs of higher-order multiples test relationships, commitments, priorities.

I didn't feel like those three little babies were mine; instead I felt like I was watching three tiny strangers struggling for their lives, but feeling no maternal instinct whatever. I've come to understand since then that it is normal for parents of critically ill newborns to delay bonding — a barrier against the possible pain of their loss. Nevertheless, it is upsetting and difficult to experience that vacuum of feeling for babies you've waited so long to love.

They looked like little red aliens or skinned chickens. The heads seemed huge and the veins were popping out of their shriveled skin.

conceived with medical intervention. For those women who conceived their supertwins naturally, the Caesarean rates were lower — 67 percent for quads and 59 percent for triplets! There is always an unexplained higher Caesarean rate when technology has been used, perhaps from an attitude that the babies are "premium babies" (are not *all* babies premium babies?) and doctors who put the babies inside prefer to bring them out.

Coping Postpartum: Organize Help, Help, and More Help

Along with the rewarding smiles and joyful experiences of raising supertwins is the daunting reality of providing for their physical and emotional needs around the clock. In addition, the needs of any other children, mountains of laundry, food preparation, cleaning, and shopping pile up. The birth of multiples changes the family's living standard and can drag middle-class families down to near poverty. The loss of the mother's income is an added financial strain, and the father may need to work extra jobs to pay the bills (frequently wishing he could be helping more at home).

Some mothers of supertwins end up with a baby at home, one in a local hospital to gain weight, and one or more in a distant NICU waiting to mature. Commuting, which can involve two or three hours a day, has to be squeezed in between feeding schedules that are both frequent and time-consuming. Janet Bleyl's story is laudable. Already the mother of six when her triplets were born at 29 weeks, she and her husband drove 120 miles round-trip *daily for nine weeks*. "We often returned home at 2 or 3 in the morning, exhausted, sometimes exhilarated at the progress we saw, sometimes devastated at the setbacks," she writes in her insightful article *When Bonding Is Delayed*. "Motherhood does arrive, albeit if late, even when babies are preterm," she writes. I would add "especially when preterm."

Multiply Blessed but Multiply Stressed

In a study conducted at Antoine Beclère Hospital in France, 14 mothers of triplets said they felt that having multiples was a source of psychological stress. Almost half of them did not have adequate help, which is a serious problem because the mother's reaction to the triplets depends greatly on how she perceives her support. The mother needs mothering to mother successfully.

A longitudinal study of 11 mothers of triplets reported in *Fertility and*

Sterility found that four were taking medication for depression, and as a group they appeared fatigued and distressed.

A mother of quads in Illinois drowned herself five days after their birth. She was being treated for postpartum depression. *No* postpartum mother, especially one with a history of depression, and certainly no mother of supertwins, should be alone with that possibility of self-destruction. Household help may have prevented that tragedy; now the father is raising four babies without their mother.

Unfortunately, few insurance companies are willing to pay for home help. A letter from the obstetrician may substantiate the amount that can be saved on hospitalization and intensive medical care. (Parents and maternity care professionals need to lobby for these benefits as do multiples clubs and organizations.) Home help should include housework and meal preparation during pregnancy and after birth, as well as an assistant on duty from 7:00 P.M. to 7:00 A.M. postpartum. Domiciliary nursing postpartum can mean earlier discharge home for babies who need monitoring, oxygen, and other special care. This helps to bring all the infants home as soon as possible, saves traveling time and costs, and enables the mother to bond sooner with all her babies.

Mothers need even more help after complications or a Caesarean delivery. Recovering from surgery interferes with a mother's direct contact with her babies in the NICU, and she may have other children at home, too. The mother needs peace and quiet to breast-feed and bond with the multiples while someone else takes care of the rest of the family and household chores.

Set up a schedule for postpartum help when offers begin to come in during pregnancy, and choose someone to organize continuity for the first year at a minimum. Most people would rather help others than ask for help themselves, but mothers of supertwins invariably wish they had let themselves ask for and receive more help. As Karen Gromada, author of *Mothering Multiples*, said, "Never deprive another person of the chance to do a good deed!" The challenge is to find reliable volunteers or paid help who will show up as arranged and coordinate with the demanding activities such as meals and baths and bedtime. The level of help required, at night as well as day, is more than volunteers can be expected to provide unless it is divided among several committed people. The mother is also not in a position to supervise the helpers; therefore, a specific person should coordinate them. It's handy if one friend assumes the job of scheduling other friends for cleaning, meals, baby-sitting,

I just wanted to be a normal mother with one baby and be able to go to the grocery store unaccosted. Instead I am known as "the mother of triplets."

With helpers taking over so much of the care of my four babies, I felt they really didn't need me — their mother — as long as there was someone to feed, change, and console them.

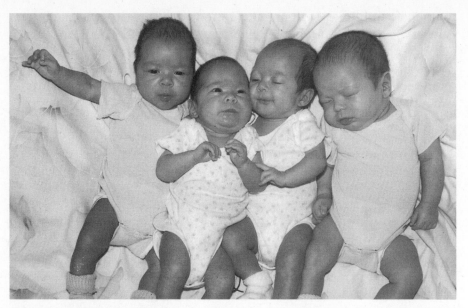

Four happy faces to start the day.

bathing the babies, and so forth. This kind of gesture is worth more to the parents than expensive gifts.

Civic help is not forthcoming today as in the past. The parents of the St. Neot quadruplets born in England in 1935 were provided with four nurses from the Great Ormond Street Hospital gratis for six months (the four babies were born at home). Their doctor allowed them to move from their small house to live in his home! Later, with money raised by the townspeople and fees paid for publicity and viewing them in their prams, the family was able to buy a larger house.

Mr. Morlok was unemployed at the time of birth of his spontaneously conceived MZ quads (1930). He was given a rent-free modest house by the city of Lansing but no personal physician or nurse. The Badgett quads (born in 1942) eventually moved into a house with money raised by their local town, but they would have appreciated help much earlier.

Hints for Home

Before you leave the hospital, ask for extra name bracelets if you need them to tell your babies apart. Car seats are usually designed for babies weighing five pounds or more, so you may need to make some modifications to secure your babies.

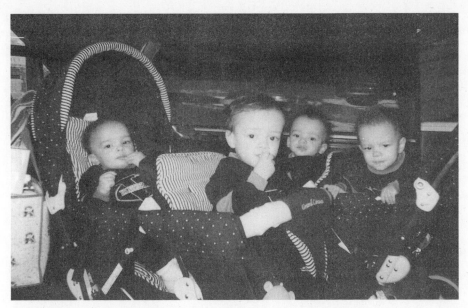

Quads can fill two twin strollers.

The multiples are happiest if they sleep together, but remember that three or more babies generate plenty of body heat; clothe and cover them lightly. It is simplest to put a (covered) mattress on the floor: there is nothing to fall from.* (The same is true of a changing area; make sure you kneel or sit to spare your back.)

Triplets need about 24 cloth diapers per day, for burping as well as for bottoms. Five dozen usually are sufficient if you will be doing laundry every day. Diaper service is less costly than disposables, without the ecological hazards, although there is still a lot of work in the rinsing. Disposable diapers are handy for traveling and when you are sick but will eat up your money if you use them all the time, and they pose a disposal problem.

Mobile Equipment

A triplet stroller is absolutely essential so that you can all get out of the house. Janet Bleyl was never able to afford the triplet stroller she needed when her babies were young, but now she is a distributor, making this critical item available at the lowest cost. Strollers are your key to libera-

*See pages 305–306 for a discussion on preventing crib death by covering the mattress.

You must get a break from the constancy of caring for three babies, even if it is just for an hour or two.

When they came home we were quite unprepared for the never-ending marathon of meeting the needs of these tiny, still-sick infants who required feeding every two hours (each feeding taking more than an hour to accomplish) around the clock.

I breast-fed all three for about six months. I expressed milk in between nursing to give to the third baby while I was breast-feeding the other two.

I didn't venture out much in the early months because I feared that breast-feeding two babies together would give offense.

My doctors never discussed breast-feeding during my prenatal visits, as if no one had ever nursed quadruplets. We were preoccupied with the medical care they might need and overlooked the subject of what they would eat to survive.

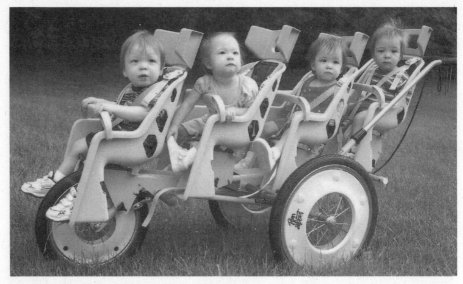

Stadium seating for four.

tion; therefore, you want sturdy ones that will last through the wear and tear of several same-aged babies and that have good resale value. Perego in Italy makes a Triplette, and the seats can be facing or in single file (maximum weight 40 pounds per seat). The Runabout is made in the United States and offers "stadium" seating for three or four on an incline with large wheels and airless tires. It is only 24 inches wide. The maximum weight per seat is 55 pounds and the Runabout is unconditionally guaranteed for five years (whereas the guarantee for the Perego is 30 days, against defects only). There is an optional weather canopy and a car carrier to attach the stroller to a car's trailer hitch, which is a great help with the bulk of three and four-seaters. All seats are removable and can be reclined: the front seat can face in either direction and the height of the handle is adjustable.

From the babies' point of view, it is ideal if you can alternate the use of a baby carrier as well sometimes. This gives you some time with each baby singly.

Breast-feeding Supertwins

The breast-feeding-challenged are those well-meaning outsiders who try to reassure you that formula is just as good, or make you anxious that your babies are not getting enough, or cause you to feel selfish for nursing them! Every mother has to do what feels right for her and her babies, and to stand resolute when others are incredulous at what you are doing or not doing.

Mothers of triplets and quads can nurse exclusively, or nurse and give bottles of breast milk. This way, even if the multiples cannot be breast-fed exclusively, they can be fed breast milk exclusively. Some mothers nurse and/or give bottles of formula; this is discussed in Chapter 13. Many mothers aim to get the infants on a schedule where they wake and feed together. Others feel that because it takes so long to feed three or more, it is better not to disturb the sleeping baby or babies who may have quite different eating patterns. Bottles are more likely to be accepted by babies if given by someone other than the nursing mother. Bring some bottles and nipples from the hospital so that you can sterilize them and keep them for storing breast milk or formula. Some mothers may choose one of these arrangements temporarily, when they are ill themselves. Supertwins may need pacifiers because they don't have as much time to satisfy their need to suck.

Triplets need up to 36 bottles and nipples a day — breast-feeding is so much easier. Ready-to-feed formula can cost up to $12,000 a year for triplets and $16,000 for quadruplets!

Breast-fed babies are much healthier — they have fewer doctors' visits, hospitalizations, and long-term illnesses — saving you much additional time and money. Mothers of triplets breast-feed 24 to 30 times a day for the first few weeks, even months! You provide 8 to 12 feedings a day per baby with each infant taking 10 to 45 minutes per session. Occasional growth spurts may go unrecognized when a baby suddenly demands more. Luckily, the more the babies suck, the more you produce. The milk supply can certainly meet the needs of all your babies; the problem may be limited access to the breast by the number of babies and your ability to stay awake for so many hours. Positioning and tandem nursing are personal choices, but it clearly saves time to nurse two at the same time, although at first you may need to develop your confidence and get to know your babies individually.

Quadruplets can be nursed in pairs so they need not take any more time than triplets. Jeri Chandler, mother of quintuplets whose babies' hospital stays ranged from 38 to 50 days, breast-fed for nine months. She wrote, "The pump became my best friend and my worst enemy. I felt attached and tied down to a machine, not a baby."

The quads had to be fed every three hours, as they were preterm. This meant that every forty-five minutes, around the clock, another feeding would have to begin. We hired a night nurse for the first few weeks. Now we have a girl who comes to help during the worst hours of the day — four to six, Monday through Friday.

The biggest mistake made by mothers is that we underestimate the amount of work. Looking after quintuplets meant nineteen hours of baby care a day. We had to prepare forty bottles every day.

I always nursed two at a time; otherwise I felt my whole existence would be breast-feeding.

Breast-feeding provides important "holding" time, which is very different from (often assembly-line) changing and washing.

Just decide that you are going to breast-feed and see what works best.

I really didn't like expressing milk and I felt a little like a cow doing it, but I just kept thinking of the babies, that I wouldn't have to do it for too long and that it was just one of those things that has to be done.

It didn't seem fair that my triplets should be bottle-fed just because they arrived at the same time.

Nursing three babies wasn't easy, but I'm sure it had to be easier than bottle-feeding three babies. Having to prepare just three clean bottles and nipples a day was hard enough. I can't imagine doing it all day, every day.

There once was a young gal
  who begat
Three babes named Nat, Pat, and Tat
'Twas fun in the breeding
But hell in the feeding
When she found there was no tit
  for Tat!

Those first few months, I just napped an hour or two at a time between feedings. A recliner suited me better than a bed.

I was able to nurse my four babies exclusively until they started on solid food, and I weaned them at 10 months, even though my original goal was just to "do all I could."

Breast-feeding Preterm Infants

Breast-feeding a preterm infant can be a challenge. With supertwins the problem is often multiplied. However, many mothers who had planned to bottle-feed supertwins, like Janet Bleyl, often change their mind when they see how desperately their tiny babies need their mother's milk. It takes much planning and effort to feed the babies when they are in the hospital. An electric pump can be used on leaving and arriving, as well as every three hours or so at home. Electric pumps (hospital grade) can empty the breasts in less than ten minutes. (See Chapter 13 for a complete discussion of breast-feeding, including using an electric pump to express milk.)

The first challenge is getting the preterm baby to stay awake to feed. The second is getting the infant to suck strongly enough to stimulate the milk to let down. If the mother has other children at home, she might be able to go to the hospital only once a day, which limits the time each baby can spend at the breast.

Each baby may have different skills and needs with regard to latching on, settling down, and burping. There may be challenges with nipple confusion, "nursing strikes," and sore nipples, which are not unique to multiples and are covered in the breast-feeding books recommended in the Further Reading.

You may find yourself nursing much longer than you ever thought you would, or becoming sad when your babies wean themselves. Usually, they do it individually so you are not suddenly dropped as milk-woman for the team!

Care of Supertwins

Mothers of higher-order multiples often advise new mothers to stick to priorities, do what works, let go of counting diapers and bottles (which is a reminder of the tedious part of parenting), and just enjoy the babies.

However, some mothers prefer to keep a log of fluids in and out, bowel movements, and of course medications, especially if babies are on different regimens. Growth can be documented here, too. Some parents like to keep track, with a blackboard or colored pins, of the infants who were fed, because sleep-challenged mothers can easily mix up the babies. Having a schedule for who has had what and when is helpful when fathers or others come to help. You can use colored pens or colored paper to code the information for each baby.

An oft-quoted Australian study revealed that a mother of six-month-old triplets spends an average of 198 hours a week (out of a possible 168!) between herself and paid/volunteer assistance on the care of the children and home. This did not include any allowance for the mother's time to bathe, dress, sleep, eat, relax, or converse with her partner!

◉ Support Organizations for Higher-Order Multiples

Twins clubs also offer information and support for parents of triplets and more, but in addition there are groups and Web sites that specialize in higher-order multiples. Triplets will experience different issues than twins because of the dynamics of a group rather than a pair. Triads are less stable than dyads, and the intragroup pairs change from time to time, just as twins reverse their behaviors. Quadruplets are often paired for social dynamics: indeed, most children choose to play in pairs.

The Triplet Connection has a Web site with chat forums and a quarterly newsletter with listings of expectant and new parents. An information packet is sent to expectant parents and there is a telephone hotline. Also available is a lengthy list of names and phone numbers of parents of higher-order multiples who are available to provide support for every condition and issue you can imagine — truly networking at its best. Please complete the group's medical questionnaire as this is a crucial source of information for you and other parents of multiples (1-209-474 0885, www.tripletconnection.com).

Mothers of Supertwins (M.O.S.T.) also has a research database and a quarterly publication. Through their Member Only on-line networks and forums, families gain pregnancy and parenting support and information. M.O.S.T. also coordinates special on-line networks for grandparents, families with quadruplets, quintuplets, and sextuplets and special needs children (1-877-434-MOST, Info@MOSTonline.org).

Finding Our Way: Life with Triplets, Quadruplets and Quintuplets is a collection of experiences published by the Triplets, Quads & Quints Association of Canada. It also covers topics outside the scope of this book, such as returning to work and stories by supertwins themselves. A similar book is *From Twins to Quints — The Complete Manual for Parents of Multiple*

The most I ever pumped in one sitting was 30 ounces and about 120 ounces in 24 hours, almost 5 times what a mother of a single baby will produce in that time!

I never kept track of nursing or had a schedule. I always had enough milk. Time, not supply, was the problem. I always seemed to have a baby at the breast, enjoying the closeness but always feeling tired.

Ironically, parents of singletons often have to defend their decision *not* to breast-feed whereas mothers of multiples, especially supertwins, often have to defend their decision *to* breast-feed.

Nurse your children in public. You will get out more and nurse more, and the public will learn that MOMs (mothers of multiples) can and do nurse!

I was back to my pre-pregnancy weight before I knew it! I'd read that breast milk has 20 calories per ounce, so all the calories I took in were quickly recycled.

I felt so shut out of the community with triplets. Baby-sitting groups didn't work out because I had three children, I wasn't invited to visit friends and I couldn't even take them to the swimming pool because each child had to have an adult for supervision.

Birth Children by the National Organization of Mothers of Twins Clubs in the United States.

The ABC Club is an international organization serving higher-order multiples primarily in Germany and reaching into Switzerland, Austria, and Liechtenstein. Expectant parents and new parents learn from the experiences of others, while adult multiples enjoy sports and social activities. The club is also committed to educating the public, making long-term observations about preterm infants and family dynamics, and lobbying for the health interests of preterm infants. Volunteers collect data, provide phone counseling and contacts for parents, send brochures, translate articles, write a quarterly newsletter, organize conferences, and mediate the buying, selling, or renting of strollers.

Even in countries where social services are more available, such as the United Kingdom, mothers often have to threaten (or occasionally come close to) a nervous breakdown to get their health visitor or family doctor to act on their behalf to arrange help. Sometimes the doctor prescribes antidepressants when the mothers ask for domestic help! One mother refused to take her babies home from the hospital until she was promised home help at a reasonable cost. That tactic may work in the National Health Service, but not in the United States, where the parents have to pay per day. The valid point has been made that more services exist for the elderly who are housebound than for mothers of multiples who are also housebound and experiencing much more stress.

The Australian government pays parents of triplets $A106 a fortnight and $A141 for quadruplets for the first five years regardless of assets but subject to an income test.

In the United Kingdom in particular, restrictions and waiting lists limit access to play groups and nursery school, forcing mothers to make tough choices about which children to enroll. When the mother splits the sessions between the multiples, she doubles her transport time and costs. Distance, traveling time, and cost are major factors restricting activities for supertwins. Because of the well-known language and other developmental delays in multiples, these preschool experiences should be a priority. Supertwin families sometimes can obtain some discount on tuition in the United States.

The explosion of triplets has made them less of a novelty; therefore, publicity and donations from corporations and communities are usually reserved for quadruplets and larger sets. Such publicity can backfire, however, as more and more newspapers and magazines pick up the story, use photos without permission, and pester the family.

The Joy of Supertwins

Most passers-by are speechless at the sight of three or more babies or may make comments like "You poor woman" or "I certainly don't envy you." Children have a different perspective: "Oh Mommy, that woman has three babies — isn't she lucky!"

One mother had triplets after a stillbirth and two miscarriages and felt that God had given her back all that she had lost. Another woman had triplets first and then quads. In both pregnancies she gained 42 pounds and both sets of multiples went to 38 weeks. However, she gained 20 pounds before conceiving the quads and lost the total 62 pounds by six weeks postpartum. The triplets weighed 6 pounds; 5 pounds, 9 ounces; and 5 pounds. The quads weighed 6 pounds, 1 ounce; 5 pounds, 10 ounces; 5 pounds, 8 ounces; and 5 pounds, 1 ounce. The mother had no problems during pregnancy; she was always able to get in and out of bed by herself and could walk a little right to the end. She attributes her good outcome to encouragement and support, a positive attitude, good food, rest, an air bed, and confidence in her doctor. This mother breast-fed all her children but limited nursing the quads to a few weeks because she felt she needed to use her energy for her other five children! If they had been her first pregnancy, she would have breast-fed them for much longer, she said.

Expectant parents need to remember, as they read about all the risks and possible complications, that it is certainly possible to birth healthy triplets and quadruplets of good birth weight. Look for mothers who have done so, and maintain contact with them during your pregnancy for inspiration. The Internet makes it easy for you to find and connect with such mothers anyway. Birth, like life, means risks, but birth is one of the safest experiences. The best you can do is to be well-informed and choose the path of action that feels right for you.

17

The Older Sibling/s

Preparation During Pregnancy

Pregnancy provides months of time to talk with any other children in the family about multiples. Involve them in prenatal visits and hospital tours, and in looking at ultrasound scans, reading children's books about twins, and singing to the babies. Encourage their help in sorting baby clothes and toys. Let the sibling choose which toys to hand down to the multiples. Review your child's own infancy with photo albums. If he or she is not accustomed to infants, arrange a visit, perhaps to some new multiples from your local club. Stuffed animals or dolls with blankets and cribs can be substitute babies for the appropriate age.

During pregnancy, multiples can take up the family's time and attention if the mother is on bed rest or hospitalized, and this is an obvious source of stress. Draw out your child's feelings and concerns about the arrival of the babies. Explain that although family life will be very different, she or he will continue to be valued and nurtured.

A lone sibling may feel that he or she is the only family member without a partner; if you already have two or more children, they provide companionship for themselves. On the other hand, the sibling may adjust better to an extra baby or two, because the exclusive maternal-infant bond with a single baby is more displacing.

Before the birth, set up a special regular activity for the sibling, such as piano lessons, swimming classes, or some after-school program. Also arrange for companionship with grandparents or other adults who live

We emphasized the status and privileges of being "older," acknowledging her skills and independence.

Whenever passers-by stop to ask the twins' names and ages, I always introduce their older sister.

Every time someone says to my twins, "How cute!" I add, "Yes, and aren't Sarah's blond curls pretty?"

I didn't realize how hard Sarah would take it. She may have gotten two brothers, but she lost both her parents to their infancy.

My son is 13½ months older than his twin sisters. He learned to talk and speak up very early to make his needs known.

All the good advice about how to treat multiples as individuals helps the singleton, too.

Up to your nth year you regarded yourself as the sole and unlimited possessor of your mother: then came another baby and brought you grave disillusionment. Your mother left you for some time and even after her reappearance, she was never again devoted to you exclusively.

— Freud, 1937

Jennie didn't like it at all when people told her she was lucky to have so many babies. She wanted me to return them to the hospital!

close by, and make sure it continues after the birth, when you are preoccupied with the newborns.

A special treat would be a short holiday with your singletons before the babies are born.

Many new stresses enter the life of siblings apart from the multiples. A new baby-sitter, activity, or school can make them feel afraid or out of control. Make sure that any changes with child care, playschool, or sleeping arrangements are established well before the birth and are kept consistent to ease the adjustment before the multiples come home.

Home help is essential so that the parents can spend time with older siblings. Organize help before the birth so that a relationship can be established between the helper and the sibling. Setting routines before the birth can help provide security during the transition.

After the Babies Arrive

After the birth be sure to greet the sibling *before* you introduce him or her to the babies, and arrange this meeting as soon as possible. Set up an exchange of cards and gifts to and from each baby. Display the sibling's gifts and cards prominently. This is a good beginning for a sibling to relate with the multiples as individuals. Set up the sibling on a sofa or somewhere safe to hold a baby.

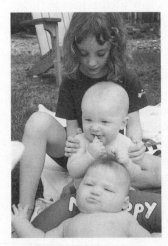

An older sister may be proud of the new responsibilities that come with a set of twins.

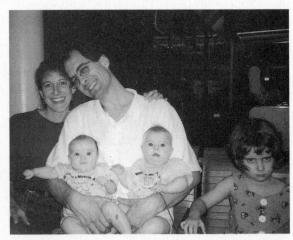

Or she may feel lonely and left out.

Let the sibling choose simple chores to develop a stronger sense of belonging and responsibility. Keep goodies hidden that you can have for the older child when visitors arrive with gifts just for the multiples.

Consider having someone mind the twins while you drive your older child to school. Make sure the child is appreciated for his or her unique qualities, not for being a big brother or sister of multiples. Use breast-feeding as a time to read a story to the sibling and help him or her feel special. A sibling likes to hear sometimes that the multiples have to wait while he or she is taken care of.

Each position in the family has its advantages and disadvantages. The single first-born is the most displaced by the arrival of twins and is often pushed into the role of "Mom's little helper" or having to act like a father. As this child lacks a sibling companion, parents need to provide extra attention and privileges to compensate. People will make a fuss over the multiples but invariably ignore the other child. This goes on for years, and parents and siblings can exchange winks and laugh together about it later to defuse the pain of being overlooked. Introduce this child to passers-by who ogle the multiples or encourage a verbal sibling to introduce the babies. Make a point of providing information on the status of all your children.

Treating multiples as individuals makes it much easier for the sibling, especially in public, and in turn the multiples are more likely to relate to siblings as individuals rather than as a unit — without ganging up. Using individual names is important for multiples and for the older sibling, who does not want to be known as the "brother or sister of the triplets." Parents can help by creating time for the singleton to be with just one multiple at a time and also to forge common interests between them. Consider letting your older child take turns sleeping with one of your multiples when the time is right.

Dealing with Regression and Resentment

Resentment and jealousy are common among siblings in any family. Often these conflicts appear not so much between the twins or triplets but between other children in the family and the multiples. A child may be afraid of expressing his anger at his mother or father and may need help in feeling safe to express appropriately those feelings about the double rivals competing for Mother's attention — and to know that you will acknowledge them. Multiples and siblings should be encouraged to vent their feelings to avoid physical abuse. Play-acting with dolls or

It was really hard on Jimmy. After the months on bed rest, suddenly his home is full of babies taking all our attention.

My daughter was worried that she would have to do a lot more around the house when the babies were born and the way the house was being re-arranged to make space for them. I couldn't deny this, it was true. Later I felt relieved when she told me that she felt stronger and more independent for the experience.

I have tried to foster the idea of five individuals, not "them and him." The fact that four happened to be born on the same day is of no real importance.

Do not continually dress them alike. When they are continually dressed alike, they are perceived as a package, a package of which your singleton child is not a part.

If you dress your singleton child(ren) the same as your multiples, you are sending the message to your singleton child(ren) that it is necessary to look like someone else.

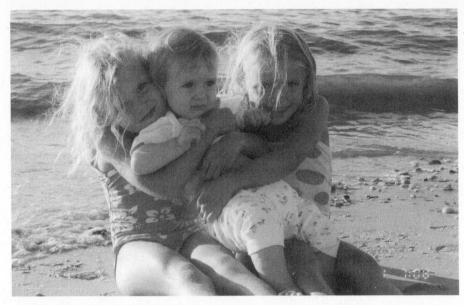

Two big sisters mean double the hugs.

puppets helps discover the child's true attitudes. Encourage family members (parents too) to hit pillows instead of each other when angry. Anger is an important emotion; it must be expressed safely. An excellent book on the subject is *Siblings Without Rivalry* by Adele Faber and Elaine Mazlish.

The La Trobe Twin Study found that two-thirds of parents reported problems with older siblings showing regressive behavior during the first six months after the twins were born. Bed-wetting was the most common, then physical aggression. Sometimes the older child will want a bottle or demand to be dressed like the twins, even in a diaper! (Playing along with this for a couple of days can satisfy the desire so the sibling can drop this behavior.) Parents have shared some funny stories about the suggestions these children have: "We could always sell one" or "Couldn't we tie them both together and make one?"

Siblings age 2 to 5 present significant problems about half as often as siblings age 8 to 11. Some siblings are outwardly hostile, but others become withdrawn or suspiciously well behaved, avoiding attention-seeking behavior and making sure they are not an additional burden. Preschool and school teachers are sometimes aware of problems that may escape parental attention at home, such as an apparently self-sufficient or passive child, who is really not independent at all but actually needs more parental care.

Include your older child in photos and in name tags you might make. However, dressing the sibling like the twins, as with dressing the twins the same (see Chapter 15), gives the impression that it is important to look like someone else.

Multiples benefit from siblings — the more the better — and this diminishes the power of the unit. When it is their turn to be older siblings, they may compete for the attention of the singleton. The dynamics change because there are so many Mother's helpers! A family of triplets, say, two girls and one boy, will become a couple with two girls and two boys, when the younger sibling is a boy. This takes the emphasis of the set of multiples and rearranges the family's interactions.

18
Some Special Features of Twinship

As we saw in Chapter 1, twinship has always been the subject of various myths, taboos, and social customs. Twin cities, twin peaks, twin beds — the idea of a matching set is appealing. As with twin objects, both twin persons must be present to make a set. Talent and advertising agencies prefer to use identical twins, most often girls, who in general as they grow up receive lots of attention and may find it hard to relate as individuals when not part of a cute duo.

Ricardo Ainslie, in *The Psychology of Twinship*, clarifies our reactions to twins:

> There is something universally appealing and fascinating about the loss of individual boundaries . . . reflecting a wish to return to a symbiotic relationship — that is, a relationship characterized by a lack of self-other differentiation in which one's needs are magically understood and met.

Parents of twins, despite the hard work, express joy and satisfaction in raising them. The challenge for the parent-multiple relationship is that every child has to first feel secure in a symbiosis with the mother, and on that basis of security, the process of separation and individuation (from both mother and co-twin) is facilitated.

Both parents and multiples learn to adjust to invasive questions and other disadvantages of being special. The assumptions of outsiders primarily concern cloning, lack of individuality, or identical behavior. Twins must tolerate the skepticism of people who, not understanding the nature of DZ twinning, may insist that children cannot be twins if

Every twin has someone special that few others have.

People see us as enviable because we are born with our soul mates, who never have to go looking to be made whole like everybody else.

— Penelope Farmer

The myth of the twin to which we are subjected creates and defines what is for us a double reality, in which any single mythical and real quality can point to, or even contain, its equally mythical, equally real opposite. And in that our whole problem lies.

— Penelope Farmer

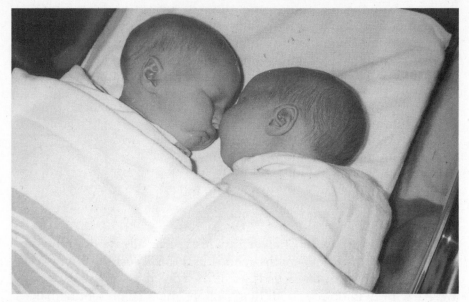

Twins prefer to sleep together, even nose to nose.

their hair is a different color or they are a different gender. On the other hand, DZ twins sometimes do look exactly alike (particularly when they are small) and they may be treated as if they were identical and sometimes under pressure to carry out a "double act."

Many of the queries and comments about twins have negative connotations because contrast implies superiority and inferiority. That is, if one twin is quick, the other twin is slow, or at least slower. Typical queries include "Is the first-born heavier?" "Which twin is the passive one?" Parents have thought up some good answers, such as "The smaller twin kicked the bigger one out" or "Why do you want to know?"

Of course, twins have confessed to their parents that they hate being twins and some remain rivals through life. The majority of twins enjoy a close relationship helping and supporting one another. Few relationships are as close or as long-lasting as the bond between multiples.

Boy-Girl and Unalike or "Invisible" Twins

Boy-girl combinations are similar to other siblings except for their shared birthday. They are, however, generally considered as a pair and may be called "the babies" rather than "the twins." Opposite-sex multi-

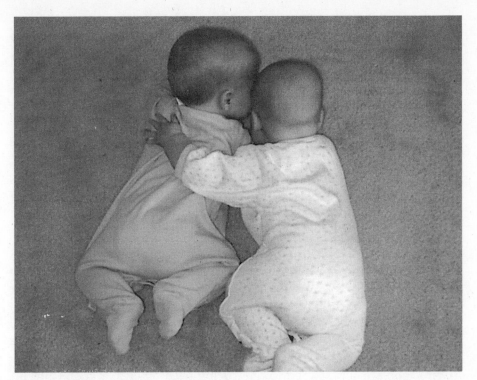

An early embrace.

ples develop at different rates, like children in any family. Girls mature first in weight, height, toileting, fine motor skills, speech, reading, and sometimes school grades. The challenge with these twins is their different developmental levels, which may reverse later. In any case, one twin should be able to move to the appropriate level in school despite a less mature or advanced co-twin.

Parents may be concerned if the twins are *not* similar enough, or they may make an exaggerated effort to treat their twins separately and differently. The view expressed by "to each according to his or her ability" may create difficulties when multiples wish to participate in certain opportunities, for example, when both twins might like an acting role or a position on a team. It is important that each child be encouraged to discover his or her own interests, rather than create an artificial situation that directs one twin to excel in one area and the other in something else, in order to balance the twinship and avoid comparison and competition. This can be carried to an extreme. For example, Dina and Melanie both

Twins help define the untwinned.
— Penelope Farmer

We had an unspoken agreement that Karen would be one way and I would be the other way so we can avoid any painful confrontation when we have to compete. Everything I do, whether failing or achieving, I think in terms of us.

Perhaps twins, especially MZs who share the same genetic makeup, are expressing individuality when they choose the same activities, the same dress or share the same mannerisms!

To what extent do parents assess their strengths and weaknesses as an individual and to what extent relative to the other multiple(s)?

When I do something with my twin, I feel full, like a complete person.

There is an unstated understanding that things will be kept equal between the twins resulting in "the twinship."
— Ricardo Ainslie,
The Psychology of Twinship

What does it mean to announce "I am a twin" or to ask the question "Are you a twin?"

like ballet, but a coin will be flipped to see which of the twins will be allowed to take classes, or Brian may be given violin lessons and Sandy piano lessons. This may be unfair to Brian if both share a talent for piano. Also, the multiples may support one another rather than be driven apart by taking up similar interests. Many twins work together successfully in the same field (see Chapter 1).

Sometimes a multiple develops low self-esteem or depression because of a discrepancy in skills and abilities when compared with the other co-multiples. Problems with language and communication make it more difficult for this child to make friends and achieve in the outside world — skills that may seem to come easily to the co-multiples. This is especially hard to bear when the twins are both the same gender.

The Couple Effect

Twins are not simply two duplicates but share and interact with each other and society as part of a *couple*.

Couples, as we all know, tend to settle into a pattern of complementary roles, which in childhood may mean that one twin may not develop certain skills because the co-twin took care of that task, whether it is practical or emotional in nature. Independent decisions may challenge twins who are accustomed to reinforcing each other's opinions and fitting together like two connecting parts.

Dr. Jane Greer defined the term "occupied zone" for the polarization between twins, and explains that it is part of the couple effect to reduce jealousy and conflicts. That is, one twin will pursue a different hobby or skill so as not to threaten the proficiency of the co-twin. Avoiding any competition where they do not both excel, unfortunately, can limit their individual development.

On the other hand, twins who do everything together are at a disadvantage. The events that would normally test one's sense of self, one's strengths and weaknesses, are not experienced independently.

Monozygotic Twins

If parents cannot tell their twins apart, they should keep it quiet; the idea may be alarming for multiples who are trying to differentiate themselves. Make sure they are clearly identifiable (even from behind in case one needs to shout a warning with the right name to avoid an accident).

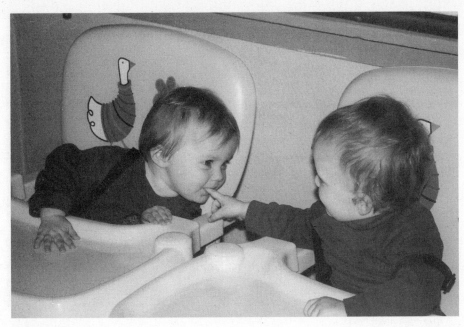

Finger food.

Monozygotic twins tend to cooperate more, whereas DZ twins are more competitive. In a study done by Nancy Segal, 94 percent of MZ twins solved a puzzle together within a given time frame, compared with 46 percent of DZ twins.

Such twins may become defensive about their closeness because all their life they have been told they must be different and be individuals. It is fun for them sometimes to dress alike or emphasize their twinship, to enjoy admiration and perhaps envy.

Twins who are the image of each other will be psychologically similar but will also show some distinguishing characteristics. The Louisville Twin Study has shown that temperament is genetically influenced but its expression in the newborn period is affected by health at birth (such as weight and Apgar score).

The outside world also will treat multiples differently when they go their separate ways, and no child in a family is ever treated equally. Children have different needs and wants. The challenge for all parents is simply to be fair in each circumstance, whether the children arrive together or separately.

For the twin ambiguities — that which unifies also divides while divided identity makes it hard to define any identity at all — is precisely the paradox that twins embody.
— Penelope Farmer

We know that our girls will always be known as "the triplets" to others and that is something special for them, but we want them to have individual friends and interests.

The Chinese are reluctant to let children see themselves in the mirror until they are old enough to have a true sense of themselves.

Twinship is a mirror. The fit of the twin is to reveal aspects of ourselves that have gone unseen.
— James Elniski, *Finding One's Twin*

I noticed my girls looking in the mirror together and using the other one's name while pointing to herself! I gave them each a different colored hair ribbon and sat with them, so we could match them up correctly in the mirror and they could start to use the right names.

We dressed our twins alike. One day we heard one say to the other, "Stand over there so I can see how I look."

The other kids in the class didn't understand about twins at first. They thought each girl was called Annie Michelle.

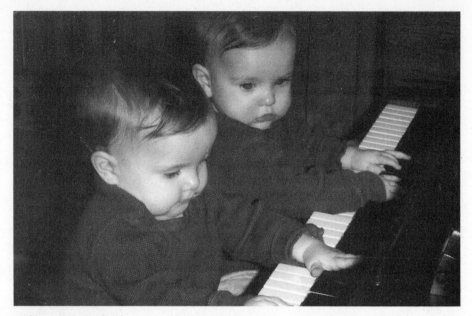

A duo enjoying a duet!

The Challenges of Twinship

It is human to make comparisons. Even during pregnancy the mother differentiates between twins and assembles a set of expectations. After twins are born, such expectations may be astute and appropriate, but sometimes they arise out of stereotyping. Parents may project themselves onto each twin: "A boy for Dad and a girl for Mom." The mother often takes the weaker, less competent twin under her wing, regardless of sex, while the father romps with the more robust member of the pair.

Schoolteachers sometimes notice that parents claim one twin is superior in a subject, whereas tests show the twins' abilities to be the same. Well-intentioned people may use motivational phrases such as " Your brother can do it and I am sure you can, too."

Each member of a twin pair or a group of multiples grows up accustomed to being part of a set. In childhood, twins may ask their parents why other children are not twins and may speculate on what it would be like to be a singleton. Similarly, single children may have difficulty grasping the concept of multiples and may wonder what it is like for MZ toddlers to look at two identical faces in the mirror and wonder who is who. Of course, they know nothing else! If twins are dressed alike, other children may isolate clothing as the key to being twins.

Sometimes twins are so dependent on each other, so interconnected, that they are actually confused about their identity. They may perceive themselves or behave almost as one person.

Emphasizing Individuality

Proper use of a person's name is especially important in a multiple's development of identity and individuality. Each of us likes our uniqueness to be validated. We sometimes resent comments that we are just like a certain family member and may be offended if mistaken for someone else.

Twins will generally correct their peers but not their teachers or other adults. It is important for parents to help each twin be recognized by name. People retain the names of unlike twins, while MZ twins tend to be called "the twins." It is more polite to ask the multiple's name rather than repeat the tiresome question "Which one are you?" Group references such as "the boys" and "the quads" only reinforce the collective entity.

Twins may also confuse their own identity at first and both may respond if one name is called. Symbiotic names like Bojo for Bobby and Joseph are confusing to other children who have not yet comprehended what makes two persons twins.

Parents can make it easier for others by choosing very different names (see Chapter 4).

Twins interact with different roles within the constant presence of each other. When each one strives to be as different as possible, it is called sibling de-identification. In contrast, sibling assimilation happens when they strive to reduce any differences and competition.

Dealing with Separation and Independence

Multiples enjoy very close mental and physical contact from conception. Twinfants play and cuddle together and may even sleep interlocked. As they learn to crawl and walk, multiples follow each other around. Later one may read stories to the other. Twins often learn skills in dressing and feeding each other before they can manage for themselves. Parents comment that multiples play together better than other siblings do. (Of course, some fight terribly as well.)

Multiples have one great advantage over singletons: they always have

---

When visitors ask about "the triplets," we keep reinforcing the names, such as "Julie and Andrea are fine, but Eleanor has a cold today."

Make sure that you take plenty of photos of each twin separately, to balance their individuality and twinship.

When we took anniversary photos of our twins, we always had them in the same position in the photo. This is a big help for recording the subtle differences in identical twins over the years.

Multiples have the jump start on singletons in personality development because they always have a point of comparison. It may take them years to find out who they are, but at least they always know who they aren't.

My brother and I always felt badly for each other if one didn't do as well as the other on a test. When people asked us how we did, we evaded the question because neither of us liked to admit that one did better. We usually did different things separately so we would not have to compete.

One of our twin boys is very good in school, but the other is the swimming star in the family.

Twins can understand if one is ready to go ahead and the other is not ready, without guilt or stigma.

It is important that parents be aware of problems that can arise without being alarmed by them.

I watched my twins at the playground, interacting very nicely. They didn't exclude the other children, but it was obvious they didn't need to include them either. And they didn't need me!

Red or blue truck? Owning two of everything went against my principles. I wanted them to have separate and different toys. But I found it was much easier if they had the same things.

Parents of multiples are lucky because of the constant companionship the children give each other. But some twins still complain once in a while that they have no one to play with!

It is truly an honor to witness the "two in the one" as their twinship so well expresses. As each paints one half of a detailed landscape, their art shares beauty of soul as well. A rare beauty of two souls so close they seem to be one.

— Jeannine Parvati Baker

each other for company and rarely need a security blanket. There is less separation anxiety when the mother leaves. Socializing is also easy for multiples, especially if they are alike in appearance. They attract attention, and people notice and remember them — at least as a unit!

Striving for independence may be complicated by rivalry between twins. Each may pair off with a parent, sometimes with a very strong bond. Brief separations should start from the very beginning. Arrange them gradually and naturally. Twins do not always have to be nursed, rocked, or entertained together. Certainly triplets have to take turns and quadruplets are often paired off. One of the multiples can spend time at home while the other children can go shopping. Friends and relatives should be encouraged to invite one multiple for day trips or overnight stays. Opportunities for social activities vary greatly with the environment: multiples who live on a farm may be thrown together much more than multiples who live in a city. As multiples become more confident and independent, their paths will diverge.

Sometimes one receives a special invitation and the parents may provide something compensatory for the excluded twin. The often-excluded singleton siblings must be remembered, too.

Although multiples have shared a womb, they learn to share their toys gradually, like all children do. First, each must develop a sense of ownership of their clothes and some toys. Once a child understands the concept of "mine," she or he can begin to lend and exchange. Parents and caregivers who lump all the multiples' clothes and toys together slow down their development of identity and self-esteem, and this may promote competition between them.

The duty of all parents is to help their children develop independence. The special attachments between multiples make this an interesting challenge. There are two normal developmental phases for the establishment of identity, occurring around age two and then again in adolescence. Twins have to define their concept of selfhood apart from their parents as well as distinct from the co-twin. Three aspects of identity need to be integrated: that of the individual, that of his or her twin/multiple, and the shared identity as a multiple. Whether the personal or twin identity is foremost depends on how the twins were raised — to function as a unit or to mix as individuals.

Singletons do not have to compete for attention with another baby at the same level of development, so their self-image develops more readily. Twins' personality development is shaped by the unique bonds they share with each other, beginning with conception, as well as by their parents and their environment. When twins tend to "specialize," parents can help them find their own friends and outlets. Alison McDonald in the United Kingdom found that "discernment" was the central task of twinship. She suggested four categories in which this takes place: "two at the same time," awareness, managing ambiguity, and defining boundaries.

Roles between the twins invariably shift and even reverse. Young twins experiment with the balance of their relationship — trading off being "leader and follower," or "bully and victim," weekly, daily, or hourly!

Triplets operate more as a democracy than twins do. Sharing and taking turns is instilled because no one can be the boss for long without the other two objecting. Mothers of triplets observe that different members pair off at certain times. Triplets are usually assumed by other people to be twins plus another sibling, especially if they differ in size and sex. In this case, the "spare" may need more support, because the MZ twins have each other.

 ## The Schooling of Multiples

If you are home with infants, school seems like a long time away. However, the preparation you make in the early years will have an impact on their adjustments in the classroom.

Although identical twins usually perform similarly, they may have different learning styles and develop different strategies when completing tasks. Teachers and parents can help them identify and utilize their own personal styles. Individuality, identity and recognition, competition, and fair and equal treatment are not always in their best interests.

Schooling is one of the major issues facing parents of multiples. This was the hottest topic in the forty-first year of the National Organization of Mothers of Twins Clubs (NOMOTC), after their 1998 survey found that little had changed in ten years. Most schools have no written policies — only anecdotes and assumptions based on their experience with singletons. Few discuss placement options with parents. Some schools always kept multiples together because of birth date or alphabetical placement. Often, multiples have language delays, ADHD, specific learning disabilities, or other special needs about which teachers should be informed. Some of these may be rationalized as "being a twin" or "typical of a boy," which delays getting the help needed. The school needs to know of influences such as preterm birth.

Our identical twins often get the same marks on a test. The first time it happened the teacher suspected cheating. But even in separate rooms they get the same answers and make the same errors.

My twin sister and I never had any problems being in the same classroom. We are each other's best friend and it was easy to do our homework together.

I think starting school is such a trauma for twins that they need each other for security until each can make other friends. After that, I think separation helps with their individuality since twins are compared so much.

We put our twins in separate classes after we found out that Elaine was doing all the work for Paul. Even in school, he'd send papers to the back of the room where she was sitting.

We both hated sharing the same class. Our teacher used to embarrass us by asking us to stand side by side and get people to try and see differences.

I decided that once a week I would keep one of my twins at home with me. This gave me some special time with each and allowed them to develop relationships with other children without the co-twin looking on. Far from being detrimental to their education, the two half-days each one missed per month enabled them to become very independent and easily establish friendships, together and separately.

Private schools may favor singletons because two may provide four grandparents who are potential benefactors whereas twins may provide only two.
— Nancy Segal

Parents who can afford it may seek out private schools with flexible programs for their multiples because they disagree with the policy of separating twins at the local school.

It wasn't just the idea of enforced separation that annoyed me, it was the belief on the part of strangers that they knew what was best for my twins.

A teacher said to me: "I know it is easier for you if they are in the same class" which had the effect of telling me that not only was I wrong, but I was selfish.

Teachers usually receive no special training for working with multiples; fortunately today there are resources, workshops, and videos to educate them (such as *More than One*, made by the Australian Multiple Birth Association). In response to the great demand for guidance about schooling, NOMOTC has created a Multiple Birth Education kit to assist teachers and parents with placement, including a position paper, a sample letter to the school principal, a research questionnaire, and a study guide for teachers. The Web site, in-services, and a special issue of the *Notebook* on education have served as resources for principals and school boards. Their best-selling booklet, *Educating Multiples*, has sales of almost 10,000 a year.

There is a special track at the International Society of Twins Studies Congresses for issues around schooling multiples.

The Best Policy Is No Policy

Research in Australia and the United Kingdom did not find evidence that separation of twins enhanced their individuality, nor is there evidence that a distinct and positive self-image cannot develop in the presence of the co-twin in the same classroom. Up to a quarter of the twins separated involuntarily are placed together the next year.

No formula for school placement fits all multiples at all times, but research supporting flexible placement is unfortunately lacking. Teachers, parents, and twins should together evaluate classroom placements for a set each year, just as classroom placement is evaluated annually for single-born children. Parents and teachers together have to find the best educational environment for each multiple, in consultation with therapists who may be involved and, of course, the children themselves. Their similar or differing abilities, social and language skills, dependence upon adults, and prior experiences of being apart are important factors. Make sure to discuss each multiple separately with the teacher to keep the focus on the individual.

Staying Together in the Classroom

Young multiples may need the comforting presence of co-multiples so they can gradually participate in separate activities with different groups by themselves. When multiples are separated before they have learned independence, they may be overwhelmed with grief and anxiety and unable to concentrate. (Best friends often want to be in the same classroom, too, which is generally accommodated by schools.)

However, multiples in the same class often build on each other's strengths to achieve academic standards. The teacher may be unaware of their individual levels since they work so efficiently together. Teachers need to pay special attention to the strengths and weaknesses of each multiple, to maximize their educational experience. Some parents have to struggle to ensure that appropriate professionals and school administrators provide the correct learning environment for the multiples.

Make sure that the twins sit apart and are clearly identifiable, with different clothes and hairstyles if they look alike. Being identified by name is important for their development as individuals. Putting them in separate study groups within the same class offers the best of both worlds.

Learning in Separate Classrooms

Some believe that twins should be separated in school in order to learn to get along without each other. There are logistical problems as well: how many schools can offer two, three, or four separate classes to accommodate a large set of multiples? However, the apparently simple idea of separating multiples into afternoon and morning sessions or choosing different schools will double the commute for the parents who may have other children who need to be dropped off or collected at the same time if there is no school bus service. Different classroom expectations, homework, projects, and field trips for each multiple in different settings become quite impractical! Parents are challenged enough to give individual attention for homework.

Twins who start school in separate classrooms face a double separation from the mother and the twin, as they did in the hospital nursery when they were born. Even when twins are kept in the same classroom, teachers recommend that two adults accompany the twins to make the first day easier.

Twin consultant Patricia Malmstrom, founder and director of the former Twin Services, cautions that twins forced apart into separate classrooms before they are ready can suffer disabling levels of anxiety and loss of self-esteem, and they may get the impression that there is something wrong about being part of a set. Malmstrom comments:

> We got many calls and letters each year from parents all over the country who are distressed because a school put their twins in different classrooms and one or sometimes both children are having serious behavior and learning problems.

Paradoxically, school policies can deny multiples the individuality and separation that schools try to promote by separating the twins.

The challenge is, as always, to respect the bond between multiples while valuing their individual needs.

The first question the teacher asked me was "Are they identical?" I was so taken back.

Individuality and independence from parents and siblings develop gradually over many years — forced separations at age four or five are unnecessary and often counterproductive.

We always had to approach the school. The teachers or principal never suggested discussions with us before they made decisions about the education of the twins. I think we were labeled as demanding parents.

It is interesting that when we ask twins about their feelings on this topic, the only twins who complain about what has happened to them are some of those who were separated.

— David Hay

Policies which require separation of multiples seem to be based on assumptions that separation will promote individuality and independence. But no school administrator has ever been able to cite to us a study or reference which supports this notion, and we find no research which validates routine separation. On the contrary, research findings and our observations support routine placement together. We feel separation should be the exception, not the rule, and that parents' opinions and twins' own desires about placement should be respected.

Malmstrom and others have observed that twins who are allowed to be together when they need to be during the early school years easily accept, and often request, separate classes in later grades.

Separation is desirable for twins in the following situations:

- They are the center of attention in a classroom and disturb the other children.

- Their twinship limits interaction with others.

- There are several "occupied zones" between the twins or a division of labor.

- Twinship is used for cheating, tricking, confusion, or entertainment.

- The twins are behaving as a "power unit."

- They are at different developmental levels, excessively dependent or competitive.

- Their abilities or developmental levels differ.

- Dominance/dependency issues exist.

- The teacher cannot tell them apart and treats them as a group.

- Twins themselves want privacy and prefer to be separated. Multiples spend a lot of time together and they may enjoy making their own friends in different classes at school.

- Appearances are so similar that the twins are always being mistaken for each other. One set of twins commented "When other kids see us, they think that we think alike, and we don't like that!"

- Separations have been started, for example, at preschool. However, many parents have not thought ahead to school in order to prepare the multiples by increasing their separations from each other.

- Separation is decided in consultation with the multiples, and the timing is right.

- Separated twins at the same school have opportunities to see each other during breaks, especially in the beginning.

- Multiples can benefit from the allocation of separate projects to build their individual abilities.

Like the rest of us, twins must learn that life is not fair. It is not always possible for parents and teachers to treat twins equally. One child may excel in sports and the other in schoolwork. Each twin will find his or her own compensations in the world. Certainly singleton siblings do not get equal treatment.

Home Schooling

Parents of twins, and of supertwins especially, may want to consider home schooling. State laws require that you provide your children with an education — it doesn't have to be within a school but you may need approval from your school district. Dozens of Web sites, organizations (Growing Without Schooling, a Boston organization, was founded by the late author and educator John Holt), journals, and conferences assist the more than one million children in the United States who are schooled at home.

Some mothers of multiples may look forward to sending their children to school in order to have time for themselves or to return to work. No doubt, schools do provide convenient custodial care. However, literacy rates in the United States were *higher* before compulsory schooling!

Many parents of twins have problems with school — forced separations, comparisons, ranking of different abilities, problems telling them apart, teasing, to name a few — so that home schooling makes sense for them. Multiples, like other children in the family, can learn and play happily together without developing problems with dependency or competition.

The flexibility of home schooling and the possibilities for travel out-

I never worried about who was being left out, because the roles and interactions changed so frequently.

Sometimes I let the twins get away with things that weren't fair to her older sister. It was easier to excuse their baby behavior, but she resented that.

Why shouldn't we be alike? We are identical twins; we share the same career; we think alike about most things. My brother may have done a bit better at school, but then he worked harder!

You can never tell a lie to your twin.

We experienced just about everything together, it was really nice. Whereas to be just one person, that is kind of scary.

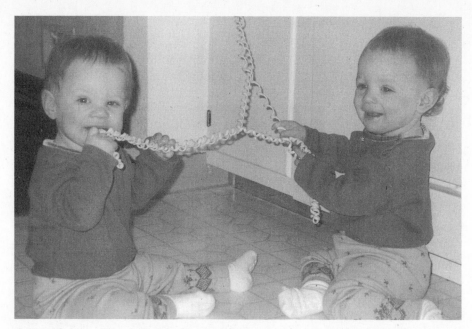

Entwined sisters: These MZ girls shared a single sac and were born with their cords entangled! (They were supervised for this photo.)

side crowded vacation periods are major bonuses. Children can socialize with other home-schooling families and participate in extracurricular activities with schooled children. Home-schoolers tend to get involved in their own projects and watch less TV — often the major attraction after a day at school. At home, learning is continuous!

Acquiring Language Skills

Language is essential for us to communicate with others and also to define thoughts and concepts for ourselves. Children learn to speak by imitation and correction. First-born singletons usually do better with language acquisition because parents, rather than siblings, are the models for speech.

The effects of twinship on speech development are being studied. Multiples spend more time speaking at the same developmental level and are slower to develop language skills. There is a limited use of words, and mistakes and mispronunciations are prolonged. Multiples reinforce each other's stuttering, stammering, and lisping unless the parents take remedial action. Pointing may also persist as a substitute for speech.

The development of language usually follows a given sequence, beginning with babbling and cooing sounds, recognition of parents' voices, and turning toward sound from age six weeks to six months. Babies at this phase also enjoy getting a parent's attention by mimicking sounds. From 9 to 12 months infants learn to understand simple commands, and at about a year they will use true speech and speak simple words like *mama, papa, dog, apple.* True speech for twins may not occur until 15 to 18 months.

Consonants near the front of the mouth (*m, d, b, t, p, n*) are the easiest sounds to make. The year-old child responds appropriately to different sounds and some instructions and enjoys imitating. Usually a child understand at least three dozen words by 14 months and by 18 months is speaking about ten words. Girls speak earlier, and a first-born girl twin born at term reaches the same standard as a singleton. Monozygotic twin boys have taken longer than 18 months (like Einstein!) before saying their first word.

Toward the second year, a child will use two-word combinations (such as "all gone") and will begin to attach adjectives to nouns: "big apple," "nice ball." At this age a child enjoys identifying pictures in books and the parts of the body. Twins may combine their names.

Between the second and third years, a child can use about 3 to 6 words in a sentence. He or she asks questions and uses negatives. Some sounds, such as *ch, sh,* and *th,* may be difficult to pronounce. From the third to fourth year, the sentence length increases, with more questions. The child can invert verbs and use plural nouns. By the age of four, according to the Cincinnati Speech and Hearing Center, the child can use all possible sentence types and has correct grammar, if not articulation, and can recount experiences and follow directions. The challenge for multiples is that their parents tend to speak in less complex sentences to them and they lag behind in speaking in complex sentences, too. Some parents are too busy to devote much time to encouraging and reinforcing correct speech.

Twin Talk

Twins sometimes exchange all kinds of sounds that they clearly understand. Their own special form of communication may develop if they are mostly left alone to play together. "Twin talk" may consist of private abbreviations, unique body language, and made-up words. This occurs more so with MZ than DZ twins, which we would expect, but the greater frequency among boys is not understood.

Twins of any sort share the curious experiences of accommodating to a peer companion even from the beginning; even in the womb; of entering the world with an established side-kick rather than alone, of acquiring speech and other basic skills à deux in the meanwhile sharing a language beyond speech and before speech — Language is for relating to Others.

— John Barth,
The Making of a Writer

Twins variably and creatively negotiate the pressures of a unitary identity whether in terms of compliance, contestation or denial.

— Elizabeth A. Stewart

Nobody had a clue what any of their language meant. The twins clearly understood it all. They even had special names for each other — Ter and Tar.

They don't really have a twin language, but they copy each other's baby talk. They clearly understand each other better than we do.

They were like alien beings when they talked to each other in their own weird sounds.

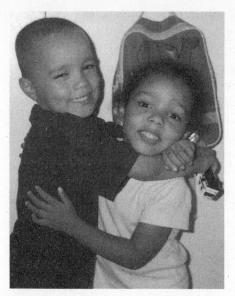

Yes, we are twins!

Malmstrom found that almost half the surveyed parents of twins reported observing "twin effects" such as nonverbal communication in place of spoken words, using a "team name" and singular verbs to refer to themselves together, and using the pronoun *me* when they meant the pair.

The medical terms for invented twin speech are *idioglossia* and *idiolalia*. Sometimes it is called *cryptophasia* or *cryptoglossia*, which means "not communicable to others." In fact, twins are aware of this phenomenon and do not use their special language with others. Nevertheless, siblings can often figure out the babble.

Development of audio-vocal skills depends very much on the home situation and the parents' social and economic levels. A study in France on language development found that twins performed less well on verbal tests (an average delay of six months with lowest scores achieved by MZ twins). However, they had better scores on perception and performance. The fact that twins scored in the normal range on motor and postural tests showed that there was no neurological deficit. The low performance on social skills and language points to environmental factors. Similarly, surviving twins score higher on verbal and reasoning tests after the loss of the co-twin.

Improving Language Acquisition

Talking and reading to your multiples is the best way to improve their language skills. Encourage the less vocal multiple to talk. Speak often and clearly to each one separately, using his or her name.

Parents need to keep modeling correct pronunciation. Intelligence tests are slanted toward language skill, which probably explains why twins score a few points below the average singleton (apart from prenatal factors such as being born preterm and of low birth weight). The

Louisville Twin Study found that while twins lagged below singletons on intelligence tests at age four, by age six they had caught up.

Parents with concerns about language delay should have their twins checked for physical problems such as hearing loss. Sometimes this is unrecognized because parents have a low expectation of language skills in the twin situation. However, Malmstrom warns against undue anxiety and suggests that parents relax and enjoy their twins' language idiosyncrasies. She also points out that their environment, which requires twins to take turns even in infancy, gives twins an edge over singletons in learning the art of conversation.

The Cincinnati Speech and Hearing Center suggests that parents seek professional help in the following situations:

- Anytime you suspect a child isn't hearing properly.

- If the child does not use two-word combinations by age two and a half.

- If by three and a half years, the child doesn't have intelligible speech.

- If the child has persistent articulation problems past age five with *p/f* and *b/v*, and distortions of *l, r, s, ch, sh,* and *j*.

- If the child had a difficult birth or illness in early infancy and you suspect any problem later.

Persistent speech difficulties can be evaluated by a speech therapist. A child may also have a mechanical problem with the tongue or palate. You can contact the American Speech-Language-Hearing Association at www.asha.org or 800-638-8255. Hearing loss may also be involved. Approximately 25 percent of children by age two have had several untreated illnesses leading to fluid in the middle ear, which can result in hearing loss and subsequent problems with language. (Milk can be the culprit; see the discussion on dairy products in Chapter 8 and the Resources.)

The Massachusetts Institute of Technology (MIT) Twins Study is a long-term study of language development in twins, supervised by Jennifer Ganger, Ph.D., and Professor Steven Pinker, Ph.D. The goal of the project is to study MZ and DZ twins to determine the relative influence of nature and nurture in language development.

> Geminate speech — wholly dictated and structured by twinship — cannot be equated with an individual language. To do so is to overlook the essence and retain only the incidental. For in Aeolian, the words are incidental, silence is the essence. That is what makes a geminate language a phenomenon absolutely incomparable to any other linguistic form.
>
> — Michel Tournier, *Gemini*

Twins are often participants in a relationship in which they are unable to communicate about what is most important to them.

— Ricardo Ainslie

Our twins once crossed the street at a time when that was forbidden. "But we held each other's hand," they said. And so they often venture off, holding hands, giving security to each other in new and strange situations.

 ## The Twin Bond Through Life

Twins share their age, uterine environment, and family life. This bond is often closer than that of marriage or of mother and child. Twinship is especially strong in MZ pairs, who usually remain very close throughout their adult life. Dependency on each other, rather than jealousy, may be a problem. Genetically the same, and more attached than friends, MZ twins sometimes choose the same career and lifestyle. If they share an apartment or a car, much of their social life may be shared.

Many teenagers and adults deeply enjoy their twinship and resent pressures on them to be different or separate. Monozygotic twins who are reared together find their own ways to become different. In contrast, if reared apart, without such influences, their likenesses can be greater, as Bouchard's research at the Minnesota Center for Adoption and Twin Research has shown.

While twins and other multiples are paid much attention as a set, especially if they look alike, twins by themselves are individuals like the rest of us. Society's belief that twins have a special relationship causes them to expect this, and whether their twinship is strong or not, they may feel disappointed when they feel and behave like regular brothers and sisters.

Ainslie points out that "paradoxically, pressures to differentiate psychologically may help undermine the sense of identity that differentiation is supposed to safeguard." This is because the degree to which twins are different is often taken as a yardstick of their normality, and this can become a goal that is imposed by the twins themselves as well as by others. In these internal and external pressures, however, "there exists a danger of creating somewhat arbitrary points of demarcation in which some potentialities are relinquished while others are appropriated." Ainslie continues:

> The characteristics that point to differentiation (whether actual or created) in intelligence, strength and sociability also constitute points of tension . . . Rather than resolving possible concerns regarding competition and identity integration, the twins generate considerable ambivalence by the sense that certain capacities or characteristics have been distributed unequally . . . the differentiating elements that might serve to avoid competition actually contribute

to increased competitive feelings, especially if those differentiating elements involve praise, acknowledgment, or other rewards.

Members of twin pairs marry less frequently than singletons. Some twins date twins and even marry twins, as did La Vona and La Velda Rowe, who married Arthur and Alwyn Richmond. All four published a newsletter, *Twincerely Yours*. Marriage between twins can be ideal because only they truly understand the twin bond.

People search for a soul mate all their lives. When you are a twin, you are born with and begin life with a soul mate. What security, what joy!

19

Treatments to Prolong Pregnancy — To Prevent Preterm Birth and Low Birth Weight

Preterm birth is the single most important challenge with multiples. About half of all twins, 90 percent of triplets, and virtually all quadruplets and quintuplets are born before the thirty-seventh week. The rate for singletons is almost 12 percent in the United States (but lower in other countries; for example, about half that rate in France). Twins may mature a couple of weeks earlier than singletons, and some studies have shown better outcome for twins at thirty-eight than at forty weeks.

While ever-younger babies are surviving at an increasing financial, emotional, and physical cost, there has been little progress in *preventing* preterm labor or accepting that nutrition and stress play a major role. I will discuss both the medical and alternative approaches to treatment of preterm labor (PTL).

Readers must understand the situation in the United States (and increasingly elsewhere) concerning litigation. In obstetrics there are two patients, the mother and infant, and more with multiples. Physicians are reluctant to step outside the established standard of care (SOC) because alternative approaches may put them at risk for a lawsuit if something goes wrong. Therefore, many long-standing practices, such as bed rest, circumcision, and advocacy of dairy products, remain in the physicians' armamentarium purely on the basis of prevalence, when in fact research shows no benefit, or even harm. This creates a bizarre conflict between the SOC and evidence! Professionalism demands evidence-based practice but inertia, vested interests, and health insurance reimbursement for out-dated procedures ensure their persistence.

All cure starts from within out and from the head down, and in reverse order as the symptoms have appeared.
— Hering's Law of Cure

The return of the repressed . . . constitutes the illness proper.
— Freud, 1896

Throughout the book, I have focused on ways to prevent complications and to improve the placebo effect. The symptoms listed in the chart on page 113 in Chapter 7 may signal that labor is beginning or may be just typical discomforts of pregnancy. You need to be well-informed and well aware of your body and babies to stay in positive health and frame of mind.

Contractions

Excessive uterine activity, cervical effacement (thinning out of the cervix), or dilation (opening of the cervix) prior to 36 weeks, especially with a multiple pregnancy, increases the likelihood of preterm birth. Contractions alone are a poor predictor of who will actually deliver preterm. Twins often settle low down in the pelvis earlier than singletons do and the increased pressure may cause contractions, without dilation.

Unfortunately, many mothers of twins, and almost all mothers of supertwins, cannot detect contractions at all; when the uterus is stretched so taut, any additional hardening may not be felt. "Silent labor" may occur. Also, they may not be able to distinguish labor contractions from the normal contractions of pregnancy (Braxton-Hicks contractions, which are often increased) or they may confuse contractions with extra fetal movement. The significant difference between the two types of contractions is that true labor contractions will cause the cervix to open. The only way to detect changes in the cervix is by vaginal examination or vaginal ultrasound: cervical shortening seen on ultrasound is a predictor in singleton pregnancies but is less reliable where multiples are concerned.

Predictors of who will deliver preterm include a previous preterm birth, salivary estriol (a type of estrogen hormone collected from maternal saliva), fetal fibronectin testing (see below), and bacterial infection diagnosed from vaginal secretions.

Sometimes uterine contractions compensate to keep blood flowing to the mother's vital centers when she is standing. The heart works the hardest to pump blood when we are standing still — this is why soldiers faint standing at attention — and mothers of multiples whose jobs require prolonged standing often develop preterm contractions. The cardiovascular dynamics for the expectant mothers are far worse than for the soldiers, because in pregnancy, especially with multiples, there is more blood to pump and more pressure from the uterus to challenge its return to the heart.

An expectant mother of multiples must be keenly aware of her body and babies in order to maintain mutual health.

Home Monitoring of Contractions

Mothers can observe and record their uterine activity at home with either palpation (feeling with their hands) or a home uterine activity monitor (HUAM). It is important for each woman to be aware of her normal uterine activity so that she can recognize changes that may signal the onset of labor. If you feel different sensations at any time, lie down on your side and time the contractions. If you have more than five contractions an hour, you need to take action to calm your uterus.

When preterm labor is detected before the cervix has undergone significant changes and before the membranes have ruptured, it can sometimes be stopped with rest and increased fluid intake. Just as a marathon runner drinks frequently to prevent muscle cramps, so hydration must be adequate in pregnancy to prevent falling blood volume and the onset of preterm contractions. Often, just drinking several glasses of water will take care of the contractions. Take omega-3 fatty acid supplements as well.

Palpation

Lie on your left side, relax your abdominal wall, and wait; then use your hands to feel your uterus tighten, become hard, and then relax. Contractions can last from half a minute up to two minutes. Time the intervals from the beginning of one contraction to the beginning of the next.

Monitoring

A HUAM, prescribed by a physician, is an electronic sensor on a belt that is wrapped around the abdomen to record contractions. The data is transmitted by telephone to a medical center, open twenty-four hours, where a nurse or physician interprets the data and decides whether the mother should come in for further checking. Recording is usually done every other day for one hour, or if necessary, twice a day.

Home monitoring can also educate expectant mothers to detect contractions and to balance their daily periods of rest and activity. The beneficial effect of rest and fluids on contractions can be shown with a HUAM.

The effectiveness of home monitoring has not been proved but there is some evidence of cost benefit with higher-order multiples. Janet Bleyl of The Triplet Connection recommends that mothers expecting higher-order multiples start at 18 to 20 weeks and use the home monitor twice a day or until they become aware of contractions without it. Chalmers, Enkin, and Keirse, in the 1989 and 1995 editions of *A Guide to Effective Care in Pregnancy and Childbirth*, reviewed the evidence and put HUAM in the "unlikely to be beneficial category" but allowed that it "may reduce the incidence of babies born weighing less than 1,500 gms but the small trials available have high potential for bias and home uterine activity monitoring should only be adopted within adequately controlled trials."

Any reduction of preterm labor is associated with the personal support and communication mothers received from the medical staff. The daily communication initiated by the medical center (that is, a doctor or nurse calls the mother rather than the other way around) reduces the isolation that many mothers feel.

Routine Bed Rest Does Not Prevent Preterm Labor in Twins

Physicians have been recommending bed rest since it was first suggested in 1910 and promoted by Bender in the 1950s. Many orthopedic surgeons recommend bed rest, too, sometimes prolonged, for patients and pregnant women with back pain. (Such patients should seek physical therapy or other kind of manual treatment to address the cause.) Bed rest is not a treatment! It is recommended when no better ideas are available and can be as harmful as prolonged standing. Also, about half the perinatal mortality associated with a multiple pregnancy happens before thirty weeks. According to the editors of *Double Talk*, Karen Kerkhoff Gromada and Mary C. Hurlbert, "a post traumatic stress disorder has been identified among women who were on prolonged or strict bed rest during pregnancy." An article published in *Western Journal of Medicine* in 1991 compared bed rest to aging in its effects on the human body.

Studies done for the National Aeronautic and Space Administration (NASA) on preventing the aging effects of space travel have shown that just *one week* of bed rest is equivalent to *one year* of aging on the skeleton. Twenty-eight days of total bed rest caused a loss of two years worth of calcium from bones, and staying in bed for 180 days will cause loss of up to 90 percent of muscular strength. Many of the Russian astronauts have never regained their bone density in the 20 years since their journeys into microgravity — conditions very similar to bed rest.

Definitions of bed rest vary greatly, from sitting up in bed for a few days to lying down (sometimes with your head lower than your feet) continuously for weeks without even "bathroom privileges." Increased rest for an acute episode of elevated blood pressure or spotting makes sense, but prolonged bed rest for an expectant mother is a catastrophe. Often a woman goes for a routine prenatal check-up and is suddenly told to make immediate arrangements to quit work, stop care of other children at home, organize household help, and budget for reduced income. For a story of this typical scenario, see Chapter 1 of *The Brewer Pregnancy Hotline* (a CD, on-line text, and book).

Negative Effects on the Mother

Prolonged bed rest has many bad side effects, such as anxiety, guilt, anger, isolation, depression, low self-esteem, poor body image, sexual abstinence, financial stress, and need for (often expensive) help in the house, along with being labeled "sick." Common discomforts of pregnancy such as heartburn, constipation, swelling, loss of appetite, thrombosis, backache, disruption of circadian rhythms, and generalized weakness, as well as bone demineralization (osteoporosis), are made worse by inactivity. There are mental effects, too, such as impaired recall and decreased verbal fluency, concentration, and perceptual motor skills. McFee et al. in 1974 compiled a list of neuroses that resulted from bed rest. At the 2001 International Society of Twin Studies Congress, researchers in Aberdeen reported a very significant 3.25 percent incidence of thromboembolism (blood clots that travel) in cases of bed rest.

Furthermore, there is loss of protein, plus reduced glucose tolerance and insulin action. The muscles most affected by bed rest are postural because bedridden people are no longer upright. Eventually, of course, all the muscles are impaired. In addition to a loss of power, the number of small blood vessels (capillaries) supplying muscles are reduced as is the ability of the muscles to use oxygen.

There is a report of fracture of both heel bones (calcanei) in the postpartum period that resulted from iatrogenic (caused by medical treatment) osteoporosis. A thirty-five-year-old woman with a triplet pregnancy of twenty-five weeks gestation was admitted in preterm labor. Bed rest, intravenous magnesium sulfate, and intermittent subcutaneous terbutaline were implemented to control contractions *for 65 days*. The pa-

One of the hardest things about bed rest in the hospital was the feeling of isolation that came with it. Most of my family and friends didn't see the need to visit me because I wasn't sick.

— Patricia Harber (mother of triplets born at 34 weeks), *Finding Our Way*

Bed rest is anything but "restful": it is often a very stressful situation.

Bed rest for six months is hard on the body; I feel I've atrophied. Even eighteen months after the birth, I still haven't recovered my strength.

I was not just sitting at home, waiting for a due date. I wondered every day, all day, whether I would birth one, two, or no babies, alive or not, and when. It was emotionally grueling, and it seemed never to let up.

tient received weekly Betamethasone for six weeks to speed fetal lung maturation. However, the tocolysis was ultimately not successful in stopping contractions and the patient underwent a Caesarean delivery at 34 weeks gestation. Walking after the birth broke the bones in her heels!

In the British study of triplet and higher-order births, *Three, Four or More*, a table of obstetric data revealed the overuse of bed rest in the United Kingdom. For example, over 70 percent of mothers expecting quads were admitted twice for bed rest, yet only 18 percent had suspected preterm labor on the first admission and none had suspected preterm labor for the second! The only symptom for the entire group was bleeding (14 percent) for the second admission. Yet they stayed an average of 54 days, and mothers of triplets spent 30 days!

The food in a hospital may be inadequate in quantity and nutrients for those who pass their weeks or months of bed rest in that location. A falling basal metabolic rate due to lack of physical activity also results in a loss of lean muscle mass. A reduced appetite and decreased food intake further accelerate loss of muscle tissue.

Negative Effects on the Offspring

One would think that after almost a century of prescribing bed rest for various complications of pregnancy, its effects on the offspring would have been extensively studied. That is not the case. The first such study I found is from 2002 and as yet unpublished! A group of physicians in Italy found that children of women who had been placed on bed rest developed vestibular disorders. There was an increased incidence of motion sickness, the need for rocking in order to go to sleep, and increased allergies. The increased rate of allergies might be due to the common combination (in the Italian population studied) of bed rest and tocolytic drugs, which disturbs the intrauterine environment.

On the plus side, there was increased musical interest and mothers confirmed that they had listened to music while on bed rest.

Despite the risk of more complications, one in seven pregnant women in the year 2001 was put on bed rest in the United States! Most mothers expecting multiples are put on bed rest, especially those carrying larger sets.

Concurring with much earlier research, a 1996 study in Saudi Arabia found that a hospitalization for bed rest showed no effect on the length of the pregnancy or reduction in preterm delivery. The Cochrane Review states:

There is currently not enough evidence to support a policy of routine hospitalization for bed rest in multiple pregnancy. No reduction in the risk of preterm birth or perinatal death is evident, although there is a suggestion that fetal growth is improved. For women with an uncomplicated twin pregnancy the results of this review suggest that *it may be harmful in that the risk of very preterm birth is increased.* Until further evidence is available to the contrary, *the policy cannot be recommended for routine clinical practice* (italics mine).

A study of 107 women concluded furthermore that "there is not enough evidence to evaluate the use of a bed rest in hospital policy for women with suspected impaired fetal growth." Interestingly, the report noted that women's opinions about the care they received were reported rarely. I hope these reviews will "put to rest" decades of controversy that have immobilized expectant mothers and created adverse outcomes!

Chalmers, Enkin, and Keirse in the 1989 and 1995 editions of *A Guide to Effective Care in Pregnancy and Childbirth* reviewed the evidence for bed rest and put it in the "unlikely to be beneficial category" for twins and "unknown" for higher-order multiples.

Alternatives to Bed Rest

Expectant mothers of multiples need moderation of activity through reduced work hours and workload, and regular rest in different positions. Ask your doctor about going on disability to reduce the physical demands of work and household maintenance, or seek a second opinion if bed rest is recommended to you. It is better to boost your nutrition and hydration and to consult some of the practitioners who offer telephone hypnosis for preterm labor contractions before opting for immobility and drugs. Remember the well-nourished mothers of multiples who carry their babies to term.

I advocate *plenty of rest* for all pregnant women, especially mothers awaiting multiples. Ideally, after drinking water (two liters a day) they should lie down on one side (the left side has a slight advantage for return of blood flow to the heart, but either side is fine) to rest at least two or three times a day. A foam wedge to support your belly when you rest on your side is a necessity and its firm incline works better than pillows (see Spurlin in Resources). Lying prone (on the front) in pregnancy is now possible and comfortable with the invention of the Bodycushion® designed by a massage therapist. The various foam parts can be stacked

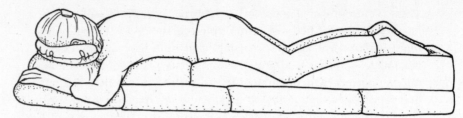

Blissful comfort lying prone.

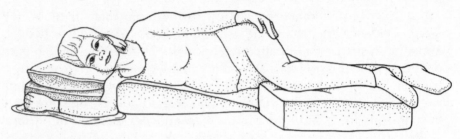

Or on your side.

to create a nice hollow for your belly, however large. The Bodycushion® can increase your comfort in all positions.

Regular massage will help your circulation and swelling as do swimming and sensible exercise. It is important to change position frequently — movement of the feet and legs generates a venous pump to return blood to the heart.

Exercises for Expectant Mothers on Bed Rest

If you do end up on bed rest, I advocate an individualized exercise program. Mobility is natural for the body. My original training was in physical therapy, and I have helped many expectant mothers admitted to the hospital for prenatal complications to exercise during their stay. Since I founded the Obstetrics and Gynecology Section (now called the Women's Health Section) of the American Physical Therapy Association in 1977, we have gained more than two thousand members across the country. You can call 800-999-APTA to find a physical therapist who has experience with pregnant women or you can do the exercises described here.

Curl-ups are the only exercises on the Essential Prenatal Exercise Chart in Appendix 4 that may increase pressure on your uterus and cervix. They are fine if you breathe correctly. *You must exhale with each movement*. Exhaling will reduce pressure in your abdomen and the fluctuations in circulation that occur with straining.

Always pay attention to your body. If contractions, blood pressure, or bleeding increase, ease off. Instead do frequent head raises on *outward* breath, supporting your abdominal muscles if necessary with your hands, as described on page 216. Pelvic tilting on hands and knees is an alternative way to exercise your abdominal muscles that will also give you a welcome change of position.

However, on bed rest, your arms and legs also get progressively weaker from lack of use. Bones lose calcium when they bear no weight. Take the longest route to the bathroom and consider lifting weights or using resistance ropes or Theraband® for your limbs.

A partner can also provide manual resistance, or you yourself can resist, for example, extension of your right elbow by placing your left palm on the back of your forearm. This will also strengthen your left biceps; such exercises work the muscles of both the resisted and the resisting limb. For the hip, you can rest your right ankle on your left thigh. Push down to resist the raising of your left foot onto the toes. You can feel this work important muscles of your right hip as well as your left calf.

Think "navel to spine" during all movements. This will help to stabilize your pelvis and lower back.

I cannot emphasize enough the importance of proper breathing during exercise. Without it, you may do more harm than good.

Also do frequent movements with your limbs. Slide your heel up and down the bed to bend and straighten your knee and hip. Circle your ankles and pump your feet. Stretch your arms over your head. Circle your shoulders, twist your trunk with your arms outstretched, clasp your hands behind your back. These exercises will improve your posture and open your chest. Remember to tighten your pelvic floor muscles frequently, too (as if you were stopping the urine flow).

Suggest to your doctor that you swim in a pool to maintain mobility. A 1990 article by Katz et al. in *Obstetrics and Gynecology* found immersion more effective than bed rest in treating edema of pregnancy. Being in water also decreases contractions, which is why those planning to give birth in a tub do not get in it until labor is well established. You may find access to a pool at a health club or hotel spa.

My family brought in so much stuff for me to do — it took 2 days to get it all home! I had made friends with a woman having triplets through a multiple births class. She and I were in and out of the hospital at the same times so I would get a wheel chair ride into her room and get to visit with her for a few minutes every few days.

Activities During Bed Rest

Here are some hints to lighten the sentence. Contact other mothers of multiples who were put on bed rest; multiples clubs, such as The Triplet Connection, maintain such a list. These women, as well as doulas and physical therapists, may visit you at home. Use this time to catch up on reading and other hobbies and to learn more about multiples. A laptop computer, if you can afford to buy or lease one, will connect you to the Internet and many sites have chat rooms. Subscribe to a flat-rate long-distance telephone service. In the Resources, you will find organizations with information for pregnancy, birth, and postpartum. Join some of these groups and send for their literature and newsletters. Learn about child development. Prepare the birth announcements.

Some women are very intimidated by bed rest and don't even think to ask their doctor about going out for a quiet dinner with their partner, which in most cases would be a welcome boost to their morale.

Bed rest provides plenty of time for communicating with your unborn babies through touch, visualization, and meditation. In this stressful situation you want to communicate your feelings to them, even of frustration, impatience, anger, or fear. Explain to your babies what is happening.

Daily singing is a joyful activity that deepens breathing and provides some toning for your abdominal muscles. It also exposes your babies to a wide range of pitch that will benefit their later learning skills. This helps to compensate for the lack of prenatal movement that your babies will experience when you are stationary.

Psychological Issues with Prenatal Complications

Preterm labor can result from emotional or economic stress, poor nutrition (especially inadequate essential fatty acids), an undetected infection, or simply work overload. The following comments are intended to increase awareness of the psychological aspects of prenatal complications such as preterm labor and hypertension. Women tend to feel guilty when such problems occur; and new insights can increase understanding and acceptance and thus decrease this guilt about what they did or didn't do.

Unless the cause is understood, only the symptom is treated. As mind and body are one, our dysfunctions and diseases also have a symbolic role — they are telling us something. Holistic health care providers ask why a person has the symptoms she does, at this point in time, and at a particular location in the body.

We have known since the 1989 Congress of the Pre and Perinatal Psychology Association of North America (now called the Association for Pre and Perinatal Psychology and Health), when Ann Evans presented new information about preterm labor, that if a woman had experienced sexual abuse by a caretaker prior to the age of eighteen, she was twice as likely to deliver before 34 weeks of gestation and two and a half times more likely to have a newborn with a medical problem. This occurred regardless of the number of previous babies, education, race, alcohol or cigarette abuse, or history of other physical abuse in childhood. Considering that sexual abuse is estimated to affect 60 percent of girls, this topic should be reviewed with every woman.*

Obstetrician David Cheek was a skillful hypnotherapist (he assisted the FBI) who considered preterm labor "a preventable disease — *if* you can talk to the mother." Before he learned to ask his expectant mothers about fear, he had a 7 percent preterm birth rate in his practice and the low-birth-weight babies often did not survive. After he helped mothers in preterm labor bring unresolved issues to their conscious minds, his incidence of preterm births dropped to 1.6 percent.

Cheek believed that doctors unintentionally arouse anxiety in pregnant women by comments that may seem benign, such as "well, your cervix is a bit soft" or "you're not very tall" or "your pelvis is on the small side." He was one of the first to recognize the nocebo effect and to avoid it in his practice. Cheek observed that when there is a haunting problem in a woman's life, a stress response begins to build. She dreams at a level that precludes recall, and tuning in to the normal contractions of her uterus, she now experiences them as painful. This in turn leads her to worry about preterm labor . . . more tension . . . more painful contractions . . . more risk. Cheek also taught that a baby who is afraid may trigger preterm labor. He found that if mothers would reassure the babies verbally that they were safe and should remain inside, the labor would stop.

Such psychological influences are not included in typical studies on preterm labor that look at the effects of drugs or bed rest. It is time to acknowledge the brain! Research by Candace Pert at the National Insti-

---

*Psychohistorian Lloyd deMause includes the prison population, the mental health population, and those for whom the memory is still unconscious to reach this figure.

tutes of Health in her book *Molecules of Emotion* has shown, its effects are everywhere in the body and one thought can set off a chain of distant reactions through substances called neurotransmitters.

The more pregnancy and birth are managed by technology, the less mothers trust their bodies and their intuition. Some women go into preterm labor because they may unconsciously believe that it is easier to deliver smaller babies or they worry about carrying such a load to term. Other women have such financial and emotional stress that they feel they are "falling apart" and the babies are falling out symbolically. The former Twin Services in Berkeley, California, published a report with the apt title *Twinshock* that discussed the often staggering physical, nutritional, emotional, and economic demands on the parents. Black teenage girls having their first pregnancy and carrying MZ twins (although this is not always known before birth) are at greatest risk for preterm labor.

Hypnosis

Cheek, pediatrician Marshall Klaus, and social workers Phyllis Klaus and Gayle Peterson all have successfully used telephone hypnosis in cases of preterm labor. When a woman calls with preterm contractions, she is almost in a trance with fear. Over the phone, she is asked to go back to the time when she was comfortable and nothing eventful was going on and then to move forward to whatever can tune her in to her uterus to discover what led to the contractions. (Contact information is listed in the Resources.)

Body-centered hypnosis developed by Gayle Peterson (see the Web site www.askdrgayle.com) has proven to be a powerful tool for increasing the likelihood of normal delivery and developing the bond between mother and unborn child. It addresses the mother's fears and concerns through vocal techniques, intonations, and symbols to encode messages aimed at decreasing anxiety and increasing confidence and well-being. Techniques for reaching the unconscious, such as tonality, phrasing, and cadence, are embedded in language and images — a lovely form of labor poetry. Gayle will make a customized tape in person or over the telephone, but if neither is possible you can buy a generic tape. Side one provides thirty minutes of relaxation with suggestions for enhancing your enjoyment of pregnancy and to help you carry to term. Side two is for use in the last two weeks of pregnancy to prepare for birth. It continues the relaxation and includes birth visualization with suggestions woven in to help you in labor.

When I train graduate physical therapists in Women's Health (including the care of high-risk pregnancies at home and in the hospital), I advise them to encourage the pregnant women to share their emotional concerns while they do their exercises. Hospitals are often understaffed and personnel are overworked, making emotional support scarce. Physical therapists visit with mothers for a longer time than other health care providers, helping them move, stretch, and change position. Active listening (rephrasing statements, encouraging elaboration) has helped mothers identify and resolve personal issues, reducing their symptoms.

A key question is "Perhaps your body is expressing something your mind may be repressing?"

An expectant mother needs to share her feelings about her pregnancy without judgment by others. Even reassurance is a put-down: listening is what she wants. Feelings are different from behavior, but they are just as real and must be recognized and validated. Expectant parents of multiples need even more support, education, and counseling, and these should continue throughout the first few years after birth.

Hospitalization

If you are admitted to a hospital for preterm labor, the standard of care includes monitoring for contractions, examination of your cervix, and ultrasound to check the babies, placentas, amniotic fluid volume, and cervical length. You may be put on an intravenous drip for hydration. If contractions increase and cause changes in the cervix and you are less than 34 weeks pregnant, IV magnesium sulfate (epsom salts) may be used to sedate the uterus. Once the contractions have decreased, it can be stopped and other agents may be given orally (see below).

Fetal fibronectin testing, salivary estriol testing, and a culture for Group B streptococcus may be done. Antibiotics may be prescribed prophylactically ("just in case") because with preterm labor there is a risk of infection. It is important to test the multiples after birth for this Group B infection, because on rare occasions one baby appears to be in perfect health for a couple of weeks but death can occur as "late onset" infection. One mother who wrote to me lost one twin at three weeks from this infection after a very easy pregnancy. She was tested and treated, but not the babies, and the one who died was the second-born, who was exposed longer to her infection.

Tocolytics

Tocolytic medications (beta-mimetics) are used in the attempt to sup-press preterm labor and were administered in 2 percent of all pregnan-cies in the United States in 2000. Ritodrine (Yutopar®) was approved by the U.S. Food and Drug Administration by the end of 1988 but has since been taken off the market for reasons explained by Gail Krebs in *The Brewer Pregnancy Hotline*:

> Any drug powerful enough to subdue established uterine activity has to have equally powerful side effects and ritodrine was no ex-ception. Ritodrine did not work selectively on uterine muscles. It also interfered with the normal activity of the heart, intestine, blood vessels, and lungs. For this reason, women receiving ritodrine expe-rienced frightening disturbances in heart rate, blood pressure, and breathing. Large numbers of women treated with ritodrine felt as though they were about to collapse because of shortness of breath and a racing heart. These are not merely psychosomatic reactions to the stress of finding oneself unexpectedly in labor. Reports of mater-nal and fetal deaths attributed to ritodrine therapy began to rise in the medical journals.

The Brewer Hotline received calls almost daily from women who were being given ritodrine despite the manufacture's contraindications, which included diminished blood volume (hypovolemia), ruptured membranes, preeclampsia, overactive thyroid, heart disease, diabetes, and hypertension.

Today ritodrine has been replaced by terbutaline (Breathine®, used for asthma), which has very similar side effects such as increased heart rate for mother and babies, palpitations, tremors, anxiety, and low blood pressure. It has not been approved by the FDA but it is widely pre-scribed, given intravenously or by mouth or under the skin — a method that is called subcutaneous terbutaline pump therapy.

Indomethacin/Indocin may be given as a rectal suppository or by mouth: it is actually an anti-inflammatory drug used mostly for arthri-tis. Magnesium sulfate is given by IV. Nifedipine or Adelat with the drug name Procardia is used for high blood pressure but will also slow labor. In the United Kingdom, Salbutomal (Inspiryl) or Ventolin (medications like terbutaline for asthma) are used. On the Web site http://www.pneumotox.com/pneumotox/geppix.html, I found ten ar-

Contraindications to Tocolytic Drugs for Preterm Labor

ABSOLUTE	RELATIVE
Severe pregnancy-induced hypertension	Mild chronic hypertension
Severe abruption of the placenta	Mild abruption of the placenta
Severe bleeding from any cause	Stable placenta previa
Infection of the amniotic fluid	Maternal cardiac disease
Fetal death or anomaly incompatible with life	Hyperthyroidism
Severe intrauterine growth restriction	Uncontrolled diabetes mellitus
	Fetal distress
	Fetal anomaly
	Mild intrauterine growth retardation
	Cervix dilated more than 5 cm
	Pulmonary edema (congestion)

ticles on pulmonary edema. They are in English but the group was founded in France in 1995 to provide information regarding individual cases, collect and update literature on drug-induced lung disease, publish updated lists of offending compounds, and formulate warnings when new side effects of drugs become known.

Chalmers, Enkin, and Keirse, in the 1995 edition of *A Guide to Effective Care in Pregnancy and Childbirth*, reviewed the evidence for oral beta-mimetics and wrote that the health gain was "unknown" because of an inadequate number of controlled trials.

A steroid drug such as Betamethasone, Metamethasone, or Dexamethasone is usually given two to seven days before the birth, between twenty-four and thirty-four weeks, to speed maturation of the babies' lungs and prevent respiratory distress after birth (see Chapter 18). These drugs, however, can mask infection in the mother. Betamethasone is used more frequently, because fewer doses are needed. Two shots, usually twenty-four hours apart, are injected into a muscle. The ACOG recommends the same dose as for singletons although others advocate higher dosages in the case of multiples.

Sometimes repeat shots are given after one week. These steroids will not cause growth of facial hair or muscle development, but women with diabetes often have very high blood sugars after the steroid shots. Therefore, blood sugars will need to be tested frequently, and more insulin may be needed.

Controversy surrounds the use of steroids before and after birth because repeated doses can cause brain damage in the newborns. The number of repeat shots needed, or even the necessity of repeat shots, is unknown. The Cochrane Review found that "there was not enough evidence to evaluate the use of repeated doses of corticosteroids in women who remain undelivered, but who are at continued risk of preterm birth."

Administration of Tocolytics

Usually the drugs are given by IV or injection to stop the contractions. After the contractions have been controlled for at least twelve hours, the mother will be given pills to take every 2 to 4 hours, even at night, if her pulse is less than 140 beats per minute. This oral medication may be continued until the thirty-sixth or thirty-seventh week.

Intravenous treatment requires hospitalization, often long term, and has significant side effects. The subcutaneous terbutaline pump (SQTP) allows medication to be infused under the skin very slowly and continuously in very small doses. Additional larger doses can be programmed for automatic delivery during periods when the mother experiences strong uterine contractions — often in the late afternoon or early evening. The total dose over a 24-hour period is less than 4 mg compared with up to 30 mg with oral medication. Side effects are reduced and the treatment can be more effective over a longer period of time — about eight weeks on the pump versus a couple of weeks orally.

Management of the pump is easy to learn, but a few days of hospitalization is necessary to determine the appropriate doses and to allow the mother to feel comfortable. Together with home monitoring, you can be followed outside the hospital and there is no need to awaken at night because of the automatic continuous infusion.

Side Effects

Your pulse may increase up to 30 beats per minute above normal. The medication also stimulates the nervous system, making you feel jittery, and you may develop tremors.

Possible fluid buildup in your lungs (pulmonary edema) will be monitored by checking your weight daily as well as your fluid intake and urine output. Nausea, vomiting, and constipation result from the gastrointestinal system becoming less active. Blood vessels expand as a result of this medication, causing you to feel very warm, and headaches can develop. There may be an increase in your glucose level and a decrease in your potassium level as measured by blood tests. All these side effects are more pronounced with the initial treatment but diminish when the medication changes to pills. All medications cross the placenta, and the babies' heartbeats or blood sugar values may be affected.

Karen Sundfors, a mother of preterm twins, has two Web sites to educate others about her experience with bed rest and terbutaline: http://www.geocities.com/HotSprings/Villa/3604/ and http://pages.ivillage.com/bh/twins73/. She says:

> I had a bad experience with terbutaline and magnesium sulfate in 1997 when I was pregnant with my daughters. I developed some complications, including a heart problem after delivery, that I attribute to my 5 weeks on the terbutaline pump and a potentially dangerous combination of terbutaline and mag sulfate in the hospital.
>
> In researching at a medical library, I was stunned to discover that these drugs are used "off label," that there is little evidence that they work after 24–48 hours (or sometimes even at all), and that they can cause a host of serious side effects and complications. I was never informed of the risks. The FDA warning against using the terbutaline pump was released about 3 months after I delivered my daughters. I had not been told the pump is experimental.

Tocolytic drugs are used frequently in multiple pregnancies in the United States because according to the standard of care, it is better to do something than nothing. This does not pass muster with evidence-based practice demanded today. In 1979, a British Medical Journal editorial, "Drugs in Threatened Preterm Labor," observed:

> The tacit assumption that inhibiting preterm labour is necessarily beneficial should not go unchallenged. Indeed, preterm labour may often be nature's best option in that the precipitating cause may be acute or chronic impairment of placental function.

Krebs explains that a uterus trying to evacuate the babies may actually be a life-saving measure (depending on the NICU) and to paralyze the uterus does a disservice to mothers and babies.

There is currently no FDA-approved medication for outpatient tocolytic therapy.
— Fung Lam, M.D., F.A.C.O.G., 2003

Other Drugs Used to Stop Preterm Labor

Indomethacin inhibits prostaglandins, hormone-like substances that can trigger the onset of labor. This medication, given orally, has a side effect of initiating the closure of the ductus arteriosus, which allows blood circulation in an unborn baby. However, this effect appears to be reversible when the drug is discontinued.

Magnesium sulfate — MgSo4 — was on the vehicle license plate of the physician who first promoted it. It is used to sedate expectant mothers with high blood pressure and threatened convulsions (preeclampsia) as well as preterm labor contractions. This medication may cause you to feel warm, nauseated, sleepy, flushed, or confused. The babies, if born soon after you take the medication, may have decreased muscle tone.

Progesterone has been shown to be effective in preventing preterm labor in some research but has not been taken seriously. Presently there is a study underway at University Hospitals in Cleveland. The most promising research concerns omega-3 fatty acids as described in Chapters 7 and 8.

Readers are encouraged to follow an optimal intake of nutrients (especially omega-3 fatty acids) and fluids and to have plenty of rest to *prevent* preterm labor and thus avoid tocolytics.

Cervical Stitchery (Cerclage)

An "incompetent cervix" dilates without contractions, usually in mid-pregnancy. It is diagnosed (and often overdiagnosed) after a woman has lost a pregnancy at 18 to 22 weeks without having labor. Cerclage involves closing the cervix surgically and removing the sutures around 37 weeks prior to labor so that the cervix is not damaged. There is a risk of infection, preterm rupture of the membranes and bleeding, and even preterm labor, which it is supposed to prevent!

The cerclage, also known as the Shirodkar or MacDonald operation, involves inserting a thread, descriptively called a purse-string, around the cervix to hold it tightly closed. The intent is to prevent the lower uterine segment from being distended by the extra weight and stretching of a multiple pregnancy. But research continues to show that it has no effect in preventing preterm labor. A true incompetent cervix (which is associated with fetal loss because it opens during pregnancy) is not caused by a multiple pregnancy. This condition can result from a laser procedure (LEEP) or a cone biopsy of the cervix or an anomaly related to the use of the drug DES (diethylstilbestrol) taken by the mother's mother to prevent miscarriage. Other causes are prior obstetric or abortion trauma, curettage of the uterus, or treatment to dilate a narrow cervical canal (stenosis).

This vaginal procedure is usually done in the hospital under spinal anesthesia, and the risks of cerclage include

- Rupture of membranes at the time of cerclage placement

- Precipitation of labor due to uterine irritation during cerclage placement

- Infection of the uterus and bag of waters

- Further damage to the cervix if there are uterine contractions that tear out the cerclage

- The chance of increased complications if the cervix is very dilated or very short when the cerclage is placed

One study reported that among women who had a history of cervical incompetence and subsequently conceived twins, 66 percent of the 43 cases were successfully carried to term following a surgical suture. However, cerclage does not prolong pregnancy in women who do *not* have a history of prior pregnancy loss and may actually cause preterm delivery and pregnancy complications.

The doubled hormones produced during twin pregnancy soften the tissues, and it is normal for the cervix to be dilated before labor — up to 5 centimeters for mothers who have previously given birth. On finding that the cervix is already well dilated, some physicians fear that it is "incompetent" and panic unnecessarily. If the woman is also experiencing strong and frequent Braxton-Hicks contractions, which mothers expecting twins often do in late pregnancy, it may be incorrectly assumed that she is in preterm labor. In 1987, O'Grady stated:

> Neither routine cerclage nor prophylactic administration of tocolytics in fixed doses appears effective in reducing preterm delivery or neonatal death in twins. In the absence of cervical incompetence or preterm labor, don't use these measures.

Chalmers, Enkin, and Keirse, in the 1989 and 1995 editions of *A Guide to Effective Care in Pregnancy and Childbirth*, reviewed the evidence and found that "neither the routine use of cervical cerclage or oral be-tamimetics has been shown to reduce the incidence of preterm labour."

Delayed Interval Delivery

In recent years it has become more common to keep as many babies in the uterus for as long as possible after one has been delivered, although most physicians do not aggressively manage the pregnancy to save the remaining ones. Kurzel's study from Chicago indicated that 10 percent of second twins may be saved with cerclage, tocolytics, and antibiotics.

Amniotic fluid mechanically dilates the air sacs (alveoli) in the babies' lungs and an adequate amount must be present between 22 to 26 weeks to avoid problems (pulmonary hypoplasia). At times amniotic fluid may leak for a while, but then the hole seals over; even when it doesn't, the amniotic fluid keeps being produced and the baby can sometimes remain in the uterus a few more critical weeks. Infection is also a risk now that the baby is no longer in an enclosed sterile environment.

Tocolytic drugs do not work well when the membranes are ruptured, so bed rest in the hospital to prevent a cord prolapse may be appropriate. I summarize accounts of some cases below.

One mother had preterm rupture of the membranes (PROM) at 18 weeks and delivered a triplet who soon died. Three days later, a cerclage was done and after being dosed with terbutaline and antibiotics — Procardia, Indocin, and Metamethasone — she carried two surviving triplets to 34 weeks, who needed oxygen for only the first day after birth. She was in and out of the hospital many times and at home was using a HUAM and taking her temperature twice a day to watch for fever, a sign of infection.

Another expectant mother of triplets delivered one who was stillborn at 21 weeks and was given a cerclage and a week of IV antibiotics in the hospital. She was admitted five more times until the birth of the remaining two at 27 weeks, who then spent three months in the hospital. Her drugs included Augmentin (antibiotic), magnesium sulfate, Indocin, the terbutaline pump, and she used a HUAM.

A third mother gave birth to one infant at 18 weeks and two surviving triplets at 34 weeks. A fourth gave birth to one triplet at 26 weeks and the other two 11 days later, but the extra days made the difference between 66 and 84 days in the NICU. The first-born required oxygen for two and a half months and later needed laser surgery for eye problems.

A delayed interval delivery (also known as iatrogenic asynchronous birth) in quadruplets from Saskatoon, Canada, claims to be the second reported case of delayed delivery intervals in quadruplets who were born on three separate days. Preterm delivery of the first infant occurred at 26 weeks gestation. Active uterine contractions ceased and ultrasound showed the remaining triplets to be in separate amniotic sacs with satisfactory heart rates. With bed rest and tocolysis, the delivery of the second infant did not occur until eight days later. After a further 36-hour delay, placental abruption prompted Caesarean delivery of the remaining two. The first infant died of complications of preterm birth at seven months, while the remaining three survived and were neuro-developmentally normal one year after delivery.

A 2001 Belgian study published in *Lancet* found that girl-boy twin pairs tend to have a longer gestation period than same-sex male twins. Also, the male twin was heavier than male newborns in same-sex pairs. This suggests that the female twin is more influential in determining the duration of pregnancy, notwithstanding total fetal mass; and, further, that females may have a greater risk of fetal undernutrition in late pregnancy, which could predispose to metabolic problems later in life. The average gain in birth weight in males of mixed-sex twins was 78 gm. Their gestation length was just over 37 weeks compared with 36 for same-sex males.

The 2002 *Guinness Book of World Records* reports that Peggy Lynn gave birth to Hanna on November 11, 1995, and twin Eric on February 2, 1996, 84 days later, the longest interval between twins. The previous record was held by Mrs. Danny Berg of Italy, who gave birth to Diana on December 23, 1987, and her twin Monica on January 30, 1988, 38 days later.

The current methods for stopping preterm labor are costly and invasive, and statistically do not improve outcome. I hope by the next edition of this book, the benefits of nutrition in general, and of fatty acids in particular, as well as a sensible, balanced lifestyle with minimal stress will have been accepted as the best course for mothers and their multiples.

I had never heard of anyone whose waters had broken but whose baby was not delivered until six weeks later so if any of your readers ever happen to be in my situation, I want them to know that although it is important to be aware of the risks, there is most certainly a chance, however slim, that everything will be OK so never give up. If we had listened to the negative attitudes of others (both medical professionals and the general public), and not followed our own instincts, I doubt we would have Angus and Lockie today, and that is incomprehensible.

— Kirsten Winspear

20

The Care of Multiples Born Too Soon (Premies)

I have emphasized ways to prevent complications in bearing multiples with excellent nutrition and prenatal care. However, some congenital anomalies, handicaps, and preterm births occur without any apparent reason.

The National Institutes of Health report that the rate of preterm and low-weight births has increased in recent years, contrary to expectations, and now exceeds 11 percent of all births in the United States *despite more women seeking prenatal care*. The huge increase of multiples is blamed for the increases. It bears repeating that 57 percent of twins and 93 percent of triplets and more are born preterm, with a perinatal mortality of 74 percent and transfer rate to neonatal intensive care units of 95 percent. Second-born twins (who are more likely to have a stressful delivery) are more at risk than first-borns.

In the 1990 study on triplets and higher-order births in the United Kingdom, medical problems in the neonatal period occurred in 32 percent of twins, 53 percent of triplets, 68 percent of quadruplets, and all higher order multiples. Nearly one-third of triplets and two-thirds of quadruplets had lung problems.

Emotional Reactions of Parents to Preterm Babies

Preterm birth is a crisis in the parenting process as well as a disturbance in the development of an infant. Both mother and father are deprived of the last few weeks of pregnancy to further their psychological preparation. Mothers may go home totally empty-handed or with only one multiple or even have different babies in different hospitals.

There is no ritual or ceremony for the "ambiguous" loss of a normal pregnancy.

It is difficult to describe my first experience of holding these tiny babies who were connected to tubes that branched off in countless directions. Most of their weight came from the machines and the blankets . . . a facecloth beside them seemed the size of a blanket.

— Candi Cuppage, *Finding Our Way*

No one ever explained about NICU and it was a shock! I walked in and cried. Wayne was below his birth weight, lying face down with tubes, needles, and oxygen in and around him. If it weren't for the last name on his bed, I wouldn't have known he was mine. Looking at him I felt I had delivered an alien. His ears were transparent, there were no eyelashes or brows or shape to his body. The monitors beeped but the babies didn't cry. Although alive, they all looked lifeless.

Bonding is a challenge with one preterm and low-birth-weight infant, let alone two or more. Parents need time to identify with their babies moving jerkily in an incubator with a maze of tubes, wires, and electrodes covering their tiny bodies.*

What parents see is markedly different from the "ideal" picture of a healthy baby. Looking like little old people, preterm babies are often scrawny and wrinkled, with disproportionately large, long heads. Sometimes they are still covered with fetal hair (lanugo). An arm may be the size of your finger and a cup could fit on the head.

Mothers often chastise themselves that they did not deliver a full-term baby. They struggle to believe that the infants are real and will both survive, especially if one is very sick or has a potential handicap. Maternal love is supposedly instant and boundless, according to our conditioning, and the mother who finds little appeal in babies who sleep most of the time, react very little, or cry a lot and never smile must also battle with diminished self-esteem. This is heavy-duty pressure on a first-time mother who is creating a concept of herself as a parent.

Generally, the more babies there are, the smaller each individual member of the set is. Parents may take heart from the example of the Dionne quintuplets (born in Canada in 1934) of whom the smallest weighed 2 pounds. These babies were born and cared for at home with simple measures, such as the warmth of the open oven.

The Mauss triplets, like the Dionne babies, weighed less than 3 pounds each at their birth in 1900 and were kept in a shoebox in the warming oven of a coal stove. The *Guinness Book of World Records* lists the lowest birth weight for surviving twins as 2 pounds, 3 ounces *combined* weight. They were born in 1931 in England.

Prematurity is a risk factor for child abuse and so is multiple birth. Sheer exhaustion and feeding problems add to these factors to create a situation needing urgent support.

Ocean Robbins (the son of author John Robbins) describes how deeply saddened he and his wife were when their babies came nine weeks shy of term, weighing 1,518 grams (3 pounds, six ounces) and 1,349 grams (2 pounds, 15 ounces), causing them to spend six weeks in an intensive care nursery.

> This has been one of the great lessons of parenting, right from the start. We have been asked to love all we can, with everything we

*Most of these are external, however, so the set-up often looks more invasive than it is.

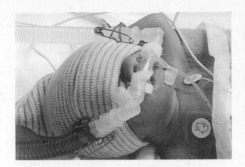

Angus on a ventilator in NICU, birthweight, 1125 gm.

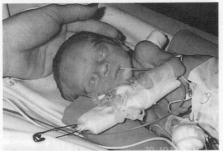

Away from his co-twin, Lockie, who weighed 1350 gm.

In the beginning, I felt cheated that I had eaten all the right food, taken vitamins and even the steroid injections, yet my babies were sick. But they survived, they are beautiful, and I now count my blessings instead of feeling sorry for myself.

The nurses kept reminding me that they were my babies but I never felt free to handle them. I was afraid. Their fragile condition made it difficult for me to do the usual mothering.

Neonatal care can sustain life . . . but it does not always restore health. Used indiscriminately, it can inflict and perpetuate dreadful suffering.
— Helen Harrison,
The Preterm Baby Book

have, and surrender. Our children come through us but not from us; they are our children and yet they are also and even more fundamentally children of God; we give them everything we have, and leave their destiny to the hands of a higher power. Sometimes, things go well, sometimes they are more difficult. Our task as parents is to love unconditionally, and to bring forth the highest and best we can, regardless of the circumstances we are given. We do not control what life brings us. We do choose how much love, intention, and purpose we bring to the choices we make.

That's where our power lies. That's where we live from. I am profoundly broken open, in awe, in grief, and in love. I feel like the rain is pouring, and the sun is shining, and rainbows are filling the sky, all at the same time.

Neonatal Care

Neonatology is a subspecialty of pediatrics that is about thirty-five years old. Technological developments in this field have dramatically affected the survival of very-low-birth-weight (VLBW) infants — those weighing less than 1,500 grams (3 pounds, 5 ounces). Twenty-five years ago only 40 percent of these babies survived. Today, the survival percentage has more than doubled, and most VLBW survivors grow up without major handicaps. However, infants born weighing less than 750 grams (1 pound, 10 ounces) still have an overall mortality rate of 20 to 30 percent. Among the survivors, approximately one-third have handicaps serious enough to be diagnosed in infancy.

Parents should expect to be fully informed of the risks and benefits of proposed treatments, of alternative treatments, and of no treatment at

I had two tiny blankets for my son during his NICU stay, and I would sleep with one next to my chest each night so it would smell like mommy, and I would trade them off in his Isolette.

Even though I feel like a stranger to these babies, I do feel that after 3 miscarriages and being over 40 years old, God has given me twins! What a tremendous gift!

Snugly and Wuggly had been in separate Isolettes (a form of incubator) until the moment of transfer. But now, two days after birth, they were brought together for the first time outside the womb. Snuggly was put in their transfer Isolette first, on his back, wrapped in blankets. Wuggly came in second, also on his back, to Snuggly's right. Both had their arms fully wrapped up in their blankets. Wuggly somehow managed to dislodge his right arm from the blanket, and immediately reached it across his body and straight over to Snuggly's face, which he tenderly stroked. Snuggly turned his head to face Wuggly, opened his eyes for just the second time I had ever seen, and gazed at his brother. Wuggly continued gently touching his brother's nose. I burst into tears. I could feel the love between them, and their joy at being reunited, and was utterly overwhelmed.

— Ocean Robbins

all. They should question the evidence supporting neonatal therapies, consult the medical literature, or seek a second or third opinion.

Involved, informed parents can have an important influence not only on their own babies' care but also on the care of countless others. Activist parents have been at the forefront of campaigns to reform nursery policies, to humanize the NICU environment, and to alert the public and medical community to dangerous or inhumane medical practices. For example, it was NICU parents who first called attention to the hazards of AIDS-infected blood transfusions, to the potential dangers of high-intensity fluorescent lighting, and to the cruelty of unanesthetized infant surgery in the United States.

Parents of a premie suddenly have many pressing questions. What are the chances of survival for their infants? Will there be any disabilities? What about medications, procedures, and treatments in the NICU? What happens after the NICU? When can the babies go home? Anxiety is a normal reaction and motivates parents to seek information and support at this time. The neonatologist will be able to give you the best estimate of your infant's chances because he or she can take into consideration many of the above factors. But no estimate is perfect. Some babies suddenly get sick and die unexpectedly; others defy all odds.

Ten Basic Questions to Ask Your Neonatologist When Your Premie Is Admitted to the NICU

1. What are my baby's chances for survival, of facing various degrees of handicap, and of having long-term health problems?
2. What medical problems are affecting my baby now?
3. How can I get more information about my baby's problems?
4. How are those problems being treated?
5. What side effects could those treatments have?
6. Are there reasonable alternative treatments we could consider?
7. How can I get more involved in my baby's care?
8. What can I do to best nurture my baby?
9. How do I find emotional or spiritual support?
10. Can the NICU's social worker help me with transportation, local housing, financial aid, or other practical problems while my baby is in the newborn ICU?

(Courtesy of Dr. D. Derleth and Preemie-L, the Web site and e-mail support group for parents of premies)

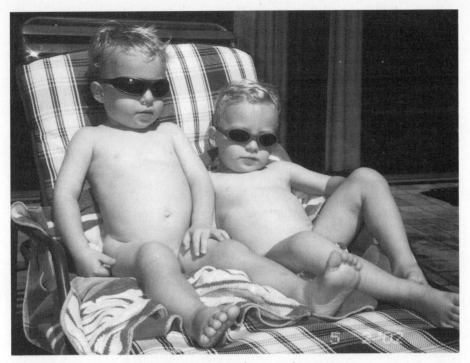

Angus and Lockie, healthy and happy at age 2¹/₂, were born at 28 weeks.

You see your baby suffering. You worry about lasting problems. You wonder if death might be better. You think you shouldn't feel this way when doctors and nurses with machines are working so hard to maintain your child's life. But the feelings of attachment were always there. The baby seemed like a part of myself, yet it was painful for me to be with him. I wanted to end his suffering.

Three of the quads soon joined the "Kilo Club" (2.2 pounds) but the fourth took much longer.

Find out if your NICU provides resources for parents such as books, videos, or articles for loan. If you have other children, check if any in-hospital support exists, such as a sibling room or day nursery with toys.

The Neonatal Intensive Care Unit (NICU)

Not all hospitals have the technical equipment and trained personnel to provide advanced life support for a "bulk delivery" of preterm infants. Level II nurseries are for infants requiring minimal oxygen support as well as intravenous therapy. Level III nurseries provide neonatal intensive care; such units are often in a regional center to which high-risk expectant mothers and babies are brought by ambulance or helicopter, if necessary.

Modern hospitals now have 24-hour visiting and encourage parental contact with the babies. Babies need their parents' care, feeding, and handling in order to thrive, just as the parents need to perform these nurturing activities to bond with their offspring. Such contact may be difficult if the mother is recovering from a difficult labor, a Caesarean, or

Make sure that your premie babies get your breast milk. Don't let the staff tell you it is not calorically right; on the contrary, it is better for the babies than the breast milk of a term mother.

One of my triplets was fed formula because the doctor thought my milk had too many calories. The two babies who received my milk thrived, but the one on artificial nourishment did poorly. Yet the doctor argued that my milk would harm him. I insisted on breast-feeding him, and in a short time that baby's health turned around.

other complications. Mothers miss the body contact that follows a normal delivery but soon they can do kangaroo care, described below.

Preterm babies usually stay in the hospital until 36 to 37 weeks gestational age (GA), although babies with very complicated medical problems remain longer. Each day costs about $2,000 per baby just for residence in the NICU. Medications and consultations are additional charges.

Feeding Preterm Babies

Start to express colostrum from your breasts, several times a day, within 24 hours after the birth (milk itself will be produced three days after the birth). Colostrum and breast milk contain white blood cells, antibodies, and other valuable properties that help a preterm baby resist infection as well as important nutrients. Recent studies have shown that such breast milk is higher in certain nutrients and infection-fighting antibodies than the milk of mothers of full-term babies. Also, breast milk improves the neurological development of preterm infants and helps prevent necrotizing enterocolitis (discussed under "Surgery" later in this chapter). No matter how small an amount is produced initially, emptying both breasts at once effectively builds your supply.

Parents often feel detached and helpless beside the high-tech equipment and professional staff who are caring for their infants. Mothers who breast-feed or provide milk for their preterm babies find that the emotional satisfaction helps compensate for the anguish and separation of a preterm birth.

Before 32 to 34 weeks GA, preterm babies often have difficulty coordinating sucking, swallowing, and breathing. Until this coordination is developed, they are fed via a tube into the nose or mouth. The tube may be removed between these gavage feedings. Whenever babies must be fed by tube or bottle, mother's milk remains the food of choice. Supplemental vitamins, minerals, protein, and calories may be added to meet the growth requirements of very sick or tiny babies.

Sometimes the digestive system of a preterm baby cannot handle breast milk, and a nutritional solution is given intravenously through a scalp tube (which is less likely to be dislodged) or via the navel.

After tolerating oral feedings, the baby can begin nursing or may drink from a special bottle for premies with a very small, soft nipple.

Even tiny preterm infants suckle better at the breast than the bottle. They breathe better, absorb more oxygen, stay warmer, and remain physically more stable than during bottle-feeding. However, unless you are able to be at the hospital for every feeding, some bottle feedings will be necessary. Make sure that your babies are fed your expressed breast milk.

The NICU usually has an electric breast pump (which is much easier than a manual one if you're pumping for twins or more), or you can buy your own or rent one from La Leche League, a pharmacy, or a medical supply house. You can also nurse one baby and pump milk for the other at the same time, which helps your let-down reflex. As discussed in Chapter 13, the breasts work on a supply and demand principle. The more you nurse, the more milk your breasts will produce — and the more weight your babies will gain. You just need to eat very well, drink lots of fluid, sleep whenever possible, and *pump*.

Request the nursery's guidelines for expressing, storing (in sterile bottles), and transporting breast milk. Refrigerated breast milk is best used within 2 to 3 days, but it can be frozen for a couple of months. To defrost, thaw under warm water. (Hot water and a microwave oven can destroy some of the milk's benefits.) Breast milk also separates so gently swirl to remix.

If you need help, contact the lactation consultant or breast-feeding specialists who work in the NICU. If help is not available, contact La Leche League or the International Lactation Consultants Association (see Resources).

Learning to Breast-feed

Whether your babies are first fed by breast or bottle, early feedings may be frustrating for both mother and babies. Consider these first feedings as learning sessions for you both and a time for closeness. A private room and an experienced nurse to assist with positioning your babies are helpful. Even if the babies cannot suckle yet, give the bottle during skin-to-skin contact and use the occasion for eye contact and voice stimulation. If possible, feed your babies when they are alert and hungry rather than according to a schedule.*

---

*Dr. Susan Ludington-Hoe, in her book *Kangaroo Care*, distinguishes three different states of alertness: (1) the baby is awake, (2) the baby is awake and attentive, and (3) the baby is hyperalert and slightly fearful. Obviously the second state is optimal for interaction.

It helped my let-down reflex to look at photos of my babies when I was pumping at home.

Breast-feeding was the best thing I could have done for my premies. Being the sole source of their food made me feel essential to their early existence and survival.

The staff seemed surprised that I was planning to breast-feed and just left me alone to figure out the pump by myself.

I fed one baby at a time on my breast and then would pump out any remaining milk to increase my supply.

When I first saw my babies covered with wires, it never occurred to me that I could hold them.

A premie twin who sucks weakly can be stimulated if the co-twin nurses at the same time. The strong let-down reflex will cause some milk to squirt into the weaker twin's mouth. Some babies will cough or sputter a bit at first.

You are giving your child the gift of life, the "milk of human kindness." Expressing also helps to maintain your milk supply and is a valuable contribution to your infant's welfare that only you can make. If only one multiple is receiving special nursery care, breast-feeding the other helps to keep up the supply. Donor breast milk can also be used, especially with higher-order multiples. (You may need to find this on the Internet if there is no local milk bank.)

If you have other children, it is a heavy chore for you to pump your breasts, transport the milk to the hospital, and be available for breast-feeding in the nursery. Your local Mothers of Twins Club or NICU parent support group may be able to help you handle all these responsibilities.

Kangaroo Care

Research has shown that kangaroo care is a potent intervention, treatment, and point of contact.

Skin-to-skin contact has been shown to enhance a baby's development and survival. Babies benefit from the touch, smell, sound, and warmth of their mother, father, or other caregiver. The Cochrane Review found reduced risk of infection, severe illness, and respiratory tract disease at six months follow-up after such care. The infant gains more weight per day by discharge. (There was no evidence of a difference in infant mortality.)

Preterm twins are small enough to both fit in one pouch, and the father can create a kangaroo pouch also. This keeps the babies together as well. Kangaroo care gives them a break from the high-tech equipment. Babies need soft vocalization and sensitive touch — especially by the family.

Be sure that each parent takes turns with each baby. The mother can kangaroo both babies together, lying down, each one reclining on a breast. A nurse will help you position the babies to get you started.

Two very useful videos about kangaroo care are available from http://www.kangaroomothercare.com, where you can also find KangaCarriers. These are wrap-around garments in different fabrics that can be worn by either parent to keep constant skin-to-skin contact regardless

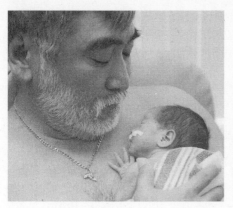 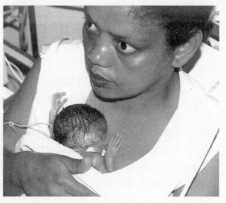

My way of coping was not to let myself realize how sick my babies were. Deep down, of course, I knew.

Fathers as well as mothers provide premie kangaroo care in the NICU.

of where you go. Keeping the babies' body temperature constant by this method helps them to conserve energy that they can expend on stronger sucking to grow faster. As I write this, there is a photo story on this Web site of Baby Stohm, who weighed 700 gms, made remarkable progress, and was eventually brought home.

An Australian site for a baby carrier is http://www.hug-a-bub.com.au.

NICU Equipment

Isolettes, also known as incubators, are closed, heated beds with transparent sides and top for observation and portholes for staff to tend the baby. Open warming beds heated with overhead infrared heat lamps give the staff easier access to a baby who requires frequent procedures. Tiny babies have little body fat and a large surface area for their weight so there is a lot of heat loss through their skin. Preterm babies also have immature sweat glands, highly permeable skin, and cannot regulate their body temperatures or hydration and require care in a constantly warmed, humid environment. Because the babies' skin color and appearance need to be monitored day and night, babies are usually naked or wear only diapers. Head caps minimize loss of body heat. Proper positioning of the babies is important. A flat-on-the-back, spread-eagle position can be highly stressful and cause problems with oxygenation. Premies are more comfortable and stable lying on their sides with arms and legs flexed close to the body. Blanket rolls provide support and a feeling of containment.

The first time I saw my twins after birth they were in their incubators. The staff wanted me to touch them, but for some reason I didn't want to; everything seemed too unreal. Pumping my breasts and reading kept me busy, but the next six weeks seemed like an eternity. Then one twin came home, followed by his sister three weeks later.

I found it helpful to keep a daily journal of events and my feelings. Knowing that we were visiting the babies, giving them expressed breast milk, plus the knowledge that they were receiving excellent care, made us feel that in time we could bring home two healthy babies, and we did.

When I walked into the nursery I was horrified at all the tubes I saw going into my babies. When the sickest baby was being ventilated she had an arterial line, a venous line, and an intratracheal tube. Ask the staff what these tubes are for; some of the leads and wires are on rather than in the baby.

Monitors continuously record vital signs such as heart rate, oxygen levels, temperature, and blood pressure, and deviations set off an alarm. Monitor alarms may be frightening at first to new parents (the leads are attached to the baby's skin and may trigger the monitor if they are accidentally disturbed). Such loud noises may also disturb the babies, causing the very disruptions of breathing (apnea) and heart rate (bradycardia) that they are intended to monitor. Request that monitor alarms, telephone bells, radios, and conversations be as quiet as possible. In particular, isolette portholes should be closed gently and a blanket should cover the top before any objects are placed on it. This blanket will help buffer noise as well as shield the baby from bright nursery lights; it is not known if their eyes are damaged by prolonged exposure to them.

The Ideal NICU

This is the vision of neonatologist Linda Cooper, M.D., who has achieved much of the following at the St. Elizabeth Health Center, in Youngstown, Ohio, where she works:

- Multiples placed together: co-bedding in isolette or cribette

- Rooming-in adjacent to the NICU for parents and babies to stay together

- 24-hour parent visitation

- Sibling visitation

- Kangaroo care

- Colorful individual clothes made especially for premies and isolette covers. (Dr. Cooper's daughter Vita makes these for her mother's NICU and won an award for community services. Tiny babies look much better in fitted clothes rather than diapers that reach to their armpits).

Complications of Prematurity

An ultrasound scan of the brain is done during the first three days. If no severe bleeding is seen, a major hurdle has been successfully cleared. If severe bleeding is seen, the chances for handicaps are much higher. The likelihood of future surgeries for hydrocephalus (excessive fluid accumulation within the skull) or for complications of cerebral palsy is greatly increased if severe bleeding occurs.

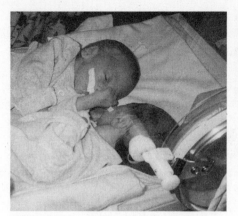

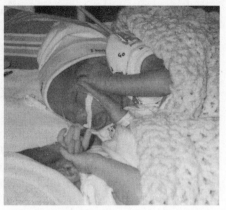

While there is usually one baby per incubator, it is important for multiples to be together where possible.

Hats prevent heat loss.

We insisted that an order be written for pain medication for the twin in the NICU. I was amazed when a staff member told us that three-month-old babies don't feel pain. I know they do. I knew that the surgery, fever, IVs, diaper rash, and diarrhea had to make her feel uncomfortable. She rested much better once she had been given an analgesic.

Even though an ultrasound of the brain is currently the best predictor of permanent handicaps while a baby is in the NICU, it is still unreliable.

Very preterm babies, if extremely ill, may be kept heavily sedated with morphine. Catheters (IVs known as "lines") are inserted into the baby's cord stump blood vessels (which have no sensation) and reduce the number of needle pokes. A central catheter may be placed in the artery of the umbilical cord stump, so blood can be withdrawn and blood pressure measured. Venous catheters bring in fluids, blood, medication, or nutrients. Oxygen monitors track saturation and ventilators assist with breathing.

Premies have poorly coordinated sucking reflexes and an immature digestive tract, which means tube feeding (gavage) or intravenous nourishment. Immaturity of the lungs, brain, liver, kidneys, and circulatory system can lead to other problems.

Their immature immune systems make them very vulnerable to infections — from the uterus during labor (especially after prolonged rupture of the membranes), or in the nursery. Careful hand washing by the staff and parents before handling the babies is important. Antibiotic treatment is begun once an infection is identified or suspected. Diuretics may be given if fluid builds up.

Breathing is the most critical function for preterm babies because their lungs are underdeveloped or do not function adequately for oxygen exchange. Assistance from a ventilator until they can breathe on their own may be needed for days, weeks, or months. Their lungs are monitored by chest x-rays, listening to their respiration, and blood analysis of oxygen and carbon dioxide levels. Mucus in the lungs is suctioned frequently.

Apnea spells — when the baby doesn't breathe for longer than fifteen seconds — are prevalent. The heart rate may slow down (bradycardia) too, so these episodes are known as "A and B spells." Gently touching the baby is usually enough to stimulate breathing again; otherwise an oxygen mask and ambu bag are used for resuscitation.* Premies who continue to have apnea at the time of discharge are often sent home with an apnea monitor and medications such as caffeine or theophylline to regulate breathing.

Jaundice

Jaundice is a condition of excessive bile pigment that gives a yellow tint to the skin and the whites of the eyes. It is caused by bilirubin, the pigment that comes from the RBX breakdown, old red blood cells in the circulation that the immature liver cannot break down. Fetal bilirubin is unstable when the baby is being given high concentrations of oxygen. High bilirubin levels can lead to brain damage. Jaundice is very common — occurring in about 80 percent of preterm babies — because there is a low concentration of the enzyme in the liver that clears bilirubin.

Phototherapy with "bililights" is the first treatment used for high bilirubin levels. Blue and white fluorescent light shine on the baby's skin to convert the bilirubin to a form that can be easily excreted by the kidneys. Eye patches protect the eyes of jaundiced babies during treatment. Bilibeds are now available and allow the baby to lie on the light source.

Anemia

Preterm babies are born with insufficient stores of iron and their blood is frequently drawn to test for anemia. Blood transfusions are sometimes required to correct this condition, and supplemental iron may be given. Breast milk contains the most absorbable form of iron, and breast-feeding is encouraged throughout the first year of life to prevent or alleviate anemia. All premies require supplemental iron during the first year of life. The last eight weeks of pregnancy is when most iron stores are laid down.

*Blood circulation problems are common in preterm babies. The ductus arteriosus (the blood vessel that directs blood away from the lungs before birth) often stays open in a premie instead of closing after birth as it would in a term baby. Indomethacin is used to close a patent (open) ductus arteriosus.

Respiratory Distress Syndrome (RDS)

Respiratory distress syndrome, formerly known as hyaline membrane disease, gained widespread public attention when President John Kennedy's preterm son died of the condition in 1963.

The syndrome develops if the baby's lung tissue is too immature to produce sufficient amounts of surfactant, a foamy fluid that coats the lungs' tiny air sacs and prevents them from closing and sticking together after each breath. Without adequate surfactant, the air sacs collapse every time the baby exhales and breathing becomes progressively difficult. Mechanical respirators assist with the lung ventilation and replacement surfactant may be given. Preterm babies who respond to the surfactant can be quickly weaned off oxygen, and the number of deaths has dropped impressively. A robust baby of at least 30 weeks will recover from RDS within about three days and be back to normal. But not all babies benefit from this treatment.

Complications of RDS

Up to one-third of the (very preterm) babies who survive RDS have some kind of residual deficit — physical, sensory, or intellectual. While eye and lung problems are the most prevalent, other side effects include damage to the vocal cords and trachea (from prolonged use of tubes in the nose and throat), hearing loss (from use of diuretics, some antibiotics, viruses, and the noise of the NICU environment), liver damage (from IV feedings), and infections (from blood transfusions).

Retinopathy of Prematurity (ROP)

Retinopathy of prematurity is a disease of the blood vessels that supply blood to the retina. The blood vessels of preterm babies have not grown all the way to the iris and they grow abnormally after birth. Bleeding and scar tissue stretch the retina, impairing vision. The condition is most common in infants with a birth weight of less than 1,250 gms and a gestational age of less than 28 weeks. The disease occurs at the time when normal blood vessel growth would approach completion, at 32 weeks of the adjusted GA.

In the 1940s, it was discovered that treating preterm babies with excessive amounts of oxygen could damage the blood vessels in the retina. Musician Stevie Wonder's blindness resulted from this condition, which is the most common cause of blindness in children today. Cases of ROP are increasing despite sophisticated oxygen monitoring, and some suf-

I had a really hard time producing or increasing my milk supply while I used the pump. I used massage, warm towels, pictures of my babies, and a tape recording of their hunger cries to stimulate my milk to let down. I was able to pump enough milk for half of the gavage feedings a day.

It took one look at my babies' tiny struggling bodies when they arrived ten weeks early to realize that if ever babies needed the benefit of their mother's milk, they did.

Every other day, I pumped my breasts to take the milk and drove three and a half hours to my surviving twin, for the two months he was in the NICU. Then I found out, like other mothers discovered, that the hospital staff just threw it away and gave her formula.

ferers actually never receive oxygen, which challenges the conclusion that oxygen causes ROP. Fluorescent lighting may have an effect.

To treat this problem, laser cryotherapy (freezing) ablates the abnormal blood vessels before they cause problems or else surgery is done to reattach the retina.

All preterm babies weighing less than 1,500 gm who receive oxygen and all VLBW babies, whether they receive oxygen or not, should be examined by an ophthalmologist at 30 to 32 weeks of adjusted GA and routinely checked until oxygen therapy is stopped. Further assessments should be made at 3, 6, 9, and 12 months of age, and later if indicated.

Bronchopulmonary Dysplasia (BPD)

Improved and more sophisticated neonatal critical care now makes it possible for the majority of infants weighing at least 500 grams to survive. This increased survival of very-low-birth-weight infants is a major factor contributing to the growing incidence of BPD, also called chronic lung disease.

This chronic lung disease occurs in preterm babies, typically with birth weights of less than 1,500 grams, who needed intensive oxygen therapy to survive RDS beyond 36 weeks adjusted GA. Approximately 20 to 30 percent of babies treated with mechanical ventilation for RDS develop this damage to some degree and require respirator treatment for a month or longer. The incidence varies greatly with birth weight, and survivors may have chronic respiratory problems because of lung scarring.

In many cases, BPD symptoms go away rapidly but other infants with BPD may have breathing difficulties for months or years. Symptoms improve with age because the lungs can grow healthy new tissue up to the

Rate of BPD Based on Weight (grams)	
501–600 gm	74 percent
601–700 gm	62 percent
701–800 gm	50 percent
1,001–1,100 gm	25 percent
1,401–1,500 gm	8 percent

age of eight. Adequate provision of calories, protein, fat-soluble vitamins, and trace elements is crucial for lung growth and healing of damaged lung tissue.

Brain Hemorrhages

Fluctuations in blood pressure may cause breakage of the fragile blood vessels in a preterm baby's brain, resulting in hemorrhages. Major hemorrhages can lead to a fluid buildup on the brain (hydrocephalus) or future developmental handicaps. Ultrasound beamed through a fontanelle (open area at the top of the skull) is used to detect hemorrhage or hydrocephalus. If hydrocephalus develops, a surgically implanted tube will drain fluid to the circulatory system or the abdominal area. This shunt usually must be kept in place for life. Sometimes a small drainage reservoir is placed under the scalp and tapped as needed.

Vitamin K is routinely given to premies to enable their liver to produce prothrombin, until their intestines can absorb it from breast milk. This supplement enhances clotting factors in the blood and reduces the probability of hemorrhage. (Vitamin K injections are often given to a woman in preterm labor, every five days until delivery. A single injection of vitamin K even just hours before the birth helps prevent bleeding.)

Surgery

Sick newborns, both term and preterm, may require various kinds of surgery such as closure of the ductus arteriosus, repair of congenital heart or spinal cord defects, installation of shunts for hydrocephalus, or repair of hernias. Chest tubes may be surgically implanted to correct pneumothorax (collapsed lung).

A serious but rare surgical emergency in premies may result from necrotizing enterocolitis (NEC) — inflammation of tissues in the intestines and colon. A baby with NEC is not fed by mouth and is treated with antibiotics. (The antibiotic Augmentin is associated with a statistically significant increase in NEC. Usually, Ampicillin and Gentamicin, Penicillin (and sometimes Metronidazole Flagyl®) are given.

If these measures fail, a portion of the damaged intestine is removed, often with the creation of a colostomy or ileostomy (an artificial opening to the outside of the body). These ostomies can usually be reversed and normal bowel function restored. However, in very rare cases, babies with severe NEC are maintained for months and years on intravenous

We always made a tape recording of sessions with the doctors. It was helpful to replay the tape as needed and listen to the tone and implications of their voices.

While the boys were in respiratory distress, they were a mass of tubes, wires, tape, and patches. It was frightening to see them at first, but the nursing staff helped us understand what all the attachments were. As we understood what the equipment was doing, we began to see more of the babies and less of the gadgets.

We kept our hopes up after the first few days, but were crestfallen with every weight loss or other setback. Most crushing were transfers back under the hood, from the intermediate nursery back to intensive care.

I regret not following my instincts as the mother of twins. I should have pursued the matter of Jason's eye problems when I first noticed the difference in their development. He seemed clumsy but had eye problems not recognized by doctors. I've learned not to be intimidated by professionals who may not recognize problems outside their field.

nourishment, only to die eventually from liver damage caused by the IV feedings.

Until recently, these procedures were often performed without anesthesia because of doctors' mistaken assumptions that babies don't feel pain. Babies were usually paralyzed for procedures with curare (Pancronium), a drug that left them unable to move or react in any way but able to feel everything that was done to them. In 1986, parents of preterm babies, led by Jill Lawson, the mother of a baby who died after unanesthetized ductus surgery, called public attention to this barbaric state of affairs. Recent research has shown that unanesthetized surgery is not only cruel but also dangerous. Stress from surgical pain can lead to a high incidence of complications that can cause disability or death.

Nevertheless, the practice of unanesthetized surgery continues (circumcision is a regrettably common example that happens every 26 seconds in the United States). Clearly, parents have to supervise their babies' pain management and advocate pain relief. Before any surgical procedure, parents should discuss their concerns with the surgeon and especially with the anesthesiologist.

Hospitalization of Multiples

Sometimes one baby may be transferred to a high-risk center for additional special care, or one twin may need readmission after discharge. Often, the NICU doesn't have enough room for a large set of multiples and some or all may be transferred to different hospitals. Dividing mul-

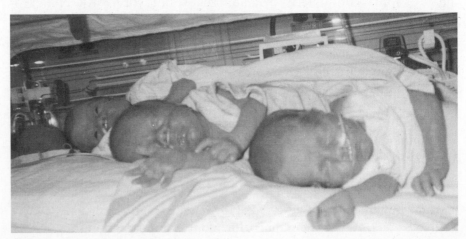

Multiples fare much better when kept together.

tiples between locations means added stress and anxiety for the parents. Sending photographs of the baby by e-mail can help to keep the bonds strong when you are separated.

If you have other children, your parenting resources will be stretched even further. Sending the child away to stay with a relative could make the child feel guilty that she or he caused the problem with the babies. Children often blame themselves if they had not wanted the multiples. Allow the sibling to decide if he or she wants to visit the hospital. Visiting the nursery helps to make the baby or babies real for the siblings, who have observed their parents' preoccupation. Children are more afraid of the unknown than of hospitals and their equipment. Give simple explanations for everything. Explain how the tubes help the baby to breathe and eat and that the machines signal if anything is wrong. Encourage the sibling to help with the birth announcements and to bring drawings and photos to the NICU.

Caressing of preterm babies by parents and other family members is top priority. Single mothers and couples whose extended families live elsewhere benefit from having friends accompany them to the NICU.

Survival Statistics

Many factors determine an individual baby's chances of survival. The most important of these are gestational age (GA), birth weight, breathing status, congenital abnormalities or malformations, and other diseases, especially infection.

In the smallest infants, GA is critical because the infant's organs, particularly the lungs, need to be sufficiently developed to allow the baby to live within the limits of current technology. Betamethasone to speed lung development is most effective when given more than twenty-four hours before delivery.

Many babies at 22 to 23 weeks are not resuscitated because survival without major disability is so rare. Only about one-third of 23 weeks GA babies given intensive care survive. Girls do better than boys and individual babies from multiple pregnancies do better than singletons. About 60 percent of 24 week GA babies who receive intensive care will survive. For a given weight, black babies have a slightly better survival rate than Caucasians; other races are intermediate between the two. Infants of diabetic mothers are at risk for slower organ maturation and a higher mortality. Severe maternal high blood pressure may have reduced placental function and the supply of oxygen and nutrients.

It would have been helpful for us to have kept a copy of our doctor's order permitting all of us to stay with the baby. That way mix-ups in communication among shifts and part-time staff members could have been avoided.

The United States is among the most aggressive societies in treating extremely small premies, although intensive efforts to save babies before twenty-two weeks GA remain controversial because of the low survival percentage and very high incidence of severe disability among the survivors.

Infants with serious medical problems who are born in Level III hospitals with large and advanced NICUs have a 38 percent greater chance of survival than those born in hospitals with little or no neonatal care available.

General Estimates of Survival for U.S. Live-Born Infants Receiving Intensive Care

WEEK	WEIGHT (LBS/OZ)	WEIGHT (GM)	SURVIVAL
22–23	less than 1 lb, 1 oz	less than 500 gm	less than 1 percent
24–25	1 lb, 1 oz–1 lb, 10 oz	501–750 gm	57 percent
26–27	1 lb, 10 oz–2 lb, 4 oz	750–1,000 gm	84 percent
28–29	2 lbs, 4 oz–2 lb, 12 oz	1,001–1,250 gm	93 percent
30–31	2 lbs, 12 oz–3 lb, 4 oz	1,251–1,500 gm	94 percent
>32	>3 lbs, 4 oz	>1,500 gm	>95 percent

(Courtesy of Dr. J. Brazy, University of Wisconsin)

A baby's chances for survival increase 3 to 4 percent per day between 23 and 24 weeks of gestation and about 2 to 3 percent per day between 24 and 26 weeks of gestation. After 26 weeks, survival is higher so increments taper off. A baby needs at least 24 weeks in the uterus for the pressure of the fluid in the lungs to increase their growth. Without this development, hypoplastic lungs result that will never mature — a disaster.

Other factors may influence survival by slowing the rate of organ maturation or by reducing the supply of oxygen to the developing fetus. Rupture of the membranes before 24 weeks GA with loss of amniotic fluid markedly decreases the baby's chances of survival even if the baby is delivered much later.

The 2002 *Guinness Book of World Records* review of preterm surviving multiples states that twins Devin and Dorraine Johnson, born in Ohio in 1996, were 119 days premature (about 23 weeks). The most premature triplets, born in Manchester, England, were 108 days early. In Australia, the Tepper quadruplets were born 105 days early — the smallest was 685 gms and the largest was 790 gms.

The world's lightest twins — 14.8 ounces and 15.5 ounces — were the Morrison girl-boy pair in Canada, born in 1994. Another set, born in Australia in 1993, also had a total birth weight of 30.3 ounces. The previous record was held by two girls, born in England in 1931, who weighed 16 ounces and 19 ounces. Like the Dionne quintuplets, very early premies have survived before the advent of the NICU.

Discharge of Preterm Infants

Discharge home is based on the stability of a baby's vital signs and the ability to suck properly, as well as weight gain. Make sure that you know infant CPR.

Formerly, it was believed that the mother would have an easier time bonding with each baby singly, as they matured and came home separately. However, on the contrary, the mother fares better adjusting to the pair or group from the beginning.

If the mother established a home routine with one or more babies and deepened her attachment to them during this time, it is a challenge for the "additional" baby or babies to be integrated into the family circle. Home is also a big contrast after weeks of constant attention, broken sleep, and bright lights in the NICU.

In the United Kingdom, for example, where the National Health Service bears the cost, the babies may stay in special care until they can come home together. An increasing number of hospital nursery units in the United States have facilities for a parent to live in, particularly prior to discharge, to ease the transition. Spending several days and nights in the nursery learning the routines helps parents feel comfortable providing total care themselves. Some parents make notes about eating and sleeping patterns, medications, and so forth.

The 1990 study of triplets and higher-order births in the United Kingdom noted:

> Both parents and professionals reported that discharging the babies home from hospital without any anticipatory planning with their parents for practical assistance often had very costly long-term consequences in terms of the effects of heightened stress and anxiety and possible later crisis management.

I couldn't believe that I was capable of caring for my baby after three months in the NICU. I wasn't a stranger to her of course, but I was always second in command (the nurses were first!).

I felt I had to earn my right to take my babies home, that the nurses treated them as if they belonged to the hospital.

I felt such pangs of anguish when I would look at those empty cribs and wonder if they would ever be occupied.

The hospital had a "care-by-parent" room down the hall from the special care nursery. There we could care for Amber ourselves, yet have the medical staff and technical equipment nearby. The doctor recommended that we stay two days and nights.

Once all my babies were home, they began to feel like mine, finally.

Outlook for the Future

Developmental studies have shown that most preterm babies catch up to normal milestones, but it may take up to eight years. In the beginning, parents need to subtract the prematurity interval to appreciate more realistically the babies' age and abilities. That is, if the babies are now two months old and they were born two months preterm, they should be at the developmental level for a newborn. This calculation is done up to two years of age, after which the gap between real age and the age corrected for prematurity become less significant. However, parents may still want to correct their children's ages for prematurity when considering placement in school.

Developmental delays, handicaps, and learning and behavior disabilities are more common among preterm babies than among babies born at term. Very-low-birth-weight babies have a 20 to 30 percent incidence of handicaps serious enough to be detected in the first 2 to 3 years of life. These include cerebral palsy, retardation (IQ below 84), hydrocephalus, seizure disorders, and vision or hearing loss. By ages 8 to 11, an additional 40 to 50 percent of very-low-birth-weight children are diagnosed with milder problems such as borderline retardation, hyperactivity, coordination difficulties, or learning disabilities. Fortunately, these "milder" problems respond to therapy and an independent and productive life can be anticipated. Supportive parents make a crucial difference for these children and their outcomes.

It is only around the age of eight, when the child is working with letters and numbers and is part of a more complicated social setting, that one can finally begin to estimate a child's adult potential with reasonable accuracy. There are more normal survivors now than years ago, but there are also more survivors with handicaps. Helping multiples with special needs is discussed in the next chapter.

Motor development tends to parallel corrected age and by two years, most preterm children have caught up. However, parents need to trust their intuition when others dismiss their concerns with the "common knowledge" that multiples are slower to develop. Most therapists would prefer to work with children at a much younger age than after the usual evaluation at two years.

Approximately one-third of preterm infants will need professional assistance to develop more muscle tone. It is important to promote trunk control first (and thus to avoid "Jolly Jumpers" and walkers). During the first 6 months, babies who were born preterm may stiffen or "fix" their arms, legs, and back muscles to compensate for their poor abdominal muscle and trunk strength.

By six months, all infants should be able to bring hands, legs, and feet to the midline of the body and roll in both from front to back and the reverse. Sitting usually occurs by eight months. When starting to stand, a child should use the legs, not the arms, with the feet kept flat. If these milestones have not been achieved, an evaluation is recommended.

A hearing test is also important before 8 to 12 months of corrected age.

Be sure to discuss with your pediatrician any developmental concerns you may have. If you suspect that your child may have a problem, follow your instincts and request a full investigation by a qualified specialist.* Early diagnosis is often the key to successful adjustment and rehabilitation. However, problems related to prematurity also may show up much later, such as changes in muscle tone, erratic eye contact, or irritability.

How to Help Your Preterm Babies

1. Observe your babies carefully to learn their (often subtle) ways of showing distress and contentment. For example, falling blood oxygen rates (as observed on the monitors), apnea (disruptions in breathing), mottled or dusky coloring, sudden changes in muscle tone, grimaces, and gaze aversion can be signs that the baby is overwhelmed. Always respect a stressed baby's need to rest and suggest that the staff do likewise. Preterm babies show physical stability and contentment by maintaining a steady normal rate of oxygenation, good color, and a calm, alert gaze (or a calm sleep). Take advantage of the times when your baby is stable and alert for care-giving and interaction.

2. If your babies respond favorably, touch or hold them as much as you can, in spite of the "lines." Gentle rocking and swaying soothe many babies and may help compensate for some of the uterine experiences they missed because of their early delivery. Premies are extremely sensitive to noise, bright lights, disturbances, and sometimes even gentle touching. Hold your hands a couple of inches away from their

*A therapist trained in Infant Developmental Movement Education can be found at www.bodymindcentering.com. Also, you can contact 1-800-999-APTA or www.apta.org and request the name of a pediatric physical therapist.

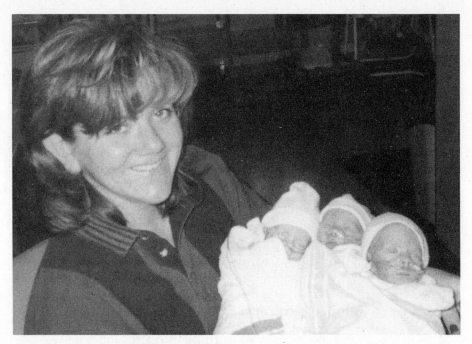

It is important for the mother to hold all her babies together as soon as she can.

bodies and stroke their energy field or aura until they can tolerate light massage. As soon as the babies are medically stable, cuddle them skin-to-skin to enhance their sense of touch and smell — important parts of bonding. Physical and occupational therapists can show you other ways to gently position, stretch, and move your babies.

3. Explain everything to your babies. It is normal and real for you to express your emotions about your baby's appearance, condition, and prognosis. Babies sense these things anyway.

4. Place a tape recorder inside each incubator or warming bed so the baby can hear your voice. Tape your normal speech as well as singing (which gives a wider pitch variation).

5. Decorate your baby's cot with personal items. Hang a mobile for your babies to watch. (Research on infant stimulation has shown that babies respond most to geometric shapes and to high-contrast colors such as black and white.) For your babies' sensory, emotional, and intellectual stimulation, change the scenery, using different fabrics

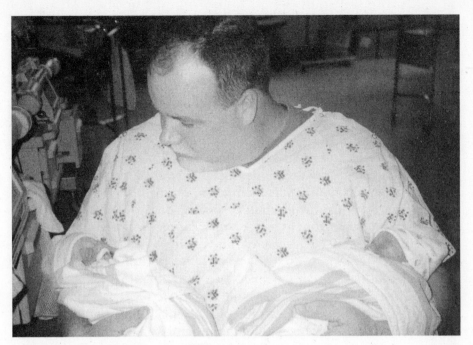

Each parent needs to learn how to hold them both.

I felt very isolated during my twins' first six months. It seemed no one could understand the difficulties of having preterm twins. I suffered severe postpartum depression. I had really wanted a baby, but the arrival of two at one time and their marathon feedings were overwhelming. If my parents hadn't sacrificed by coming 1,200 miles to help me, I wouldn't have made it.

Jim and I feel we developed a stronger sense of family togetherness because of our twins' prematurity. It made us more dependent on each other for moral and emotional support.

and assorted soft, colored toys. A "crib gallery" is now available that can be placed inside the isolette to display pictures and other items of visual stimulation. Always offer such stimulation carefully and assess and reassess your babies' reactions. Initially, your babies may seem disinterested or stressed by novel sounds, sights, or sensations. Some babies find even eye contact stressful at first. Be patient. What a baby may find overwhelming one day, he or she may find fascinating the next.

6. Learn to hold a baby "by the base" to facilitate midline head control (demonstrated in my video *BabyJoy*; see Resources).

How to Help Yourself

It takes time and a lot of support to adapt to this abrupt interruption of the pregnancy, and there are organizations and Web sites to help you through the ordeal. Some hospitals have parent support groups; and parents of twins and supertwins clubs can link you with a "graduate parent" who has been there and understands the anger, confusion, and depression. Such volunteers provide support and may accompany parents to the NICU to help explain babies' progress reports. Some units have a full-time nurse for parent communication.

Keeping a diary helps not only to document reports given by hospital staff but preserves a record of your feelings and observations. This journal gives some structure to this disoriented time and makes a precious keepsake for the multiples.

Complications and problems related to multiple birth, and prematurity in particular, put tremendous tension on the marital relationship, as well as challenging your attachment to your babies. The increasing number of films, books, and Web sites today can educate members of the obstetric and pediatric team to better help a couple work through their understandable feelings in a sensitive and caring way.

Parenting Premies is a quarterly newsletter published by parents for parents faced with the consequences of a preterm birth. Parent Care, Inc., offers information, referrals, and other services to parent support groups, families, and professionals concerned with infants who require special care at birth. These organizations support families with critically ill newborns, help parents create and maintain local groups, and encourage communication between perinatal professional and health care organizations (see Resources). Web sites include http://www.prematurity.org.

21
Multiples with Special Needs

An infant with a congenital defect or other handicap can be a tremendous shock to a mother and father. Nevertheless, parents need to see and hold a baby with anomalies in a private setting. The earlier you do this, the easier the adjustment. If a twin is whisked away while the parents are told "something is not quite right," the parents feel out of control and may envision far more serious defects than are actually present.

Parents typically go through the same stages with the loss of the idealized child as they do with a death. Shock, denial, anger, and guilt can drive the parents to isolation. It is natural to want to know why the disability happened — even if there is no answer — and to look for someone or something to blame. Friends and relatives do not know what to say, so they may avoid calling or visiting. Insensitive comments like "Well, at least you've got one normal baby" let you know which individuals cannot acknowledge your grief.

The writings of Albert Solnit and Mary Star, as well as those of Marshall Klaus and John Kennell, describe the sequence of events that help prepare parents to adjust to a child with special needs. The parents first grieve the loss of the ideal infant whom they visualized before birth. Then they can take the next step of becoming attached to the real child.

Sometimes the anomaly can be observed prior to birth with ultrasound, but seeing it in the flesh may be shocking. Some defects, such as heart anomalies and cleft palate, can be surgically corrected. Others, such as Down's syndrome, are irreversible, but our current understanding of appropriate stimulation means that children with this condition

People tell me that I must be "chosen" or "special" but I feel neither. It is very difficult dealing with the general public who stare or ask ignorant questions when my child behaves differently.

The joys have far outnumbered the sorrows, and the love our family has for these two little girls, handicapped or not, has bound us closely together and given us increased realization of those things in life that are truly important.

When I realized that my beautiful girls were "extraordinary" instead of "not normal," my entire attitude changed. Other children simply do things automatically; everything that ours have accomplished is a miracle.

Annie came into my world and taught me many lessons at a very high price. I wish it had never happened. I wish she didn't have special needs, but she is also exactly the daughter I wanted . . . As I scooped her up in my arms, Annie smiled and reached up to stroke my face. Annie makes me wonder, at times like that, just what everyone is so afraid of.
— Allison Bourne, *Finding Our Way*

I discovered that I compared them less and thought of their twinship less as their second birthday approached. I know they're twins and I always will, but the comparisons have finished and the pain of adjusting to the one twin's handicap is easier now.

Treat each according to their abilities.

now learn more successfully than seen in previous generations. (Nutritional therapy has been able to keep some Down's syndrome children on par developmentally with their peers.)

With premies, some handicaps may not be apparent until later — at least five years for cerebral palsy and eight years for the detection of intellectual deficits. Their special needs may call for help with intellectual, physical (sensorimotor), or psychological challenges.

One or more multiples may have a disability and the disabilities may be different. One may have a visual impairment, for example, and another may have cerebral palsy. Growth discordance makes one twin seem like a younger sibling and can strain the twinship, especially around puberty, even with DZ twins, who can be as different as any siblings.

Twinism (emphasis on twinness) in such situations is counterproductive, as in a photo I saw of one twin in a tutu and ballet shoes and her identically dressed co-twin, who was in a wheelchair.

It is very important to have your questions answered by the doctors; some may try to protect you from the details. Also, parents may perceive a problem to be less serious than the doctors see it, especially if normal attributes and good features are emphasized. David Hay points out that the "perception of disability can matter more than the actual disability." He explains the four dimensions of perception — diagnosis, causation, intervention, and prognosis — as parents come to terms with the problem. The last two steps result in formal recognition of the challenge and the gathering of resources to address it.

Preterm Birth and Low Birth Weight

Minor disabilities occur in about 15 percent of children born at term and more frequently in preterm infants. Children with minor disabilities usually lead normal lives.

Very preterm infants of 24 weeks GA or less at birth have about a 50 percent risk of disability. Impairments may include learning challenges, below-average performance in school, and visual problems. Although many problems are not observed until school age, early identification facilitates learning. An individualized program to stimulate and educate children with special needs will maximize their potential and minimize developmental delays.

As GA increases, better outcomes increase dramatically and are similar to the chances for survival. For example, if the survival rate is 80 percent, then about 80 percent of those who survive will be free of major disability. Thus, with 80 percent surviving, 20 percent will die, about 64 percent will be healthy, and 16 percent will have major disabilities.

Unfortunately, the higher rate of disabilities in multiples and the complex dynamics that characterize families with multiples are poorly recognized. A notable exception is the work of Hay and his colleagues in Australia. Their research into attention deficit hyperactivity disorder (ADHD) has shown that it is slightly more common among multiples and is associated to some extent with speech and reading problems. They found, however, that twins become more similar in their hyperactivity symptoms as they grow to adolescence, but do not necessarily become more similar in their inattention symptoms (which do not disturb a co-twin). Hay recommends that parents keep requests simple to avoid the frustration of attempting multitasking.

Learning to Cope

Many children with significant disabilities enjoy life and are a source of pleasure to their parents. Much has to do with parental expectations and enthusiasm. Most neonatologists explain the benefits and risks of resuscitating and treating extremely small premies and involve parents in medical decisions. However, some parents whose children were very preterm and who are severely impaired have complained that they did not fully appreciate the consequences of taking heroic measures to preserve the lives of their preterm babies. Some have said they would have decided to withhold some treatments had they known the likely result.

Well-intentioned friends and professionals may advise parents of a twin with a handicap not to compare the two or even to think of them as twins. This is very difficult to do after all the preparation and anticipation with twin furniture, paired clothing, and double gifts. The mother is unrealistically expected to act as if the babies had been born a couple of years apart!

Parents of children with handicaps, like parents of preterm infants, need to adjust their expectations with regard to the time that the child takes to reach developmental milestones. Assess each baby with a disability according to parameters that are adjusted for any prematurity, rather than comparisons with the co-twin or other multiples. Having said that, evaluating a disability is often easier in multiples because parents do make those comparisons. For yet others, saying the child was

They always have each other to keep themselves amused . . . AND distracted!

For a while the twin with Down's syndrome and the normal twin were developing similarly. But as they get older the gap is widening. One prints letters and the other can't even hold a pencil. I feel bad about comparing them, but I get trapped in it.

I'll never stop wishing that my son with Down's syndrome could be as bright and active as his twin sister, but we're doing all we can by providing a preschool experience and stimulation at home. I know he'll do the best he can. Besides, he's really cute.

It gets more difficult not to compare the two when the differences are striking, and sometimes heartbreaking.

We rejoice at every new accomplishment each little boy achieves! They continue to surprise us with their ever-increasing capacity to grow and learn.

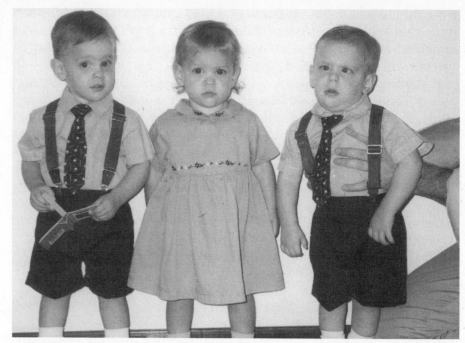

Each multiple has special needs — and special gifts to bestow.

born early or too small, or the fact that twins often create their own language, may serve as a form of unconscious denial.

Unlike a singleton, the multiple with the disability has the companionship and example of the co-multiples, although he or she will develop at his or her own pace. However severe the handicap, the affected child will nevertheless have special attributes.

If both twins are affected, the parents have the burden of raising two children with disabilities. More commonly, however, one infant is affected (even in an MZ pair) and this imbalance creates complex family and social dynamics discussed in the section "Supporting the Unaffected Twin."

Getting Help

The risk of mental illness rises for the mother of a twin with a handicap. Life is more difficult because of the pressure to balance parental attention between children of the same age and, in this case, very different mental and physical needs.

You need family members and others to help you on a regular basis and especially when you are ill or otherwise unavailable. Many services support families and children with special needs. A team may include a physical therapist, an occupational therapist to improve self-help skills and activities of daily living, and a speech therapist for language challenges. Psychologists and social workers help with school and psychosocial issues. In the United States, support for children with reading disabilities or ADHD is mandated by federal law. The March of Dimes, United Cerebral Palsy Foundation, organizations for parents of children with Down's syndrome or cystic fibrosis, state or local human services departments, and hospitals and clinics in your area can be approached for assistance with early intervention.

The Association for Pre and Perinatal Psychology and Health can provide names of therapists who help individuals of any age, especially infants, to relive and release early trauma. William Emerson, himself a surviving twin, in Petaluma, California (see Resources), is probably the most experienced psychologist in this field. This level of healing is an important dimension of recovery and adjustment.

Gatherings organized by twins clubs tend to be attended by happy mothers of healthy twins. This can increase the isolation for both a mother and a twin who cannot interact with others in the same way. Some mothers feel awkward that their serious concerns effectively trivialize the discussion of the other mothers. For mothers of multiples with disabilities, the Internet chat rooms are the best support. There is a Web site for the most rare conditions linking parents across the globe. If you do not own a computer, you can access the Internet at your local library.

Supporting the Unaffected Twin

In some families, the child with a disability may become the center of importance. It is important that the unaffected twin understands that he or she is not going to have the same affliction and is not responsible for the co-twin's disability.

Frequently, small achievements by the twin with a disability tend to be praised while the unaffected twin's skills and accomplishments are overlooked because for him or her they are "normal." As the twins develop, explain to the unaffected twin the capabilities and limitations of the affected twin in order to justify the extra attention and expense.

The unaffected twin may resent limitations imposed by the condition of the co-twin on family life. He or she may be embarrassed to bring

I was emotionally isolated in those early months. The concerns of other mothers seemed so inconsequential to me. I couldn't relate to one teething baby when I was coping with two, and one baby having cerebral palsy. Other mothers didn't know how to respond to my problems either.

The healthy twin may languish while parents focus on why things had gone so wrong with the other one.

I made sure to keep telling Brad that it was no one's fault that his sisters were sick.

friends home for fear of being teased. Sometimes the unaffected twin sets up "accidents" or regresses in behavior or deliberately lowers his or her performance level. At other times, he or she becomes jealous of the attention the co-twin receives or may experience "survivor guilt."

The way the parents accept the disability influences how any older children in the family will respond. Young siblings of a child with disabilities are generally resilient and patient with outsiders, who have more trouble dealing with the situation. Adolescents, however, may feel shame, especially if the co-twin behaves in an unsocial or even aggressive way. It helps when the unaffected twin develops enough confidence to explain how his or her life is affected by the co-twin without blaming the situation for every little mishap.

Dr. Martin Levison, who has a son with a developmental disability, recommends holding family meetings during which each child talks about the things he likes and doesn't like about all his siblings, including the sibling with a disability.

Make sure that you use "people first" language and correct others who do not. For example, say "Helen has a disability" or "Nathan is visually challenged," instead of "Helen is disabled" or "Nathan is part blind."

A child with special needs may not be able to live independently as an adult, so your commitment may be much longer than you anticipated.

It is important to involve both twins in any decisions, such as the co-twin's move to a remedial school. The unaffected twin can "play a caring role but should never be obliged to be a caretaker." However, sometimes he or she chooses the role of rescuer. In such cases, it is helpful if the parents arrange for the child to meet privately with the affected twin's therapists. Professionals who care for children with disabilities are cognizant of family dynamics as a critical context for rehabilitation.

22
The Death of a Multiple: Parents' Perspectives

Death and disability are more common in families with multiples, and the adjustments are complex for both parents and survivors. A twin has a greater chance of death from conception through the first ten years of life than a singleton does.

Early human development, observed with the tools of reproductive technology, has been described as "remarkably imprecise." With losses more frequent in humans than animals, up to 70 percent of spontaneously conceived embryos fail to implant and only 10 percent of transferred embryos produce full-term babies. Despite developments in obstetrics and advances in neonatal care for various types of high-risk pregnancies, the risk of loss in the perinatal period for twins remains about five times that of singletons and ten times for triplets. For MZ twins the incidence is two and half times that for DZs. Females fare better regardless of zygosity. The highest rate of perinatal mortality occurs in same-sex male pairs and the male of an opposite-sex pair.

As the size of the set increases, so do the risks for disability and death. Some of these risks are increased by the use of ART, prenatal diagnostics, and fetal reduction. One study found that the "take home baby" rate after ART is 57 percent if two chorionic sacs were seen, and 87 percent for two viable embryos. With three sacs viewed in early pregnancy, the chance of a triplet birth is 20 percent; and of three viable embryos, 68 percent (see Appendix 1).

The prevalence of cerebral palsy is substantially increased for the survivors after a co-twin fetal death and twice as high in same-sex twins as in opposite-sex twins.

I always thought that somehow my two babies were guaranteed. Going to a funeral of a friend's twin changed all of that, and I see that the outcome of multiple pregnancy can't be taken for granted.

Those feelings of loss and sorrow are never truly gone — just gone a little deeper within.

All these would'ves, could'ves, should'ves — I am doing what I suppose anyone does who has lost a child and will never get totally beyond them.

The first two years were the hardest as I dealt with the simultaneous emotions of grief and joy. My initial response to his death was denial of his sister's identity as a surviving twin. I seldom spoke of her brother and mistakenly believed that if I didn't mention him, the burden of pain would magically lift from my shoulders.

This chapter explores the death of a multiple from conception through early childhood and the impact of this loss on parents. (In Chapter 23 the effect on the surviving multiples and siblings is discussed.) Expectant parents who confront the unthinkable by reading this chapter — without undue worry or preoccupation — will be at a tremendous advantage should a death occur. They will also appreciate their living twins, despite obstacles and challenges that may arise.

Parents, despite being in shock following a death, will be better prepared to create memories while the opportunity is there and to avoid later regret of things left undone. It is also very important that the partner be aware of the mother's wishes in case she is anesthetized or otherwise unable to act at the time.

Parents of living multiples will inevitably meet other parents who have suffered the loss of a multiple — this chapter will guide them to respond appropriately.

It is significant to find out whether the cause of death was (1) intrinsic to the infant, such as a genetic disease or cord defect, (2) a maternal condition affecting the intrauterine environment, such as diabetes or high blood pressure, or (3) a condition unique to multiples, such as feto-fetal transfusion syndrome. The cause of death cannot always be determined, which remains a nagging frustration for the parents.

A triple loss — that of a baby or babies; of the identity of being parents of multiples; and of the relationship within the set — may occur during different stages of the childbearing year, with each stage having its own particular experiences. Grieving is different for parents of multiples than for parents of singletons; there are greater physical and emotional burdens in the recovery from multiple pregnancy and looking after the survivor (as well as any additional siblings). Parents must face the complexity of birth, life, and death coming "all in one package."

Loss in Pregnancy

Mourning is a paradoxical state during pregnancy, already a time of heightened emotions, whether an unborn baby, a sister, a friend, or other family member is mourned. Suppressing feelings about the loss for the sake of the baby or babies inside, however, can cause the mother to become emotionally isolated.*

*My mother rarely mentioned the death of my five-year-old sister during my gestation, or of her two earlier miscarriages. She did discuss being on bed rest in order to carry me to term after first-trimester bleeding.

Parents who lose a multiple have often suffered cumulative losses on their path to parenthood, such as infertility, miscarriages, and fetal reduction.

So many people want a reason for the loss of a baby — such as being poor, not eating a good diet, or not going to the doctor. When an infant dies, it's easy to think that you must have done something wrong — not eaten quite enough vegetables, gotten too much exercise or too little, not had sufficient "positive thoughts," lain on one side too much, not been "really ready" emotionally for twins, not accepted all the tests, etc., etc., etc. — not realizing that you may have had nothing to do with it.

We lost our twins to TTTS and I then went back to the chapters in *Having Twins* that I had skipped and found very useful information that I wished I had taken the time to read before our loss. Not all parents have successful twin or higher pregnancies, and the media tends to "glamorize" the successful ones while the rest of us are left to wonder if we made the right decisions or not. More needs to be available to the parents who are struggling daily to save their babies. Not all multiple pregnancies end with two or more healthy beautiful babies to bring home. But these babies do matter and do affect many, many lives and are *never* forgotten by the families that lose them.

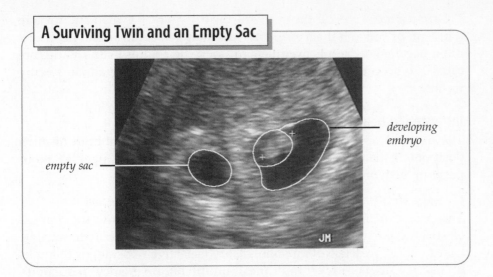

A Surviving Twin and an Empty Sac

developing embryo

empty sac

JM

They told me I was having twins at twelve weeks and now there is only one. I've been knitting two of everything, and my parents gave me two bassinets.

The doctor told me that ultrasound was inconclusive and began to list possible causes of my bleeding. When he said it could be the miscarriage of one twin, I stopped listening. I knew.

"Vanishing Twin" Syndrome (Spontaneous Fetal Reduction)

Not infrequently, twins are detected in early pregnancy but by the next scan one has disappeared, having been reabsorbed usually without bleeding, a phenomenon that was first called *vanishing twin syndrome*. The increasing use of ultrasound has shown that more multiples are lost in the uterus than previously thought — some studies estimate a rate as high as 80 percent. While the loss of a twin embryo may pass without symptoms, this type of miscarriage may be emotionally devastating.

Before ultrasound, women and their doctors had no proof of this loss, although women have sensed it. The surviving twin may unconsiously express the memory in art, choice of profession or spouse, and other behavior. (See my book *Primal Connections: How Our Influences from Conception through Birth Influence Our Emotions, Behavior and Health*.)

Miscarriage (Spontaneous Abortion)

A miscarriage is accompanied by vaginal bleeding, cramps, and decreased hormone levels. It is usually a benign event medically (up to 20 weeks) but emotionally brings a profound sense of loss.

In Japan, the number of miscarriages counted after twelve weeks (when the sex can be identified) increased from 2.52 percent in 1966 to 10.01 percent in 1996. Pesticides, fungicides, fertilizers, and fat-soluble chemicals are blamed; and it was observed that "intrauterine pollution" affects males more.

Parents find it meaningful to name the baby who has died and to have a funeral or memorial service. This also helps to confirm that he or she did indeed exist. Parents may have to assert their rights in this matter because the hospital usually takes charge of a baby younger than twenty weeks.

Intrauterine Death of One or More Multiples

The death of a multiple at 26 to 30 weeks (if delivery of both or all is postponed) means carrying the other baby or babies longer to avoid preterm birth of the survivor.

Choosing Intrauterine Survivors in Multiple Pregnancy: Fetal Reduction

This procedure involves killing one of the fetuses to improve the chances of survival for the other or others. The decision to terminate may be based on the presence of an abnormality (selective fetocide) or the risks of bearing higher-order multiples (multifetal pregnancy reduction). Often a couple has gone through years of expensive and stressful infertility treatment to conceive, only to be faced with such a decision. On the other hand, doing nothing could end or compromise the lives of equally precious children (for example, a fetus with anencephaly causes polyhydramnios, which can jeopardize the survival of the co-twin).

Multifetal Pregnancy Reduction (MFPR)

This "emergency solution to an obstetric misadventure" involves reducing to triplets or twins a larger set of multiples conceived through ART. Some women who conceive triplets choose to reduce to twins. Rarely are twins reduced to singletons.

Ending the life of a multiple because he or she has no chance of survival, or is unhealthy and would have a dismal life, is very different from decreasing the numbers of normal healthy babies to improve the outcome when the life of all may be jeopardized or because the mother feels she cannot cope with triplets or more. Each couple must explore the many "what ifs?" and ethical dilemmas for which there can be no right answer.

Selective Fetocide

This procedure is also called selective reduction. An injection of potassium chloride into a baby's heart at about ten weeks carries an 8 percent risk that the entire remaining pregnancy will be lost prior to 24 weeks, and about 75 percent of mothers who choose this option will begin preterm labor. Cusick et al. in 1995 estimated that only about 40 to 45 percent of pregnancies that undergo multifetal reduction reach term.

Other challenges include infection and incorrect selection of the "target fetus." Failure to kill the fetus has been reported.

Mothers who have undergone this experience frequently feel that the staff did not show enough respect for the dead baby and did not acknowledge the mother's feelings of anguish. Clearly, much counseling and support are necessary when this procedure is performed — both before and after.

Later comes the challenge of explaining the reduction to the survivors. Some couples may decide to keep that information secret, although this is unwise because the survivors remember, albeit for the most part unconsciously (see Chapter 23). When the news of the death comes as a surprise, perhaps from an outsider, a survivor will be justifiably perplexed and resentful that the knowledge of such an important life event was withheld.

Selective reduction of twins does not result in a singleton pregnancy, nor does the reduction of triplets result in a biological twin pregnancy. Although the mother's body will gradually adjust, the hormonal and physical changes in the uterus have been those of a pregnancy of more babies throughout the initial months.

Waiting to Deliver: One Dead and One Alive

For mothers who carry a deceased baby for the sake of another baby in utero, it is like being "stuck in the time between the death and the funeral." That raw, painful period following the death lingers until the delivery.

Cindy Joers describes how dealing with the death of one of her twins at thirty-one weeks was "beyond devastating" while her pregnancy continued to 36 weeks.

> So many questions rolled around inside my head. The agony of worrying about the other twin was excruciating: "what if he didn't make it either?"
>
> The situation I was in was called "going longer" — when a multiple dies in utero and the pregnancy continues for the sake of the surviving baby/ies. This whole concept was mind-boggling. What would I say to people who commented on my VERY large tummy? It had been such a joy to say that I was having twins, but now what? I WAS still having twins, but one of them would be stillborn. As the

pregnancy went on, what was happening to Jack? What would he look like when he was born? How was all of this affecting Brett's health? The questions were endless.

The day after we found out Jack had died, the perinatologist handed me a book titled *Miscarriage — A Shattered Dream* (or something like that) and I was totally horrified. Our boy, in my opinion, would have been a viable baby. In my mind it was clearly a DEATH and the term miscarriage seemed to trivialize it to me.

Also, during one ultrasound I mustered up the courage to ask what Jack would look like when the twins were delivered and her response was, "Well, he'll look like a baby." I was upset that she didn't ANSWER my question. As if I didn't know he would look like a baby. I wanted details — what condition he would be in — would we be able to hold him and so on.

I went in for weekly non-stress tests and ultrasounds to make sure that Brett was thriving and active, plus weekly blood tests to make sure my body wasn't reacting negatively to the demise of our one twin.

With a heavy heart I went through this routine. I knew I needed to do it for our surviving co-twin but knowing that I would only be coming home with one baby was so far beyond my realm of comprehension. I cried and cried over the loss of what we had been so excited about — raising twins. I cried over the prospect of having to leave one of my babies behind after they were born. As a mother already I knew that was going to be the hardest part of my whole experience.

Brett's first screams were hearty and I knew he would be fine. It was the silence of Jack's delivery that was deafening. My doctor proudly showed me Brett when he was born but then didn't even say a WORD when Jack was delivered. I had to ask if the other baby was out and the anesthesiologist told me that he was. That irritated me. A very sensitive nurse brought Jack to us and unwrapped his blanket so we could see his whole body — it was perfect. He was my baby and I thought he was beautiful. He had that same red hair as Brett and the nurse cut a locket of it for us to keep. Although I was a bit apprehensive about how he would look physically and having no knowledge of what to expect, I just remember thinking, "He looks so perfect, but his legs are so straight. A baby usually has his legs curled up." His skin was starting to decompose and he had vernix and a bit of blood on him, but they dressed him in a hat and gown so he looked more like he was sleeping. He was just over three pounds and 17 inches long — a little peanut who felt like a feather in my arms.

As hard as it was to hold him and take pictures I cannot imagine doing otherwise. Holding him validated his existence to us and the pictures will be something to share with his brothers when they are older and want to know more about the delivery.

An autopsy was inconclusive in determining why he may have died, but I have to think it was a cord accident since Brett is a healthy, vibrant five-year-old.

As awful as it was to have to carry my baby knowing he wasn't alive, it did give me and my husband time to plan for what to do when they were born. We had a month to think and read and sift through how we wanted to handle all this. We included Jack on the birth announcement and we had a chance to spend time with him at the hospital. My heart breaks reading about other parents who chose not to see their stillborn babies and now they regret it because they were in shock and couldn't think straight.

It is very important to personalize the dead baby. Family and staff can help by saying "your baby" rather than "it," by using his or her name, and pointing out characteristics, likenesses — behaving exactly as they would if the baby were alive.

When my doctor told me "one of the babies did not make it," it just seemed so unreal to me. I didn't even get a chance to try to save her. I never thought she would die, especially not before she was delivered. I always thought I would at least get to hold her. I considered medical problems, but not death. My husband and I were both in shock. One of the most upsetting things was that I did not even know when she died.

Loss During Labor (Stillbirth)

A pregnancy that ends at 20+ weeks or of 350+ gms is termed a fetal death. The shock of a stillborn baby is especially hard for a mother who thought she had finally made it to term. As British psychiatrist Emanuel Lewis observed, birth involves a transition from the "inner" to the "outer" worlds with many accompanying changes. In the case of a still-

Cecelia was very much a baby. Her body was macerated from being inside me for several weeks. I saw her beautiful little body, her hands, her feet and I cried and cried . . . she was my baby. The nurses helped us to perform a baptism. This was the only time I would ever have with my daughter, and it was special. Afterwards I spoke with the nurses for about an hour about everything that had happened. It was important for me to talk through all of this.

The nurses were wonderful and have since become friends. They took pictures and prepared keepsake boxes with lockets of hair, footprints, handprints, and preserved their footprints in plaster. They allowed us uninterrupted time with our girls. We then invited family members to join us. It was very special.

Although I had three months to prepare for this month, the tears were quick to flow from a well I thought I had buried deep inside. Over the last few weeks I had been so careful not to allow myself to think of this moment, and when it came I found myself quite unprepared for it.

I was doing everything I could, so what could go wrong?

birth, both an outer and inner void remain, and even though a birth has occurred, the anticipated transition fails to takes place. This leads to a deep emotional confusion (greatly underestimated by outsiders) that becomes all the more confusing when there is also one or more survivors.

Stillbirth to many people means no history, no known cause of death, and no name. Birth or memorial announcements for stillborn babies also rarely state the length and weight of the baby. (See Appendix 4 for advice about how parents can retain decision-making power at this vulnerable time and avoid additional losses.)

Recovering on the maternity floor can be extremely painful and the mother should be transferred to another area where there are no babies.

The Collision of Multiple Realities

With advances in neonatal care today, ever-younger multiples are rescued and parents often find themselves caring for one, two, or more survivors, who are often fragile, with special needs and disabilities, while at the same time suffering the death of one or more other children. In many ways this is the worst of both worlds.

The death may disrupt plans to breast-feed, which becomes another loss. Breast-feeding can be difficult to establish and maintain at this particularly painful time, and mothers need much support so that the experience can be rewarding and comforting.

Marriages may be at risk because of the impact of bereavement combined with the demands of parenting tiny sick babies. After a long period of hospitalization and the mother's stress related to commuting and pumping breast milk, the baby may return home to begin a new series of challenges: monitoring, medications, and therapies. This fragile child may survive the early weeks only to die later. A great number of such families in this predicament contact the Center for Loss in Multiple Birth (CLIMB), a support network for parents who have experienced the death of one or both twins or higher-order multiples during pregnancy, birth, or infancy/childhood, including death from SIDS.

The Double Bind of the Double Bond

The death of one multiple presents a totally different situation from the death of all or the death of a singleton. Yes, the mother has at least one survivor and for that she is considered "lucky." Having gone through

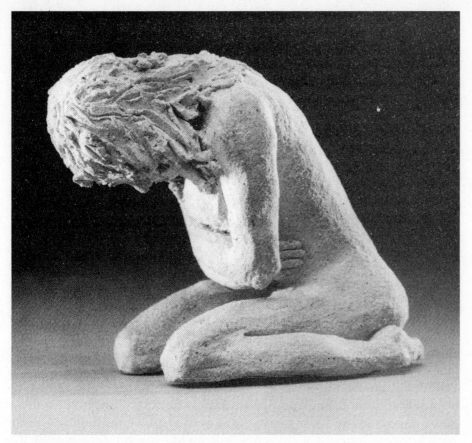

The Anguish of Loss, *from the book* The Anguish of Loss *by Julie Fritsh with Sherokee Isle.*

Many times the doctors told us to go home and take care of Corey and forget about Katie. They said they would let us know when she died and not to really love her. That's hard. How do you not love your own baby?

Unfortunately, outsiders do not give unborn and small babies much value for their brief existence.

I resented comments like: "Maybe it is for the best — two would have been a handful" or "She wouldn't have had a normal life." She was *my* baby.

several months proudly pregnant with multiples, she is suddenly thrown into the bizarre situation of having one living baby and one dead baby (or more), or perhaps one who is struggling to live. Flooded with conflicting feelings, a mother of twins, for example, must face the daunting task of nurturing and bonding with the living baby while grieving for the baby who died. These feelings, which polarize her reaction to each baby, are in direct conflict: bonding and separation, attachment and detachment, pride and guilt, joy and regret, excitement and disappointment, happiness and grief.

Just as any survivor never replaces those who are gone, the tragedy in this case is not lessened because the mother has one or more babies born

The possibilities for insensitivity are so much greater in multiple birth losses; we parents have to be ready to stand up for our rights at a very devastating time.

We were very upset when Anthony died and the nursery removed the sign that said Twin A, as if he wasn't a twin anymore and there was no need to make a distinction.

Recently at a family gathering they took a photo of all the family twins — three sets. But they didn't include my daughter because her twin had died.

If Sarah's early death did anything, it made me focus on the moments she was alive.
— Craig Mahood

I wanted to dress the baby for the funeral but they advised me against it because of the autopsy. I was saddened not to be able to make this small motherly gesture.

at the same time. The shock and confusion subdue not only parents but sometimes those who should be there to help and are stunned and can only speak trite words of reassurance.

Saying Goodbye

The few days between the death of the baby or babies and the burial or cremation are critical because this is the only time to be shared with that child or children. There must be time to say good-bye. This period is especially significant if one preterm baby has died and the other is struggling to live, and indeed may die also. Holding and viewing the dead infant are important so that the mother, especially, can concretely recognize which baby lived and which one died. Parents need to feel that they did enough for the baby who died. This in turn makes it easier to celebrate the life of the survivors and attend to their future care.

Parents and siblings can grieve and talk about the dead baby later if they have formed a strong memory and clear image of that child, and a clear image of their set. Time is usually short; therefore, every tangible experience and item of contact is crucial. Photographs, or videotapes if possible, especially of the babies together, are particularly important. Take shots with them together touching hands, being held singly and together by each parent, naked as well as dressed in something the parents chose. Include them in a whole family shot. Take black and white as well as color photos in case discoloration occurs later. Artists can render twins together if such a photo was never taken, and also they can create a picture of babies lost at any stage. Images like this can help the parents through any confusion about who lived and who died. (See Appendix 4 for a list of other mementos.) Parents of multiples who have died receive less support for these opportunities than bereaved parents of singletons do. Zygosity testing is very important for closure and to explore the reasons for death.

The several consecutive stages of grieving are now well known — shock, denial, anger, guilt, and resolution. However, they can be more complex depending on the number of multiples involved; the stages are often intermingled and recycled. Parents need to talk about their experiences and their babies and express their feelings regardless of whether they are rational. It is normal to judge, blame, and go over the "if onlys." Many have unanswered medical questions. If these components of recovery are not explored, they may be directed inward and cause depression.

A Multitude of Losses

In addition to experiencing the loss of one or more children, parents are no longer "parents of twins" in the eyes of society — a new personal and social identity they had enjoyed for a while. Of course, they will always be parents of twins, just not living ones. The great majority of women who conceive twins feel blessed, "chosen by God," and "special, because not everyone can have twins." The more they have been the center of attention in their family, community, or physician's practice, the greater their loss of status following an unexpected death. Friendships they had begun with other parents of multiples suddenly are missing the unifying factor — more than one child born at the same time. Parents need to grieve both the loss of the individual baby and the loss of the twinship in all its meanings. Take your time to deal with the double items that will dismantle the twinship.

Moving On Through Grief

Autopsies cannot always determine why one baby died and the other lived, and this uncertainty can remain a source of frustration. Furthermore, the living baby may have a permanent disability or medical problem needing immediate intervention. Even if this twin is perfectly healthy, parents may have trouble bonding for fear that they will lose this baby too. Sometimes parents will even avoid naming the surviving baby or taking photos in the first few weeks. However, these acts of identity are even more important in the event of death because bonding paradoxically facilitates letting go.

Parents must take time from the physical and emotional demands of the surviving baby to focus totally on the twin who died and discuss their feelings about the loss. Preoccupation with the surviving baby offers a tempting escape from the painful business of grieving, but in the absence of adequate and timely grieving, serious psychological difficulties can develop. Parents who postpone grieving (under major pressure from others to be "OK," "putting it behind them" and so on) may have problems bonding with and caring for the living twin, endangering his or her safety as well as their own.

On the other hand, preoccupation with grieving may cause parents to delay attachment to the living baby. In such cases, the mother may be functional but so emotionally distant that it can affect the behavior of the

Many parents of twins are at first more preoccupied with experiencing "my twins," somehow getting them together and being recognized as the parents of twins rather than with grieving for the one who died. It is hard to say goodbye to "my twins" without having first said hello.

— Jean Kollantai

Losing a triplet meant I was cut down a notch, because in others' eyes now I have just "twins." The hospital put on wrist bands that said Twin A, Twin B, and Baby C. What was I supposed to make of that?

It helps to have the other baby who has to be taken care of, despite inner heartbreak.

My baby was there, briefly, but gone so fast. I wonder sometimes what parts of my life are real and which are not . . . I don't care what they say about time, life is forever changed, and that's that. How I feel about the change from one day to another are the spokes on the wheel.

For the first six months I was totally preoccupied with ignoring what had happened, and then in the next six months I was totally preoccupied with it.

I can never decide whether it is harder, in a way, to have Tim as a constant reminder of Oliver's absence or whether we are luckier to have, so to speak, half left. I think it's perhaps an unanswerable question. A loss is a loss, and it has to be sustained; there are no replacements.

It is hard to try to love and care for a survivor and other children while wanting to be alone to grieve. In retrospect, I think I was extra hard on my children, resenting their needs and their wanting my attention.

Children expect old people to die, not tiny babies and it can be very hard from them to understand why.

survivor as he or she develops. It is a challenge to balance experiencing joy and grief separately to heal the pain.

If the surviving baby is very sick, the death of the other twin may seem more "acceptable." But once the surviving child recovers and begins to develop normally, mothers often find the loss of the co-twin more and more painful. For a long time, mothers may look at the living baby and "see two." While watching the survivor talk and play, they often think that there should be two little ones talking and playing together. Understandably, parents question why the living one escaped death. Depending on the circumstances of loss, some parents find peace by acknowledging that it wasn't a question of one twin dying, but more a miracle that the other twin or multiples lived. For other parents who suddenly lost a baby after a normal pregnancy and who have a healthy survivor, the feeling may be "This one is here; where is the other one?"

Grieving is a long-term process that can go on for at least two years or more. Just watching the survivor grow, as well as crises and events years later, may trigger emotional responses linked to the death. Postponed grief can emerge at any time, and parents often feel that they are sitting on a time bomb. Thus, early support for their feelings is essential.

Marital Challenges

The death of a child creates the ultimate stress on the marital relationship, and its impact varies with each couple. Sometimes tragedy strengthens a marriage, but it can also shatter it. Partners may experience grief in different ways and at different times, and this can cause conflict and misunderstanding. One partner may be at the shock stage, while the other is experiencing anger or guilt, for example, and the next day or week the roles may be reversed. Often one parent focuses on the baby who lived and the other on the one who died. Society tends to expect the father to remain composed and deal with the formalities — death certificate, burial, support for the mother — so his private grief is the more likely to be misunderstood. Fathers may feel betrayed that they could not prevent the death or protect their partner from this loss and sadness. Some hope that by not talking about it or not showing their emotions it will be easier. But the father needs to express and explore his feelings, otherwise the mother may perceive his lack of emotional expression as indifference. Mothers, in contrast, tend to seek out people with whom to discuss the loss — a healthy part of the grieving process.

In our society, many people find it difficult to discuss death and share grief, even with other family members. It is easier for people to ignore the death and fuss over the surviving baby and to assume that the parents are doing the same. Relatives, friends, and neighbors may be reluctant to call and may avoid contact or discussion of the tragedy. This encourages the parents to avoid confronting the painful reality. Silence about the death can haunt the family for years. Parents experiencing loss need to set the example for timid relatives by discussing the dead child, using his or her name, and by asking for the kind of listening they need. One woman was hurt that at family get-togethers two cousins, each with twins, would talk nonstop about "the twins" and totally ignore her and her surviving twin.

Sometimes a mother recalls how, in hindsight, she had a strange feeling that something was not quite right or an intuition that one twin was doomed. Several women have related to me that while their husband jumped up and down with excitement in the delivery room or when the ultrasound technician went out to get the doctor, a thought flashed through their minds that one twin was dead or wouldn't live. One expectant mother heard herself telling her husband to wait and listen to what the doctor had to say before celebrating.

Mothers sometimes idealize the dead baby, for example, as a spirit strengthening the life of the survivor, and the survivor may feel the wrong child died. Others may resent comments about their "angel in heaven." Outsiders often encourage the idea that the other baby was an "extra who didn't work out." If the mother has other young children, other people may say that it "didn't matter" or was "just as well." Many parents are ambivalent about the arrival of twins at first, but come to accept and welcome the event. Such comments add to their guilt feelings. The relationship with a deceased individual continues after death.

While talking is helpful, it may not be enough to release the deeper anguish. The intense anger, rage, and grief also may need to be expressed physically — by punching pillows, screaming in a private place, or undergoing a type of body-oriented psychotherapy.

Loss of Both Twins

Some parents believe that at worst, they will come out of a twin pregnancy with at least one multiple and have to deal with the problems of having one or more survivors. Few mothers ever considered the possibility and the horror of both (or all multiples) dying.

I try to forgive my family and friends since they couldn't know what it's like and I remind myself I'd have been just like them if I hadn't been through the experience myself.

Mothers who have a surviving twin, like everyone else, never think that a woman with two babies may have lost a triplet. With higher-order multiples, loss of one or more of the babies is common.

You've probably seen me out
  with my boys
I'm a painful reminder of your
  stolen joys
The joy of twins is something
  you should have had
I know when you see me, you turn
  away sad
But I share in your tears when
  you see me
Because for us there should have
  been three.
    — Terri Koelling

Aftertaste

Hollowed out
a shell ever after now
a cedar canoe of a woman
burnt and carved into
a new and terribly
empty shape.

The winds whistle
mercilessly
through the spaces
between my bones
echoing where hope
and trust once lived.

At night I whisper
the names of my daughters
to the stars
and try and try
not to notice the
constant taste
of ashes or the
glaring hole in
the universe.
— DD 12/97

My babies were in three different hospitals. I felt horribly confused and isolated and I was not able to get to two of the triplets before they died.

When we saw them, I had almost wanted there to be some type of deformity so that I could visually see that there was a reason this occurred, but all I saw were two perfectly-formed babies who looked like a combination of both of us.

One-third of CLIMB members have lost both twins. Between twenty and twenty-four weeks is the riskiest time but stillbirths can happen all the way up to term, and the risk increases with the number of multiples. CLIMB has helped more than 6,000 bereaved parents of twins with the challenge of their "multi-realities."

Sometimes both babies die with no apparent cause and the parents are left empty-handed without knowing why. The mother who undergoes labor and gives birth to babies already dead takes on an awesome task; others may not feel they can handle this and choose general anesthesia and a Caesarean. (If it is too late for surgical delivery to benefit one or both twins, the mother should have support for a vaginal delivery because her physical recovery will be much easier and the risk to her for a subsequent pregnancy and birth will be lower.) Again, the paradox exists that the more profoundly the mother experiences the death and grief, the better she can adjust and heal. Unfortunately, the shock of grieving for so many lives at the same time is so immense that one does not think these things through at the time.

The challenges of carrying on with life after total loss can be overwhelming. More than one mother has written "the stillness is deafening." Another described how the period of holding the babies, taking photos, planning a funeral, buying a casket, and burying them was such an unnatural experience that she felt completely isolated. It felt unreal, like playing a role in a movie. Parents, who were so very pregnant with babies and expectations, often after years of trying to conceive, are now left without babies and huge bills from the hospital and physicians.

While parents who lose one twin are reminded by tactless outsiders to feel grateful that they have one baby, parents who lose both may receive worse commiseration such as "Well, at least you didn't know them" or "Just think of it as a miscarriage, you'll get over it faster." Parents who experience the anguish of no survivors often resent others' reticence in acknowledging the death or the parents' grief. The comments are well intended by family or friends who don't want to see you upset and sad.

Subsequent Pregnancies

Mothers of twins are often ambivalent (yet compelled!) to become pregnant again, wondering about their chance of having another set of twins, and twins with problems (hence it is important to know the zygosity). Some do conceive a second set, and their level of anxiety depends on whether the loss was related to a random event or a maternal condition. On the other hand, some are disappointed to be pregnant with just a single baby the next time — if there is a next time. This is a huge challenge for ART mothers, having to undergo all the medical procedures again.

No surviving twin or a subsequent sibling can be a replacement. He or she may suffer a vague sense of guilt and experience some pressure to live up to certain expectations or the feeling of walking in another's shoes, especially with twins. Ideally, any pregnancy loss should be fully grieved before another conception is attempted. Some mothers do get pregnant quickly, however, in an attempt to have "virtual twins" — two children at least close in age.

A new conception three months after a loss means that the baby will be due around the anniversary of the death. Wait a little longer.

It is a difficult task for the mother to work through mixed feelings toward her dead child, whom she may still picture inside herself, while coping with hopes and thoughts about a new baby. The mother who has lost a twin sometimes had no time at the birth to grieve fully, and she may need more time before she is ready for the next baby. The birth of another baby makes final the death of the predecessor.

Conception of a Second Set of Multiples

Mothers who conceive twins again are "multiply blessed" but experience great apprehension, even more pronounced when they have undergone fertility treatments. Some, of course, are immediately thrilled to have multiples again. All realize that it is still not a replacement for the original set.

Darcie was pregnant with twins and lost her mucus plug at 35 weeks. She had no other signs of labor when she went the next day for a checkup — no movement was seen on the ultrasound screen. She had mustered her courage to read ahead of time about the potential hazards of bearing twins. Darcie understood that something could happen to one of them but she had never considered the loss of *both*. Labor was induced, and Darcie went through the ordeal of labor knowing that both her twins were dead.

> Our identical girls, Mia and Grace, were perfect, warm, plump and beautiful. We, and our families, held them, washed their bodies, took photos, and loved them while we could. The next weeks were a blur of funeral arrangements, sending birth/death announcements, too

They were so beautiful, so perfect, so peaceful . . . so quiet . . . I wanted to scream. I hated the quiet! Not ever having an explanation for the cause of death made their loss even more difficult to bear because we had no closure. Finally, we had to accept that we would never know, nor would we ever understand what had happened.

People seem to feel that if we cannot produce our children for all to see, that we are not mothers. Even though I cannot hold my babies, I am still a mother. I am still their mother. Women like myself go through all this pain, of losing their children, and then actually go through more pain, of people denying our status as mothers. We will always be mothers.

Next time I was pregnant, I kept thinking how the baby must be lonely, that there should be two inside.

Having a subsequent baby brought a joy back to my heart that I never thought I would feel again.

I was really glad to have another baby two years later. My surviving twin had a lot of problems and his body developed contractures because he lay so long in intensive care. He wasn't cuddly, so this baby has made up for that.

Unlike single pregnancies, the opportunity to do it again and try to get it right almost never occurs. Only mothers of twins, insensitive as they sometimes are, can understand better than anyone else — if and when they care enough to put themselves in my shoes — what a loss it is to have "just one."

I wanted twins again, but as soon as I found out I was pregnant I became terrified that I'd have twins.

It's not easier because you have one left; it's different. You're not lucky, but the time will come when you can rejoice in your surviving child.

We had had to learn the profound and tough lesson . . . that truly no one replaces anyone — not even a genetically identical person or people born also to you at exactly the same time.

many flowers, milk coming in unneeded, and packing up all the baby stuff, giving away all the doubles.

Her 3½-year-old son couldn't understand that the girls weren't coming home and hysterically refused to let his parents put away the crib (he had helped his father assemble it).

> We waited a few weeks and one day he suddenly said, "You can put the crib away. My babies are dead." We found it helpful to read him stories about death and stillbirth and take him to the cemetery so it could become more real for him. It was a struggle for my husband and I to attend to his needs when we were drowning in our grief but it anchored us to life and kept us going.

When Darcie found out she was pregnant with twins years later, she was horrified.

> As much as I wanted to have what I had lost (twin girls) I was so afraid to go through it all again for nothing. I no longer trusted that pregnancy would have a happy ending. I was still grieving and really was almost in denial about my pregnancy. I had lost my innocence in learning that terrible things can happen.

Her twins were born at 37½ weeks by planned Caesarean because Twin A was in breech presentation.

> I had them in the same hospital and it was very traumatic to revisit. When I heard the first baby cry it was the most joyful sound ever. It took more time to attach to them because we were still scared, even after their births, and mistrustful of happiness. We miss our first twins every day but we feel so thankful to have gotten the chance to parent twin girls again.

Bereavement Support

Support groups, counseling, and therapy, as well as family anniversaries, all ease the adjustment. The greatest help are other parents who have suffered the loss of a multiple. (A list of such individuals and support groups can be found in Resources.)

Jean Kollantai in Anchorage, Alaska, experienced the death of one of her twin sons at 39 weeks of unknown cause and as a result started CLIMB. Recognizing that some marriages break up after a death because parents grieve differently, she emphasizes how important it is for parents to talk about their loss. She edits *Our Newsletter*, issues of which provided extensive material for this chapter. (See Resources.) Through her network, parents can receive the names and addresses of others who have experienced a similar loss, self-help and informational materials, as well as assistance in locating specialized information and resources. Resources are also available for parents who have lost two or more babies, or who have lost a twin in childhood or adolescence. The support activities are not intended to take the place of counseling or bereavement groups but to help meet the special needs of parents of multiples as outlined in this chapter. CLIMB also provides ongoing support as parents reassure their surviving children of their unique individuality as well as acknowledging their origin in a set of multiples.

Some clubs for parents of multiples offer bereavement support and have taken the initiative to present mothers who lost one or both twins with honorary membership — a gesture that is deeply appreciated.

It is too bad that people think a man doesn't get really upset at the loss of a baby. We all pay heavily for this assumption. A few weeks after the birth I found I was obsessed with thoughts of death, filled with anxiety, and pretty well convinced that I was losing my mind. The sheer agony of losing a child still overwhelms me.

It wasn't until I took the time to write the story of what happened that I felt I could come to grips with it and know how to move on from there . . . I am strengthened each time I tell the story.

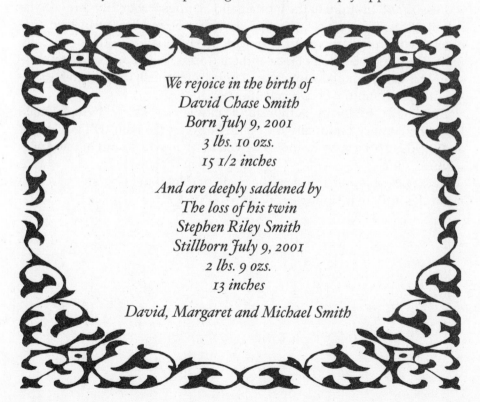

We rejoice in the birth of
David Chase Smith
Born July 9, 2001
3 lbs. 10 ozs.
15 1/2 inches

And are deeply saddened by
The loss of his twin
Stephen Riley Smith
Stillborn July 9, 2001
2 lbs. 9 ozs.
13 inches

David, Margaret and Michael Smith

We learned the folly of believing we have control over what happens in our lives and the wisdom of letting go when the time comes. We found depths of hurt and strength in ourselves we'd never known and watched the boundaries drawn between birth, life, and death blur until they ceased to exist or matter.
— Lisa Fleischer

I can't honestly say it passes. The intensity of it fades, the unfulfillment remains. It is just not possible to replace one child with another and it is this irrevocability that is so hard to accept, even to realize at first. As with a scar, the lividness slowly fades, and so does the intensity of grief, anger, and guilt. But the scar remains and nothing can eradicate it.

I reveal my situation, when appropriate, without self-pity and without minimizing my experience to comfort others.

Suggestions for Friends and Family

- Make a small gift to the parents, either a donation *in the baby's name*, a memento (appropriate for family's beliefs), or an item with the baby's name on it.

- Remember the *anniversary* of the baby's death, birthday, and/or anticipated due date. A card, phone call, or small gift will help the parents know that others do remember and care.

- Use the *name* of the deceased baby when speaking of him or her; rarely do these parents hear their child's name.

- The second Sunday in December is National Children's Memorial Day. The Compassionate Friends sponsor a worldwide candle lighting at 7 P.M. in each time zone. A card with a candle is a welcome gift to the parents on this day.

Untimely death brings about new levels of understanding of the human condition and deeper experiences of awareness and compassion. The Australian film *Some Babies Die* is a deeply moving account of neonatologist Peter Barr's support for an entire family's grief. The dead baby is dressed and brought to the mother and siblings frequently through the hospital stay. Photos are taken and put with the medical records in case parents who refuse them at the time want them later (as they generally will). The children's acceptance and comfort with the process is impressive. This exceptional documentary contributes much toward greater authenticity around the bereavement experience.

As noted childbirth author (and mother of living twins) Sheila Kitzinger wrote: "Gradually the space between the pain will get longer and the death of a baby becomes woven as one vivid strand in the whole texture of life."

In the next chapter, I discuss the challenges of parenting the surviving multiples and their siblings.

23
Survivors of a Twin Pregnancy

After the initial grieving, parents still face the challenges of having to parent the survivor (a constant reminder of the lost co-twin) through birthdays, anniversaries, and developmental milestones. Knowing so poignantly that life offers no guarantees, these parents have a heightened awareness of all the risks and hazards that threaten the survivor and a strong need to protect him or her. This is quite normal and will diminish in time as the child becomes more independent and capable. Discuss the death from the beginning so that information is gradually assimilated without the truth being divulged later as a shock or a secret.

Another issue is the question of parental identity and group participation. For example, does the mother feel more comfortable joining a group of mothers of singletons or a group of mothers who have lost a baby (many of whom do not yet have a living child and desperately want one)? How much do the parents say to others about the lost twin? Can people recognize the living baby without acknowledging the dead co-twin? Does the survivor consider himself or herself a co-twin or co-triplet even though his or her present status may be single or part of a pair? Almost all parents continue to consider the survivor as a twin or triplet and agree that it is best if everyone adheres to this truth.

Parenting a surviving multiple on these terms is more than heartbreak — it is high-risk parenting. This is especially true for first-time parents, after all the excitement of a multiple pregnancy often after many years of infertility.

It is extremely important that parents resolve their grief privately to be able to acknowledge and support their child's grief separately. Parents must let go of "how it would have been" — the icon of twinship. Sometimes a survivor goes through life feeling that the parents preferred the deceased co-twin (the "sainted other half"), especially if he or she was the opposite gender. The survivor needs room to grow up feeling that he or she is enough, without experiencing life as "half a broken set."

The Twin Bond

The twin bond has invariably been described as the closest of all bonds, especially between MZ twins (who have a greater risk of death). One study found that 49 percent of MZ twins said they would miss their twin most of all family members in the event of death. In contrast, 25 percent of same-sex DZ twins and 13 percent of mixed-sex twins said they would miss their twin most. (The rest of the DZ twins said that they would miss their mother most.) Another study found that 90 percent of MZ twins and 61 percent of DZ twins felt closer to their twins than to their mothers. Ninety-eight percent of MZ twins are intensely satisfied with being an MZ twin compared with 72 percent of same-sex DZ twins. Ninety percent of opposite-sex twins were satisfied with their relationship.

In a Michigan trial concerning the death of one adult twin, the deceased twin's co-twin was awarded the same amount as the deceased twin's husband for "past and future loss of society."

Research psychologist Nancy Segal interviewed some of the 157 twins who were released in 1945 from Auschwitz. They confirmed that the twinship was the key factor in their physical and psychological survival. Simply knowing that if a co-twin died the other could be killed, steeled their determination to survive and to develop ingenious strategies to protect each other. These twins fared better because they had the presence of their co-twin to keep human bonds intact despite their dehumanized existence.

Segal has also interviewed more than one hundred twins who were reared apart, showing both the impact of genes and strong bonds of twinship. Studies of twins who became bereaved in adult life revealed how the bond of twinship strengthens with time. In fact, especially with MZ twins, the death of one in adulthood may soon be followed by the death of the other, from similar or unrelated causes.

Acknowledging the Death to the Surviving Twin

Parents are naturally concerned about the effects of the death on the surviving co-twin, which may be substantial (in contrast with the common disbelief that babies remember nothing of their pre- and perinatal period). The living co-twin needs evidence of the reality and identity of the dead co-twin, despite the parents' feelings of loss, guilt, and anger. Elizabeth Bryan rightly warns that twins from whom information about a twin's death is hidden, or who are not allowed to express their feelings about the loss, suffer most. The child will sense a family secret (that he or she unconsciously remembers), and such secrets are potentially very harmful because they violate the child's sense of trust. If the survivor is not included in the funeral, he or she will certainly wonder why later.

If parents refer to death as "going to sleep," the surviving child may have nightmares or become afraid to sleep alone. Parents who are not comfortable explaining death to the survivor should seek help from counselors or the books and materials recommended in Further Reading and Resources.

Barb Schaack Kaminski shares some of the ways her family kept alive the memory of MZ twin Lisa, who died at six and a half months due to congenital problems. Each time Barb encountered a photo of Lisa, she pointed to it and said to Amy, the co-twin, "Lisa." Gradually Amy learned to say Lisa's name and to ask questions and express her thoughts and feelings about Lisa in many ways. As she grew older, Amy made graves with clay and when she saw an "L," she would say, "That is the letter of Lisa's name." Lisa is remembered in some way when the twin birthday is celebrated, and Amy visits Lisa's grave, always with photos taken. They also keep a candle lit through the Christmas holidays for Lisa. Another valuable treasure for Amy will be the book in which her parents wrote about the day the twins were born.

Just as parents who lost a twin like to meet other couples in the same situation, it is helpful for the co-twin to make contact with other survivors. The Multiple Births Foundation in London set up a Lone Twin Register to offer support and networking to survivors who lose a twin at any stage of their lives. Subgroups are formed according to the time of loss (birth, childhood, or adult life), whether the twin was a sister or a brother, or whether the twin died in exceptionally traumatic circum-

My son seemed to sense that something was happening with his co-twin in the NICU. He was inconsolable and we could not put him down. The nurses said a lot of twins have that experience when one of them is dying.

stances. The Twinless Twins Support Group International and clubs for multiples provide bereavement resources, too.

Reactions of the Surviving Co-Twin

Psychotherapy that enables adults to access early memories has demonstrated that multiples in the uterus are, like all fetuses, conscious and aware — most significantly, aware of each other. This has been confirmed by ultrasound. Adults, who did not realize that they had been a member of a twin pregnancy, have relived experiences with their co-twin before and during birth. Some have reported experiences of "something missing" that pervaded their life since that time, affecting their relationships, self-confidence, and even fertility.

Therefore, it makes no sense to withhold information from a child until he or she can supposedly understand. In 1986 an article in *Pediatrics* discussed the results of a questionnaire about siblings' grief reactions sent to parents who joined SIDS support groups. Parents believed firmly that their children had been deeply affected by the tragedy, even children who could not yet speak. Unusual behavior and restlessness, nightmares, other sleep disturbances, and temporary loss of speech have been observed in the child who survives.

Traumatic events make a lifelong imprint on unborn babies. Even in the hospital the newborn survivor may become very upset at the time when the co-twin is dying. Bryan writes about a baby who could not be consoled for 48 hours after the death of her sister. One mother described her infant's cry as "pitiful, a cry of sorrow." Sometimes survivors are fussy babies who calm down only when swaddled, held firmly, or have a stuffed animal close by. After months of close contact within the uterus, the loss of a co-twin is keenly felt.

Toddlers who have lost a twin at birth, or soon after, may later appear to have totally forgotten. The memory is temporarily buried, and the anecdotes at the end of this chapter strongly indicate that it is better to keep memories alive. One mother described the surviving co-twin, at the age of 18 months, "standing up in her crib and staring into space," and the mother felt intuitively that the baby was remembering her dead twin sister.

Sadness about the lost co-twin may be aroused when survivors look at themselves in a mirror, an especially common reaction among MZ twins (and the parents, of course). They may believe they are seeing the co-twin who died. Survivors may ask the mother if they were born alone or may search for their missing sibling in various ways. Even a supposedly unaware twin survivor may behave as if he or she senses that someone is missing — drawing pictures of people and objects with parts missing, or portraying two people in self-portraits.

Emanuel Lewis quoted a case of a three-year-old survivor who would habitually point out two of his animals and blocks. One day "he held up a toy car with a split windscreen, half of which was missing, and said 'Why? Who broke the window?'" Then he picked up a car with one front tire missing: "Why? Puncture?" Then to his mother, "How?" His mother then told him about his dead co-twin, to which he replied, "I am one."

Preschool children may want to set the dead co-twin's place at the dinner table, to talk to the co-twin, to draw him or her, to put out clothes for him or her and so on. This is similar to the Ibeji commemoration of a dead twin, described in Chapter 1. Subsequent children, too, may behave in this manner to integrate the death. Some older twins even talk about dying as a way to be together. Occasionally, an older survivor unconsciously puts himself or herself into dangerous situations, risking death as a way to rejoin the dead co-twin.

Although some twin survivors are held back by their grief, others experience a great acceleration in development, speech, and social skills when on their own.

Survivor Guilt

Feelings of guilt may occur when a person escapes a situation — be it a concentration camp, plane crash, or a multiple pregnancy — while others, often loved ones, die. It is necessary for the survivor to come to accept that he or she was not the cause of death.

In childhood, death of a co-twin plus parental overprotectiveness may cause the survivor to become fearful and dependent. The survivor may also react with complete denial, fantasizing that the co-twin is still alive. Survivor guilt often carries over into anger at the parents for letting the co-twin die or at the co-twin for abandonment.

Parents have to guard against their expectations that the surviving twin become a combination of himself or herself and the dead co-twin. Such expectations pressure the survivor into living a double life. Psychologists have noticed that the surviving twin may take on mannerisms or skills of the twin, unconsciously or deliberately, to please his parents.

Supporting the Survivor

A second loss is sustained by the surviving co-twin, who is now single. He or she has lost a co-twin and a future twin relationship with its special status and unique features. Fetal grieving does exist, memories do last, and children and adults who were co-multiples carry their losses forever, although usually unconsciously.

The survivor can be involved in the funeral (perhaps with a special adult as a companion) by placing a chosen object in the coffin or planting a memorial tree. Parents need to be emotionally prepared that the surviving child may respond by being indifferent, angry, or inconsolable. Young children may need time to understand what a twin is and why tiny babies may die.

When one twin is dying, it is important to let the survivor know that she or he is loved and cherished and not responsible. As well, parents must explain the illness and inform the survivor that he or she will not get it or die.

When one twin dies after an illness of several months or following a prenatal diagnosis of a fatal problem, parents experience the grieving process differently from a sudden and unexpected death. The shock may be less sudden but the parents have invested more time in the baby's life as well as more hope for recovery. Mourning can be delayed by the total involvement with the survivor and the often grueling demands of child care.

The survivor senses the parent's ambivalence at birthdays and new milestones that normally call for celebration but are also a reminder of the death. The survivor may grow up feeling guilty if he thinks he was the cause of death or that his parents preferred the co-twin and are suffering the loss of being "parents of twins."

All the recommendations in this chapter and in Appendix 9 for the loss of one twin apply, of course, to multiple losses. Teachers and kindergarten staff should know about the death so that they can comfort the child if needed.

Long-Term Effects of Unacknowledged Fetal Grieving

My interest in prenatal psychology arose from an understanding (long resisted!) that many of us who work in maternity care are motivated by unresolved emotions about our own conception, pregnancy, and birth. Since writing the first edition of *Having Twins*, I have experienced many dimensions of my prenatal existence under the guidance of Farrant and others, and I have concluded that my interest in twins stems from a personal experience of intrauterine loss.

My mother was six months pregnant with me when my five-year-old sister died, a fact that I was completely unaware of until I relived my mother's grief in my late thirties. However, it took me some time to understand that the profound grief I felt was more than my mother's emotions over that loss. I experienced other memories from that early time including a disappearing embryo and a pervasive sense of loss. Clinically, my mother, aged thirty-nine and pregnant for the fifth time, was on bed rest to avoid threatened miscarriage. In those days, bleeding was not connected with a "vanishing" twin, and it was long before the use of ultrasound. After these events during her time on bed rest were brought to my conscious mind, I understood my reasons for pioneering prenatal exercise in my professional work and why I have always rejected the stagnation of bed rest.

I have made many other connections with the loss of my twin, including feelings of being wrong, especially the wrong gender, which led me to seek opposites in my relationships. Running an after-school "kindergarten" for two sets of twins in my neighborhood when I was a preteen, writing *Having Twins* (especially my emphasis on healthy, active pregnancy), before I consciously knew of my twin, and supporting a considerable number of surviving twins and mothers who have lost a twin are further examples. Since delving into this field, I am prepared to suggest that anyone working in the field of multiple pregnancy who is an apparent singleton and not a parent of multiples probably shared the uterus with a twin at some early stage. When we consider that the most conservative estimate is that one in eight persons is a surviving twin, this is credible.

Buried Memories of Prenatal Loss

Surviving twins have had the unique experience of both intrauterine sharing and intrauterine loss. Because the frequent incidence of losing a co-twin in the womb is estimated to be as high as 80 percent of twin pregnancies, the subject of fetal grieving and its aftermath deserves more attention. While much progress has been made recently toward understanding the grief process of adults and children, fetal grieving is not widely acknowledged.

The conflict over space and survival in the uterus, especially when a multiple does not survive, may manifest itself in later life as issues of identity and creativity. A twin who sought psychotherapy from Arnold Buchheimer, in Massachusetts, for blocked creativity came to understand that as a surviving MZ twin he could not feel whole unless he gave up, or blocked, part of himself. After therapy, he was able to take possession of his self and his space in the world without fearing that harm would be done to another, and his professional work blossomed.

Christopher Millar, an Australian physician and family therapist, also concluded from his experiences during primal therapy that he is a surviving twin. In his monograph *The Second Self*, he suggests that many famous writers and artists reveal their identity as a twin survivor through their work. Examples include Edgar Allan Poe's "The Oval Portrait," Dostoyevsky's novels, Lewis Carroll's *Through the Looking Glass*, Oscar Wilde's *The Picture of Dorian Gray*, Bob Dylan's song "Simple Twist of Fate," Paul McCartney's song "Yesterday," John Lennon's "#9 Dream," Leonardo da Vinci's *Mona Lisa*, Shakespeare's *Twelfth Night* and his "dark lady" of the sonnets, and Elvis Presley's song "I'm Left, You're Right, She's Gone."

Millar concludes that such artists' creative drive results from experiencing a loss of part of themselves. Their artistic creations express their drive for reassurance that some part of them will exist after they are dead. "Each creation is at once an attempt to regain their first creation, namely a copy of themselves, and an expression of their creative spirit which produced the copy in the first place."

Millar believes that the dead twin in some of these examples was identical but female, a situation caused by a chromosomal abnormality called Turner's syndrome that could have been sufficient to cause the miscarriage. (Millar also suggests that a single pregnancy that results in the delivery of a baby with Turner's syndrome may have also started as a twin pregnancy.) He postulates that confusion about self following the death of an MZ twin in utero may result in autoimmune diseases. The gender identity of homosexuals and transsexuals may result from loss of one member of a mixed-sex MZ pair because the loss of an identical self of the opposite sex results in sexual confusion. Millar also suggests that a deceased MZ twin may influence the development of schizophrenia, "loss of ego boundaries strongly suggesting some confusion about what is Self and what is not Self."

Physician George Engel, in describing his close bond with his MZ twin, reports a "diffuseness of ego boundaries, never feeling sure who was who," and says that he experienced a profound confusion between himself and his brother in dreams. He also was very aware of family anniversaries and dates of key events shared by himself and his twin. (See "Family Time" later in this chapter.)

Unaware Twin Survivors

Although children commonly fantasize about being a twin or being adopted, increasing numbers of individuals who had never been told that they are a surviving multiple have discovered this fact in the course of various therapies. (Many psychotherapists, however, are unaware of the impact of the prenatal twin bond and may miss the opportunity to acknowledge that a client may be a twin.)

Some singletons and mothers of singletons feel "incomplete," which makes sense if a twin was lost. This quote in Kay Cassill's book is typical:

> Since childhood I've always felt very lonely, I couldn't overcome it and couldn't figure out why I felt that way. Even as an adult, I still felt this longing. It was when I was about to have my first child that my mother finally told me I was a twin and that my twin had died at birth.

Fascination with mirrors and reflections, as well as facial asymmetry, left-handedness, stuttering, and malformations have been attributed more to twins than to singletons and may lead single adults to believe they once shared the uterus. However, Boklage's research showed that not only are twins more often left-handed than the rest of the population, but so are their siblings and parents. Therefore left-handedness and twinning have familial associations.

Twin survivors may be particularly sensitive and reluctant to make deep commitments to relationships, for fear of sudden loss. And, like survivors of other tragedies, they often experience feelings of responsibility and guilt: "Why did I live and he/she/they didn't?" In the case of multiples these feelings are primal and profound. First, unlike cases of survivor guilt from accidents, the experience of twin loss is not part of the conscious mind and therefore is unavailable for discussion and integration without assistance. Second, because a co-multiple dies, the surviving twin may experience haunting feelings of being a parasite or destroyer. This is probably inevitable for feto-fetal transfusion survivors (FFTS, explained in Chapter 7).

Farrant described one patient who, unaware of her twin history, always bought two items of clothing and another who even bought a duplex house so the other side could be kept empty. Mothers of a surviving twin have reported various behaviors such as the child talking to a make-believe companion, dreaming of a twin, or setting the dinner table for the nonexistent twin.

Mariellen O'Hara, a psychotherapist and birth educator, suffered three miscarriages. All her life she experienced a feeling of "reaching toward someone" and had a recurrent dream that she was in a fog, with a piece of stretchy wall, "like plastic," between herself and the other person. She recalls trying to reach through it, wanting to grab and save the other. As a child, she often asked her mother if she had a brother; although she already had three brothers, she was always looking for another one. Her mother suffered a miscarriage six months before Mariellen's conception and six months after her birth. During Mariellen's gestation, her mother experienced bleeding and contractions between the fourth and fifth months. She had never discussed these episodes with Mariellen who, much to her mother's astonishment, was able to describe exactly how her mother felt. Her mother remembered that Mariellen had reported her recurrent dream since the age of four. She also recalled that Mariellen in childhood often played with plastic, stretching it on her face and calling out, as well as looking through glass, especially frosted glass, or any silky, shimmery material.

During regression Mariellen felt "weird sensations," and the right and left sides of her body felt different, lopsided, one side hot, the other cold. During one session she re-experienced the formation of her amniotic sac, "watching a balloon inflate and feeling it coming out of the middle of me, and spreading all around me, with each breath . . . like a parachute or a sail. I was encased in it when done, like a larva in a cocoon." In both her recurrent dream and her therapy, she felt an "intense desire to unite with the other person." She sensed that he was a male, and her grief was profound when she experienced his demise. The experience of his leaving not only meant she had to be on her own but was "earth-shaking, the deepest connection to who I was — the male part of me." She subsequently realized how difficult it had been all her life to accept her "masculine" qualities, such as assertiveness and career success. She felt that her excess weight was where she stored her grief.

Mariellen's connection with her uterine experiences allowed her to acknowledge her feeling of deep loss and realize that she could not "find" her twin. Gradually the dreams went away, as did her repression of her "masculine" qualities. She concludes, "It was a turning point for me no longer to search but to live my own life fully and to have healthy, stable, relationships with men without fear of abandonment."

Unexpected Memories by Unknowing Surviving Twins

A participant at one of my workshops described the following experience of twin loss. (Her mother later birthed two sets of twins.)

> I expected this to be another experiential process I would doze through. But midway through it, when we were those balls of cells fumbling slowly through the tube, I was *there* now. Feeling caressed by the tube, softly following toward something . . . a very secure feeling. Protected, safe, whole. But my serenity was to be short-lived. As soon as we entered the womb I split and became two. Shortly thereafter (it could have been weeks, the process was timeless), my "other" went away, forever. The vision that I have that goes with it is of a woman riding off into the darkness with her back to me, and all I see is the back wheel of a yellow bicycle, a sort of golden-yellow star rolling away into the darkness. From then on, my entire being, body and all, was bathed in sorrow — a deep, all-encompassing despair that permeated the whole universe for me. That was *all*, that was life. It was so *physical*. I was weakened by it.

She went on to describe her experiences of being born and giving birth and to discuss her lifelong aversion to golden yellow. However, as soon as she was pregnant and also postpartum, she found herself putting gold stars on everything — clothes, swing, birth announcements, and toys. She concluded, "I do believe that my daughter is that spirit who has come back to me. Ninety percent of the time when people see her, here's what they say: 'You two must be *twins*!'"

While revising this book, I received this e-mail:

> I took your Women's Health course last July. You used me as an example in the class for identifying birth trauma, and I spent the whole night throwing up, just as I had after some visceral work about 8 months earlier. (My physical restrictions had a strong emotional component!)
>
> For many years I have had 3 recurring dreams. The most frequent one is that I am running to catch a train, but I never manage to do so. I also had a dream that I was driving on a freeway cloverleaf, trying to figure out at what exit to get off. The third dream always had a different scenario, and I only had it a few times, but I was barefoot and

the floor was mushy under my feet. In the most vivid dream, I was in "jail" (interesting concept for the womb, based on my relationship with my mother) and the floor was mushy. Later in the dream I was dragging a dead body, wrapped in a carpet, down the hall and I thought I saw it move, so I slammed its head into the floor, as if to make sure it was dead.

Your class and your book helped me to identify that I was probably a twin in utero. My husband and I have the same birthday, and I believe that is part of my attraction to him — he fulfills the place of my lost twin. I caught the train in my dream a few months ago and haven't had any of the other recurring dreams. My new recurring dream is my breastfeeding a baby. My husband and I recently decided to start trying to have a baby, and I cannot tell you how good I feel about that decision now, and how your class and book helped to facilitate my journey to this point.

Resolution of Repeated Miscarriage in the Survivor of a "Vanishing Twin" Pregnancy

A woman I will call Jenny was referred to me by her obstetrician because of her pregnancy losses, having experienced one ectopic pregnancy and three miscarriages by the age of thirty.*

Her medical history included many diagnostic tests, some painfully invasive and expensive, and she was understandably very depressed and discouraged.

As I took a detailed history — including, as with every client I see, information about her own conception, gestation, and birth — I learned that her miscarriages always occurred between four and six weeks of gestation. Her mother had also had three miscarriages. Jenny had conceived her first pregnancy at the same age at which her mother conceived her. Jenny's second conception occurred around the time of her sister's birthday. (I always watch for such anniversaries that may illustrate a family dynamic being unconsciously acted out in a generational pattern.)

Intuitively, I felt that something had happened to Jenny during her own fourth to sixth week of development and suggested that she explore this possibility through regression.

*This case history was published in the *International Journal of Pre and Perinatal Psychology and Medicine*, Volume 1, No. 1, 117–120, 1989.

In place of techniques such as hypnosis, controlled breathing and the like, I use a free, open-ended approach that I learned from Graham Farrant. The client simply lies on her back on a padded floor, so she is safe from falling and is free to move, with her arms and legs apart. I then gently encourage her to become aware of bodily sensations and underlying emotions and to allow herself to go back in time to the first occurrence of those sensations, their primal origins.

During the first session, Jenny felt disconnected from her body, except for some nausea, and she expressed much victim language. Ultimately tears and anger poured forth over the myriad medical interventions to which she had been subjected. During the second session Jenny went into deeper feelings and after a half hour of inactivity she said that she was "floating, dangling with a string through my middle." (Such metaphors may be obvious to us, but the client may not make the connection of the string representing the umbilical cord.) Grimacing and grief reactions followed. She moaned, "It's leaving, and I'm moving this way," as she slid slowly to the left. I asked if it felt right to say "I'm leaving," wondering if her mother attempted to abort her. "No," she replied. "I'm staying, I'm hanging in here. But I'm so afraid and I don't want *it* to leave." I asked her if she was hanging on with her hands and feet and she answered, "I don't have hands and feet yet." Thus I knew that her embryological development at the time of loss was prior to six weeks.

Jenny had never heard of the "vanishing twin" syndrome as it was called then, but when we discussed the possibility, she noted with amazement that (1) she had always wanted twins, (2) the child whom she had occasionally fostered was "coincidentally" a surviving twin, and (3) when she is pregnant, she feels she completes a part of herself that was missing. She later asked her mother about her gestation and discovered that her mother had indeed experienced first-trimester bleeding.

During five more sessions, Jenny re-experienced many prenatal events, including her conception, which she described as a "splitting." I surmised from this description and her feeling that a part of herself was missing that she was an MZ twin. She often expressed her intrauterine existence with much grimacing of the left side of her face and body, which tied in with her feeling that her twin was to her left.

During the two months of therapy, Jenny's demeanor improved markedly, her painful periods and headaches abated, and she became calm and cheerful, a "new person," as her referring physician observed.

In her seventh and final session, she seemed to complete a stage of bereavement for her lost twin and I closed with a guided visualization of her uterus as a nest, with affirmations of her capably nurturing a pregnancy to term. Two months later she conceived and wrote to me that the turning point was being able to regard herself as a nurturer. (Surviving twins often feel that they played a role in the death of their twin.) Jenny had no more miscarriages, and after birthing two healthy children, opted for sterilization.

"Family Time": Generational Patterns and Twin Loss

Australian psychiatrist Avril Earnshaw first wrote about the re-enactment of events from one generation to the next in *Family Time: The Bridge Across the Generation Gap*, and a later version titled *Time Bombs in Families and How to Survive Them*. She suggests that the timing of family events is genetically encoded, that we inherit time-tagged messages precisely linked with emotional crises of our parents' lifetimes. These events reverberate, often as anniversaries, in our own adult lives and the lives of our children. Although the actual events may be different, related events tend to occur at the same age. This is perhaps an explanation of the amazing coincidences of twins reared apart, documented by the Minnesota Center for Twin and Adoption Research.

Psychiatrist Emanuel Lewis, at London's Tavistock Centre, described a case of compulsive generational patterns. A woman's daughter, her stillborn twins, and her first grandchild were all born on February 1. The mother also had two sons, each from a twin pregnancy, and in each case the other twin died at the fifth month. Her last pregnancy was also twins, who were stillborn. The woman's two oldest daughters experienced unplanned pregnancies, which Lewis felt were unconscious replacements for the stillbirths.

Joan Woodward, who conducted twin research in England, notes that twins who lose a twin in childhood tend to be fearful for their own children when they reach the same age. She describes one man in his forties who became ill when his daughter reached the same age as his MZ twin had been when he died in an accident.

Every situation has the potential to be resolved; the first step is acknowledgment.

It is important when a twin "vanishes" or dies at any stage that the parents affirm the rightful existence and basic goodness of the survivor.

Woodward describes various degrees of rejection felt by surviving twins. Many reported cruel comments related to the uterine situation, such as "You took all the food" or "You crushed your twin" or "You dismembered him before birth." (One child, having been told such things by her parents, made a later suicide attempt.) While these were memories of actual remarks made to children, parental emotions are always sensed by the child, even in the womb. Negative messages can be conveyed nonverbally to the unborn survivor and cause the child to grow up with such thoughts as "I was a

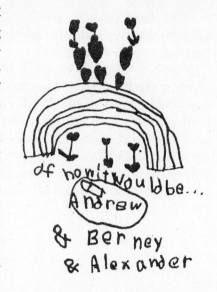

murderer in my mother's eyes." It is no wonder that such a child will feel undeserving, guilty, resentful, and alone. Many develop a lifelong pattern of trying to please Mother to make up for the loss of the twin. When the lost twin is of the opposite and preferred gender, the surviving twin may experience further loss of self-esteem. Woodward interviewed female twins who lost brothers and felt "useless as they were not the longed-for son." (I knew this feeling myself.) This is a common family dynamic, but it is intensified when death is involved.

Dealing with the Feelings of Siblings

Other children in a family with twins may have wished that one or both of the babies would disappear (jealous young children usually do), and after the death they may feel responsible and guilty. Parents feel torn that they are emotionally less available for the other children, who may also be grieving or figuring out what happened to the baby. Children will often express, verbally or behaviorally, what their parents repress. Young children are so perceptive that it is essential to be emotionally and factually honest with them at all times, even and especially on a difficult subject such as death. Also, when parents express emotion, this reassures the children that adults have feelings, too, and that it is safe to show them.

If the deceased baby was not named, the older child or children will appreciate being consulted on the choice of a name. Often an older sibling has a name ready.

It is helpful to facilitate as much discussion as possible of facts, dreams, sandbox play — whatever helps the subject to be explored and explained. When most of today's adults were children, family deaths tended to be surrounded with unresolved tension. Consequently, many adults avoid contact with bereaved families. Today, in contrast, there is a greater awareness of the benefits to expressing openly all feelings involved in the grieving process, and much more specialized information and support are fortunately available.

Appendix 1

Assisted Reproductive Technologies (ART)

In addition to hormonal stimulation of the ovaries (OI), techniques that have increased the number of multiple births include *in vitro* fertilization (IVF), gamete intra-Fallopian transfer (GIFT), embryo transfer (ET), and zygote intra-Fallopian transfer (ZIFT). These are invasive and expensive undertakings. To increase the likelihood of a successful pregnancy, two or more embryos may be transplanted into the uterus. There is a temptation to place more than two because additional embryos have to be either frozen or discarded. Some parents will store them for the future and a "conceptual twin" may be born years later as a singleton.

The process of IVF involves removing one or more eggs from the stimulated ovary and mixing them with sperm in a glass dish (not a test tube). After fertilization, the resulting embryos are placed in the uterus. In GIFT, the eggs and sperm are mixed together and then placed in the Fallopian tube, where conception would have occurred naturally. In ZIFT, the actual zygote is placed in the tube. Donor egg/donor sperm may be used in these procedures, too, ideally from known donors.

IVF versus Natural Conception

Risks are increased when babies are conceived with ART. Research has shown that:

- Some 26–27 percent of IVF births are multiple (22 percent twins, 4 percent triplets), compared with the natural rate of 1 percent.

- From 11–24 percent of births after IVF–ET were preterm, compared with 5–6 percent for natural conceptions.

- Three percent of these babies were born at less than 32 weeks of gestation (very preterm). In the general population, only 1 percent of babies was born at less than 32 weeks.

- From 9–32 percent of the babies weighed less than 2,500 grams versus 4–7 percent for all births.

- From 3–7 percent weighed less than 1,500 grams. This compares with 1 percent respectively for all births.

- Rate of perinatal mortality (19 per 1,000 pregnancies and 26 per 1,000 live births) is higher with assisted conception, compared with 8 per 1,000 pregnancies and 16 per 1,000 live births for natural conception.

- In Sweden, 5 percent of the babies had a congenital malformation (1.4 times as likely as Swedish infants in general to have a malformation). Interestingly, the overall likelihood of congenital malformation was significantly increased for singletons (risk ratio, 1.3) but not for multiple births.

- There is a 1.5 percent risk of cerebral palsy per baby with ART twins (8 percent risk with triplets), compared with 1 percent for natural conceptions.

More girls are born when hormones are used to stimulate the ovaries.

Appendix 2

Declaration of Rights and Statement of Needs of Twins and Higher-Order Multiples adopted by the Council of Multiple Birth Organizations of the International Society for Twin Studies, May 1995

Introduction: The mission of the Council of Multiple Birth Organizations (COMBO) of the International Society for Twin Studies is to promote awareness of the special needs of multiple birth infants, children, and adults. The multi-national membership of COMBO has developed this Declaration of Rights and Statement of Needs of Twins and Higher-Order Multiples as benchmarks by which to evaluate and stimulate the development of resources to meet their special needs.

Declaration of Rights

WHEREAS myths and superstitions about the origins of multiples have resulted in the culturally sanctioned banishment and/or infanticide of multiples in some countries:

I. Multiples and their families have a right to full protection, under the law, and freedom from discrimination of any kind.

WHEREAS the conception and care of multiples increase the health and psychosocial risks of their families, and whereas genetic factors, fertility drugs, and in vitro fertilization techniques are known to promote multifetal pregnancies:

II. Couples planning their families and/or seeking infertility treatment have a right to information and education about factors which influence the conception of multiples, the associated pregnancy risks and treatments, and facts regarding parenting multiples.

WHEREAS the zygosity of same-sex multiples cannot be reliably determined by their appearances; and whereas (1) the heritability of dizygotic (two-egg) twinning increases the rate of conception of multiples; (2) the similar biology and inheritance of monozygotic (one-egg) multiples profoundly affect similarities in their development; (3) monozygotic multiples are blood and organ donors of choice for their co-multiples; and (4) the availability of the placenta and optimal conditions for determining zygosity are present at birth:

III. A. Parents have a right to expect accurate recording of placentation and the diagnosis of the zygosity of same-sex multiples at birth.

      B. Older, same-sex multiples of undetermined zygosity have a right to testing to ascertain their zygosity.

WHEREAS during World War II twins were incarcerated in Nazi concentration camps and submitted by force to experiments which caused disease or death:

IV. Any research incorporating multiples must be subordinated to the informed consent of the multiples and/or their parents and must comply with international codes of ethics governing human experimentation.

WHEREAS inadequate documentation, ignorance, and misconceptions regarding multiples and multiple birth increase the risk of misdiagnosis and/or inappropriate treatment of multiples:

V. A. Multiple births and deaths must be accurately recorded.

     B. Parents and multiples have a right to care by professionals who are knowledgeable regarding the management of multiple gestation and/or the lifelong special needs of multiples.

WHEREAS the bond between co-multiples is a vital aspect of their normal development:

VI. Co-multiples have the right to be placed together in foster care, adoptive families, and custody agreements.

Statement of Needs

Summary: Twins and higher-order multiples have unique: conception, gestation, and birth processes; health risks; impacts on the family system; developmental environments; and individuation processes. Therefore, in order to insure their optimal development, multiples and their families need access to health care, social services, and education that respect and address their differences from single born children.

WHEREAS twins and higher order multiple births are at high risk of low birth weight (<2,500 grams), and very low birth weight (< 1,500 grams), disability, and infant death:

I. Women who are expecting multiples have a need for:

A. education regarding the prevention and symptoms of preterm labor

B. prenatal resources and care designed to avert the preterm birth of multiples, including:

    1. diagnosis of a multiple pregnancy, ideally by the fifth month, which is communicated tactfully, with respect for the privacy of the parents;

    2. nutrition counseling and dietary resources to support a weight gain of 18–27 kilos (40–60 pounds);

    3. obstetrical care which follows protocols of best practice for multiple birth; and when the health of the mother or family circumstances warrant:

    4. extended work leave;

    5. bed rest support; and

    6. child care for siblings.

(See References, Section I.*)

WHEREAS breastfeeding provides optimal nutrition and nurture for preterm and full-term multiples; and whereas the process of breastfeeding and/or bottle feeding of multiples is complex and demanding:

  II. Families expecting and rearing multiples need the following:

    A. education regarding the nutritional, psychological, and financial benefits of breastfeeding for preterm and full-term infants;

    B. encouragement and coaching in breastfeeding techniques;

    C. education and coached practice in simultaneous bottle feeding of co-multiples; and,

    D. adequate resources, support systems, and family work leave to facilitate the breastfeeding and/or bottle feeding process.

(See References, Section II.*)

WHEREAS 60% of multiples are born before 37 weeks gestation and/or at low birth weight and experience a high rate of hospitalization which endangers the bonding process and breastfeeding; and whereas newborn multiples are comforted by their fetal position together:

III. Families with medically fragile multiples need specialized education and assistance to promote and encourage bonding and breastfeeding. Hospital placement of medically fragile multiples and hospital protocols should facilitate family access, including co-multiples' access to each other.

(See References, Section III.*)

WHEREAS multiple birth infants suffer elevated rates of birth defects and infant death:

IV. Families experiencing the disability and/or death of co-multiples need:

    A. care and counseling by professionals who are sensitive to the dynamics of grief associated with disability and/or death in co-multiples; and

    B. policies which facilitate appropriate mourning of a deceased multiple or multiples.

(See References, Section IV.*)

WHEREAS the unassisted care of newborn, infant, and toddler multiples elevates their families' risk of illness, substance abuse, child abuse, spouse abuse, divorce, and potential for child abuse:

V. Families caring for multiples need timely access to adequate services and resources in order to:

    A. insure access to necessary quantities of infant and child clothing and equipment;

    B. enable adequate parental rest and sleep;

    C. facilitate healthy nutrition;

    D. facilitate the care of siblings;

    E. facilitate child safety;

    F. facilitate transportation; and

    G. facilitate pediatric care.

(See References, Section V.*)

WHEREAS families with multiples have the unique challenge of promoting the healthy individuation process of each co-multiple and of encouraging and supporting a healthy relationship between the co-multiples; and, whereas the circumstance of multiple birth affects developmental patterns:

VI. Families expecting and rearing multiples need:

    A. access to information and guidance in optimal parenting practices regarding the unique developmental aspects of multiple birth children, including the processes of: socialization, individuation, and language acquisition; and

    B. access to appropriate testing, evaluation, and schooling for co-multiples with developmental delays and/or behavior problems.

(See References, Section VI.*)

WHEREAS twins and higher order multiples are the subjects of myths and legends and media exploitation which depict multiples as depersonalized stereotypes:

VII. Public education, with emphasis upon the training of professional health and family service providers, and educators, is needed to dispel mythology and disseminate the facts of multiple birth and the developmental processes in twins and higher order multiples.

(See References, Section VII.*)

WHEREAS twins and higher-order multiples suffer discrimination from public ignorance about their biological makeup and inflexible policies which fail to accommodate their special needs:

VIII. Twins and higher-order multiples need:

    A. information and education about the biology of twinning; and

    B. health care, education, counseling, and flexible public policies which address their unique developmental norms, individuation processes, and relationship. For example by permitting and/or fostering:

        1. the treatment of medically fragile co-multiples in the same hospital;

        2. the neonatal placement together of co-multiples in isolettes and cribs to extend the benefits of their fetal position together;

        3. medical, developmental, and educational assessment and treatment which is respectful of the relationship between co-multiples;

        4. the annual review of the classroom placement of co-multiples, and facilitation of their co-placement or separate placement according to the particular needs of each set of co-multiples;

        5. the simultaneous participation of co-multiples on sports teams and other group activities;

        6. specialized grief counseling for multiples at the death of a co-multiple;

        7. counseling services addressing the special needs of adult multiples.

WHEREAS the participation by multiple birth infants, children, and adults as research subjects has made important contributions to scientific understanding of the heritability of disease, personality variables, and the relative influence of nature and nurture on human development; and, WHEREAS relatively little is known about optimal management of plural pregnancy and the unique developmental patterns of multiples:

IX.   Scientists must be encouraged to investigate:

A.   the optimal management of plural pregnancies;

B.   norms for developmental processes which are affected by multiple birth such as: individuation, socialization, and language acquisition;

C.   benchmarks of healthy psychological development, and relevant therapeutic interventions for multiples of all ages and at the death of a co-multiple.

Adopted by the Council of Multiple Birth Organizations (COMBO) (comprised of representatives of sixteen organizations from ten countries: Australia, Belgium, Canada, Germany, Indonesia, Japan, Sweden, Taipei, United Kingdom, United States) of the International Society for Twin Studies at the Eighth International Twin Congress, Richmond, Virginia, May 31, 1995.

*References and the complete document can be found on http://www.multiplebirth.com.

Appendix 3

Biography Becomes Biology!*

Please write what you know about the following events (each parent):

Age _____ # of pregnancies _____ births _____

Same-sex parent's age at your birth _____

Same-sex parent's age at birth of last sibling _____

Birth/Gender order (e.g., 2 sons, 1 daughter, myself) _____

_____

Your own conception _____

_____

Your own gestation _____

_____

Your own birth _____

_____

Breast-fed? _____ How long? _____

If pregnant: Conception of present pregnancy _____

_____

Course of present pregnancy _____

_____

_____

*phrase coined by Carolyn Myss, Ph.D.

Please describe previous conceptions, pregnancies, and births on a separate paper.

Your mother's health history _____

_____

_____

Your father's health history _____

_____

Episodes of childhood sexual abuse _____

Episodes of domestic violence _____

Other life crises _____

_____

_____

_____

_____

Write and attach your autobiography.

Appendix 4

Summary of Essential Prenatal Exercises

Do each exercise twice at first, progressing at your own pace to 5 times. The sequence can be repeated in reverse order. Rest and breathe deeply between each exercise.

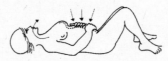

1. Abdominal Wall Tightening on Outward Breath: Bring navel to spine.

2. Pelvic Floor: Quick flicks and slow waves with vaginal muscles.

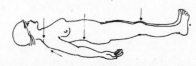

3. Stretch Out the Kinks: on the bed, against wall, navel to spine.

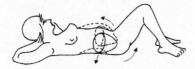

4. Pelvic Tilting: various positions, navel to spine

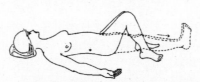

5. Heel-sliding keeping back flat.

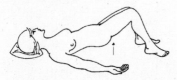

6. Bridging, hands behind head as you improve. Straighten one leg alternately.

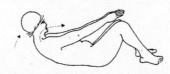

7. Straight Curl-up as you exhale.

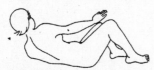

8. Diagonal Curl-up to each side as you exhale.

When **standing up**, roll over onto your knees and push off with your arms. When rising from the bed or floor, go on to one knee and straighten your legs to stand.

Posture Check (Appendix 7).

Relaxation session: Twenty minutes' complete tension release in any comfortable position twice daily.

9. Squatting, feet flat. Hold on to partner or chair.

From *Essential Exercises for the Childbearing Year,* 5th edition. ©1976, 1982, 1988, 1995, 2003. Elizabeth Noble, *New Life Images.*

Appendix 5

Summary of Essential Postpartum Exercises

Commence within 24 hours; repeat each exercise twice to start, progressing at your own pace through the phases. Rest between each exercise and continue with normal breathing.

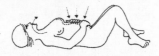

1. Deep Breathing with Abdominal Wall Tightening on outward breath. Bring belly toward backbone, in any position.

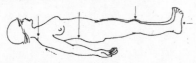

3. Stretch Out the Kinks: hold and keep breathing.

2. Pelvic Floor Contractions.

Posture check. (Appendix 7) Before standing: sit with legs over bed for a few minutes and swing your feet. Brace abdominals, buttocks, and pelvic floor when upright and walking around and especially

Relaxation: Lying on the front half an hour, twice daily. Use pillows for breast comfort.

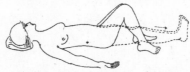

4. Heel-sliding keeping your back flat.

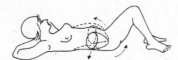

5. Pelvic Tilting pulling navel toward spine.

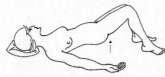

6. Bridging progress to placing hands behind head, extending one leg (alternat-

Check if you can interrupt your urine flow. Check your center seam (recti muscles) after **third** day. When center seam is back to 2 fingers wide, do #8-9.

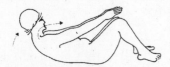

7. Straight Curl-up as you exhale.

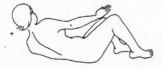

8. Straight Curl-up as you exhale.

Progressive abdominal exercises: Curl-ups with arms folded across your chest, and finally, hands behind your head.

Reprinted from **Noble, Elizabeth.** *Essential Exercises for the Childbearing Year,* 5th. edition, 2003.

Appendix 6

Summary of Essential Exercises after a Caesarean

Commence as soon as you recover from the anesthetic. Do each exercise twice to start, progressing at your own pace. Rest and breathe deeply between.

1. Breathing Exercises: Upper chest, mid-chest, diaphragmatic on outward breath.

2. Forced exhalation to bring navel toward spine.

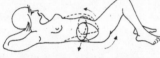

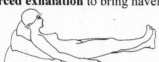

3. Foot Exercises: bend, stretch, rotate.

4. Leg-Bracing: tense and relax legs.

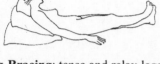

5. Bending and Straightening Alternate Knees.

6. Pelvic Rocking. Navel toward spine, combine with **pelvic floor contractions.**

Posture check (see Appendix 7. Before standing: Bend knees and use arms to roll toward edge of bed. Sit first and swing feet a few times. Brace abdominal muscles as you stand upright, walk, lift. **Check your recti muscles after day 3.** Check ability to **control urine flow**.

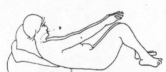

7. Reach to your Knees as you exhale,

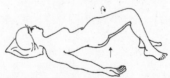

8. Bridge and Twist to prevent gas pain.

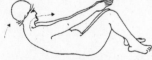

9. Straight Curl-up on outward breath.

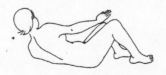

10. Diagonal Curl-up on outward breath.

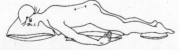

Relaxation on front as soon as you can.

Reprinted from **Noble, Elizabeth. *Essential Exercises for the Childbearing Year,*** 5th. edition, 2003.

Appendix 7

Posture Checklist

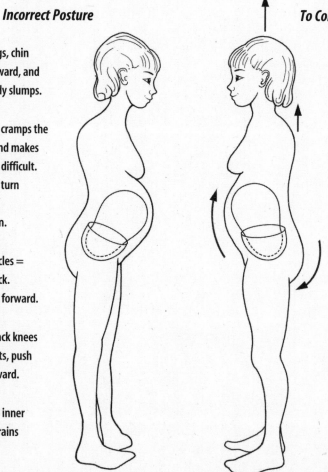

Incorrect Posture

If neck sags, chin pokes forward, and whole body slumps.

Slouching cramps the rib cage and makes breathing difficult. Shoulders turn forward, arms roll in.

Slack muscles = hollow back. Pelvis tilts forward.

Pressed back knees strain joints, push pelvis forward.

Weight on inner borders strains arches.

To Correct Posture

Straighten neck, tuck chin in so ear lines up with shoulder.

Lift up through rib cage and lower shoulders. Roll arms out.

Contract abdominal muscles to align spine. Tuck buttocks under to tilt pelvis back to neutral.

Knees soft to ease body weight over feet.

Distribute body weight through center of each foot.

Appendix 8

Medical Risks of Epidural Anesthesia during Childbirth

This is the index of complications from epidural anesthesia that can be found at the Web site of Lewis Mehl-Madrona, M.D., Ph.D. — www.healing-arts.org/

- Introduction
- Epidurals and pain relief
- Overall complication rates for epidural anesthesia
- Effects of epidurals on Caesarean rate
- Significant low blood pressure (hypotension)
- Fetal distress
- IV cannulation
- Trauma to blood vessels
- Punctured dura
- Infection
- Backache
- Broken catheters
- Abnormal uterine contractions
- Second stage labor effects
- Inadequate pain relief
- Accidental spinal anesthesia
- Maternal heart attack or spinal cord ischemia

- Asthmatics
- Medication interactions
- Interactions with other illnesses
- Malignant hyperthermia
- Respiratory arrest
- Other neurological disabilities
- Nausea and vomiting
- Allergic conditions
- Heart problems
- Headache
- Motor blockade
- Use in VBAC (vaginal birth after Caesarean)
- Technical considerations
- Herpes simplex
- Case examples: mild problems
- Permanent disability from epidural anesthesia
- Deaths from epidural anesthesia
- Critique of 3 other studies
- Does epidural analgesia protect against Caesarean section in nulliparous patients?
- Epidural anesthesia and uterine function
- The relationship of ambulation in labor to operative delivery
- References

Appendix 9

Plans for Parents and Hospital Personnel in the Event of Loss

Parents' Action Plan in the Event of Loss

1. I/we would like to hold the baby for as long as I/we wish and as often as I/we wish.

    It is now well accepted that parents need to see and hold their baby in the event of a death, unlike some years ago when well-meaning professionals thought they were "sparing" the parents by whisking a baby away unseen. When one member of a multiple set dies, it is even more important to see the baby in order that a concrete reality may be grieved and to resolve this grief alongside the presence of the living twin/s.

2. I/we would like _____ (siblings, relatives) also to see/hold the baby/ies as often as I/we wish.

    Reality is never as grim as fantasy, and death can be comprehended by small children and provides important closure. It is important for family and friends to see that this person had a body and an existence.

3. I/we want to name the infant/s _____.

    Naming the infant(s) provides identity, and by acknowledging the reality of that existence makes it much easier to talk about him/her/them later on and reduces the illusory aspects of the experience. If a particular name has been chosen for the infant, experts recommend that it still be used in the event of death. Reserving it for the next baby may confuse that baby's identity and the child may feel that he or she has to walk in the shoes of the deceased sibling.

4. The following mementos would be especially significant for us to keep:

    For example, lock of hair; handprints and footprints; photographs, ultrasound scans, videos, regardless of condition of the baby who died, including photographs of the baby washed and dressed; photographs of both babies together and also being held by the parents; ultrasound scan or x-ray; crib blanket; medical record; birth certificate; fetal monitor tracing; identification bracelet; cord clamp.

5. I/we would/would not like to have a baptism.

6. I/we would like details about zygosity.

   This is important for medical and genetic reasons as well as natural parent curiosity (and that of the surviving twin) to know as much as possible about the offspring.

7. I/we would like to know the cause of death if it can be determined.

8. I/we do/do not wish to have an autopsy.

9. I/we would like to have a burial/cremation/ or to donate the body/ies.

   For example, if a baby is less than 20 weeks or 500 grams (approximately a pound) you must express your wishes or the hospital will dispose of the body after sending it to the pathology department. A grave is an important symbol and an act of closure for the bereaved. Otherwise the dead baby is experienced like someone missing in action. Psychiatrist Emanuel Lewis at the Tavistock Clinic in England points out the existence of the Tomb of the Unknown Soldier is likewise an important symbol. However, a common grave is vague and confusing to the siblings, who can benefit from attending a burial. An open casket (which requires embalming) allows all who attend the funeral to register the actual existence of the baby. When this has not been done, mothers have regretted the ethereal nature of the loss. Some may combine a memorial service with the christening or baptism ceremony for the other twin.

10. I/we would like to notify _____ of the death by the following means _____.

    Make a list of the people whom you would like to notify immediately for support while you are in the hospital. When one twin has died, the timing of birth and death announcements may be awkward. Some couples send them out together or write a joint announcement.

11. I do not want general anesthesia in the case of a baby who dies before birth.

Well-intentioned doctors may believe that knocking out the mother "spares" her the experience of delivery. However, the "nothingness" quality that may accompany the birth of a baby (or babies) who dies before or during labor is accentuated if anesthesia is used, making it difficult for the mother to perceive the event concretely and grieve for an actual person. Death also causes confusion in the staff, who may be overwhelmed. Stand up for your rights — the baby belongs to you, not the hospital — and you will never regret having done so.

12. I wish to cancel a tubal ligation (if one was planned).

Guidelines for Hospital Personnel in the Event of Loss

Emanuel Lewis has written extensively on the subject of infant death. He observed that death in obstetric situations tends to "de-skill" hospital staff. Personnel often are unable to overcome their own reactions to the stillbirth and suppress their feelings of failure and grief. Thus, professional staff tends to avoid discussion of the loss that would be entailed by listening and supporting the parents. (Ideally, there would be opportunities to provide healing for healers, such as staff mutual support groups and private rooms for expression of feelings that mount up in a highly charged environment.) Much of the following guidelines are based on Lewis's advice.

1. Do not ask a mother/father if they want to see the baby. This unintentionally communicates the concept that they have created something that they possibly cannot bear to look at. Numerous studies have shown that mothers imagine their baby's deformities and condition to be far worse than they actually are. Rather than regretting having seen and held their baby, parents usually deeply grieve the lost opportunity to do so.

    The dead baby should be handed to the mother and/or father, wrapped, and later dressed, appropriately. Staff can help by discussing the appearance and characteristics of the baby and referring to the baby by name, thus making the birth and death real so that parents can more easily mourn the loss they are experiencing. Substantiation of these monumental life events by others is a big help. The baby should be available to the whole family throughout the mother's hospital stay as often as they wish. Respect the parents' need to examine their baby naked.

    Expect mothers and fathers to mourn the death differently and counsel them with regard to these differences. In general, mothers prefer other people to open a conversation with them about the baby who died. Depressed fathers, on the other hand, may also feel this way but worry that people avoid discussing death. Fathers usually feel compelled to suppress their feelings in order to give the mother support. Personal sadness and individual reactions to the loss may make it difficult for spouses to be mutually helpful.

2. If the mother or father cannot hold the baby until she dies, reassure them that one of the staff will. Sometimes a baby is critically ill and not expected to live more than a few hours. Remember that handing their baby back to the nurse is the hardest thing parents may ever have to do, so receive the infant with great sensitivity.

3. Never attempt to reassure the mother that she was lucky to have one live twin, or another healthy baby, or not to have a disabled baby, or to have avoided more than she could handle, or present other rationalizations of the tragedy. Even if the dead baby had severe abnormalities, Lewis points out, "her dead baby will always be important to her, and she will never forgive you, even though she may have had similar thoughts herself." Well-meaning health professionals, like others, often underestimate the grief and loss felt by parents of multiples.

4. Keep the parents together. Separating them may imply that women are stronger or that a father's grieving is less significant.

5. Ask the mother if she wishes to have a private hospital room. Sometimes it is better not to make any arrangements which may reinforce feelings of guilt or isolation or lead to feelings that others need to be protected from feeling upset over the loss. At least provide an appropriate place for private time with family members.

6. Help the parents deal with practical events. Guide bereaved parents through their haze to make whatever decisions are necessary, such as the details of burial. Help them get in touch with a grief support network. Sit down, offer parents a refreshment, and give them your undivided attention. Avoid talking over an incubator because you may give the impression that there are more important things to do than to listen to the mother's fears and worries. It would be expedient to have a copy of Appendix 9, Part 1, "Parents' Action Plan in the Event of Loss," in all maternity units.

7. Encourage the mother to focus her attention on the dead baby. Help the mother integrate the duality of her birth/death experience. Recall details of the birth before they are forgotten, to acknowledge not only the existence of the dead twin but also the need to grieve. At the same time, the mother needs to bond with the living infant(s). Multiples who are separated from mothers as a result of Caesarean section run a greater risk of rejection, especially if there are problems with the baby/ies.

8. If one or more surviving multiple remains in the hospital, write the name of the deceased co-multiple on their name card (and consider adding a photo). This alerts everyone who tends that baby to the fact that he or she is part of a set.

9. Answer questions clearly, simply, gently, and, above all, truthfully. There is nothing that anyone can say or do that will take away the loss. Instead of advice, opinions, and comments, simply listen and affirm the feelings that are expressed and ask what you can do.

Glossary

Abruptio placenta: Premature detachment of the placenta from the wall of the uterus during pregnancy or birth.

Acardia: Congenital absence of heart.

AGA: Appropriate for gestational age.

Alpha-fetoprotein: A protein produced by the fetus. High levels in the mother's blood can mean multiple pregnancy or an abnormality.

Amino acids: The building blocks of protein.

Amniocentesis: A test to screen for certain genetic disorders using cells in the amniotic fluid.

Amnion: The inner membrane of the sac enclosing the fetus within the uterus. Also called *amniotic sac*.

Anabolic: The building-up of complex substances from simple ones.

Analgesia: Medication to provide pain relief without complete loss of sensation (anesthesia).

Anemia: A condition in which the blood contains a reduced number of red blood cells.

Apgar score: An evaluation of a newborn's condition at 1, 5, and 10 minutes after birth.

Apnea, apneic spells: When breathing stops for 15 to 20 seconds.

ART: Assisted reproductive technologies. (See Appendix 1.)

Betamethasone (Celestone): A steroid drug given by injection to the mother to speed maturation of fetal lungs.

Biophysical profile: A evaluation that combines results from a non-stress test with ultrasound, heart rate, breathing patterns, movements, and amount of amniotic fluid.

Biparietal diameter: The distance between the bones at each side of the skull.

BPD: See *bronchopulmonary dysplasia, biparietal diameter*.

Bradycardia: Slowing of the heart rate.

Braxton-Hicks contractions: Normal, irregular contractions of pregnancy.

Breech extraction: Manual assistance by the doctor when delivery is not spontaneous.

Breech presentation: The lower part of the body (feet or buttocks) presenting at birth.

Bronchopulmonary dysplasia (BPD): Damage to an infant's lungs caused by the use of a respirator. Now called *chronic lung disease*.

Caesarean section: Surgical delivery of the baby through an incision in the abdominal and uterine walls.

Catabolic: The breakdown of complex substances into simpler ones.

Cerclage: Suturing an "incompetent" cervix to prevent it opening in pregnancy.

Cervical dilation: The opening of the cervix during labor (measured in centimeters; 10 centimeters is fully dilated).

Cervical effacement: Thinning of the cervix before and during labor (measured as a percentage).

Cervical incompetence: Premature opening of the cervix, generally in the second trimester.

Chorion: The outer sac enclosing the fetus within the uterus.

Chorionic villus sampling (CVS): A genetic screening test by examining cells from the chorion at 10 to 12 weeks gestation.

Chromosomes: The genetic material contained in the mother's egg and the father's sperm that combines during fertilization.

Chronic lung disease (CLD): See *bronchopulmonary dysplasia*.

Cord prolapse: A rare emergency that occurs when the umbilical cord drops out of the uterus into the vagina before the baby, leading to cord compression and oxygen deprivation from pressure by the body part coming after.

Cotyledons: Reservoirs of blood in the placenta.

Crohn's disease: Inflammation of the intestines.

Diamniotic: Twins who developed in separate amniotic sacs. They may be dizygotic (DZ) or monozygotic (MZ).

Dichorionic: Having two chorions. See *chorion*.

Dilation: See *cervical dilation*.

Dizygotic (DZ): Referring to twins who result from the union of two eggs and two sperm. Also called *binovular* or *fraternal*.

DNA fingerprinting: The most reliable form of zygosity testing that has nothing to do with fingers but looks at the similarity of DNA in cells from the inner cheek or blood.

Doppler flow study: Prenatal evaluation of the blood flow to the placenta.

Down's syndrome: A genetic disorder (trisomy 21) that results in physical anomalies and mental retardation.

Ductus arteriosus: A short vessel connecting the pulmonary artery to the aorta.

Ectopic pregnancy: A pregnancy that grows outside the uterus, usually in the Fallopian tube.

Effacement: See *cervical effacement*.

Electronic fetal monitoring (EFM): Measurement of the fetal heart rates with external monitors before and during labor.

Embryo transfer (ET): An embryo created outside the woman's body is transferred into her uterus.

Endometrium: The outer layer of the tissue lining the uterus.

Epidural: A regional anesthetic administered during labor around the nerve roots outside the spinal cord.

Episiotomy: An incision made in the vaginal opening at birth.

Essential amino acids: Parts of proteins that cannot be produced by the body and must be supplied by the diet.

Essential fatty acids (EFAs): Fats that cannot be produced by the body and must be supplied by food, for example, omega-3 and omega-6, used for vital cellular functions.

External version: A procedure in which the doctor turns the baby or babies in the uterus by applying manual pressure on the mother's abdomen.

Fetal death: Death of a baby weighing at least 350 gm or of 20 weeks gestation or more.

Fetal reduction and multifetal reduction: The selective destruction of one or more fetuses/embryos in a multiple pregnancy to enhance the survival chances of the remaining one/s.

Feto-fetal transfusion syndrome (FFTS): A rare condition in which one twin develops at the expense of the other when they share a monochorionic placenta. This can also occur among MZ members of a set of higher-order multiples.

Fetus papyraceus: A dead fetus pressed flat by the development of the living twin.

Fraternal twins: See *dizygotic.*

Fundus: Body of the uterus. Fundal height (the distance from the pubic bone to the top of the uterus) is measured at prenatal visits.

Gastroschisis: A congenital defect in the wall of the abdomen that remains open.

Gavage feeding: Infant feeding via a thin, flexible tube passed through either the nose or mouth and into the stomach.

Gestational age: Fetal age in weeks calculated from the mother's last menstrual period.

GIFT: Gamete-intra-fallopian tube technique for placing the sperm in the tube.

HCG: See *human chorionic gonadotropin.*

HELLP (hemolysis, elevated liver enzymes, and low platelets) syndrome: A severe condition of late pregnancy.

Hematocrit: The percentage of red blood cells in the blood.

Hemoglobin (HGB): The oxygen-carrying iron pigment in red blood cells.

Higher-order multiples (HOM): Triplets and more.

Home uterine activity monitor (HUAM): An electronic device that measures the frequency and intensity of uterine contractions.

Human chorionic gonadotropin (HCG): A hormone produced by the chorion; it can be measured soon after conception to confirm a pregnancy.

Hydatiform mole: A "cystic placenta," a degenerative process in the villi of the chorion which gives rise to multiple fluid-filled cysts.

Hydramnios: See *polyhydramnios*.

Hyperbilirubinemia: Excessively high levels of bilirubin in the blood during the newborn period.

Hypertension: High blood pressure. See *pregnancy-induced hypertension*.

Hypoglycemia: An abnormally low level of sugar in the blood.

Iatrogenic: Caused by the physician.

Identical twins: See *monozygotic*.

***In vitro* fertilization (IVF):** Union of egg and sperm in a glass dish in a laboratory.

Incompetent cervix: A cervix that opens in pregnancy, potentially resulting in a miscarriage or early preterm birth.

Infant death: Death in the first year of life.

Internal version: A procedure in which the doctor manually brings the feet of the second baby down to perform a breech extraction. See also *presentation*.

Intracytoplasmic sperm injection (ICSI): The sperm is placed directly into the substance of the cell.

Intrauterine growth restriction (IUGR): Birth weight of less than the 10th percentile for gestational age.

Intraventricular hemorrhage (IVH): Bleeding into the ventricles of the brain.

IVF-ET: *In vitro* fertilization with embryo transfer.

Ketones: By-products of the breakdown of fat.

Kilogram (kg): The metric equivalent to 1,000 grams or 2.2 pounds.

Large for gestational age (LGA): Birth weight above the 90th percentile for gestational age.

LBW: See *low birth weight*.

Let-down reflex: Hormonal release of milk stored in the breasts.

Leukemia: A cancer of the white blood cell system.

Linea nigra: A line of darkened pigment from the navel to the pubic bone that occurs in some women during pregnancy.

Low birth weight (LBW): A birth weight of less than 2,500 grams or 5 pounds.

Membranes: The sacs that enclose the fetus in the uterus. See *amnion* and *chorion*.

Monoamniotic (MA): Twins who have developed in a single amniotic sac. These twins are always MZ.

Monochorionic (MC): Having one chorion. See *chorion*.

Monozygotic: Referring to twins who result from the union of one egg and one sperm that divides in two. Also called *monovular*.

Necrotizing enterocolitis (NEC): A potential complication of prematurity that creates a gangrene-like condition of portions of the gastrointestinal tract.

Neonatal death: A death in the first 28 days after delivery.

Nitrogen balance: When intake of nitrogen from proteins equals its daily excretion.

Nocebo effect: An ill effect caused by the suggestion or belief that something is harmful.

Non-stress test: An evaluation of fetal movements and fetal heart rate using an electronic fetal monitor.

Nosocomial infection: An infection from the hospital environment.

Oral glucose tolerance test (OGTT): A test to determine blood glucose levels after drinking a high-carbohydrate beverage.

Palpation: Examination by touch.

Patent ductus arteriosis (PDA): When the fetal connection between the aorta and the artery to the lungs remains open after birth.

Perinatal mortality: A stillbirth, or death during the first week after birth.

Perineum: The area between the vagina and the anus.

Phototherapy: A treatment for high bilirubin levels (hyperbilirubinemia) that uses light waves to break down bilirubin so that it can be excreted in the urine.

Physiologic jaundice: A buildup of bilirubin in the blood during the newborn period, causing the skin to become yellow.

Placebo effect: A beneficial effect that occurs because of a belief that something is good.

Placenta: The organ formed in the wall of the uterus composed of maternal and fetal tissue through which nutrients and waste products are transferred between the mother's and the babies' circulations.

Placenta previa: When the placenta is attached low down on the uterine wall and partially or completely blocks the cervical opening.

Placental abruption: Premature detachment of the placenta from the wall of the uterus during pregnancy or birth.

Polyhydramnios: An excess of amniotic fluid in the uterus. Also called *hydramnios*.

PPROM: See *preterm premature rupture of membranes*.

Preeclampsia: A pregnancy complication in which there is protein in the urine, rapid weight gain, rise in blood pressure, and swelling from fluid retention; formerly called *toxemia*.

Presentation: The part of the baby's body that is against the cervix at the time of labor and delivery. Possible presentations include: *vertex* (headfirst); *breech* (lower part of the body first); *transverse lie* (baby's body across the mother's pelvis).

Preterm/Premature birth: Birth between 20 and 37 gestational weeks.

Preterm premature rupture of membranes (PPROM): Breaking of the membranes prior to 37 weeks gestation.

Prolapsed cord: See *cord prolapse*.

PROM: Breaking of the membranes prior to labor.

Proteinuria: Protein in the urine.

Q: every, as in "Q4h" — every four hours.

Respiratory distress syndrome (RDS): A common complication of preterm birth in which lung tissue collapses due to lack of surfactant to keep lungs inflated.

Respiratory syncytial virus (RSV): A viral infection of the lungs and breathing passages that can be severe for infants born preterm.

Retinopathy of prematurity (ROP): An eye complication of some preterm babies in which blood vessels of the eye grow abnormally; also called *retrolental fibroplasia*.

Retrolental fibroplasia: See *retinopathy of prematurity*.

Rh factor: A protein in red blood cells that can be incompatible with the mother's blood if she is Rh-negative and the babies are Rh-positive.

Rhogam: An immunization given to Rh-negative women after a miscarriage or birth to prevent production of antibodies in future Rh-positive pregnancies.

Selective fetocide: The medical destruction of one or more fetuses in a continuing pregnancy usually because of an anomaly.

Selective multifetal reduction: Selective reduction of one or more fetuses of a higher-order multiple gestation to improve the outcome with fewer fetuses.

Sesquizygotic (SZ) twins: Twins arising from a single egg, but after the first division each half is fertilized by a different sperm.

Small for gestational age (SGA): A newborn with a birth weight that is below the 10th percentile for gestational age.

Spinal anesthetic: A regional anesthetic into the spinal fluid surrounding the nerve roots. It is given at the end of the second stage of labor to facilitate an instrumental or Caesarean delivery.

Spontaneous fetal reduction: A fetus is reabsorbed in early pregnancy, formerly called the *vanishing twin syndrome*.

Stillbirth: A baby born dead at 24 weeks of gestation or later.

Superfecundation: Two eggs are released from the ovaries and are fertilized at two separate times.

Superfetation: Two eggs are fertilized in two different menstrual cycles, resulting in marked difference in the weight of the twins at birth.

Supertwins: Triplets, quadruplets, and other higher-order multiples.

Surfactant: A foamy substance formed in the lungs that keeps the small air sacs (alveoli) from collapsing.

Terbutaline: See *tocolytics*.

Tocolytics: Drugs that reduce uterine contractions.

Toxemia: See *preeclampsia*.

Transverse lie: Baby is lying horizontally in the pelvis.

Trial of labor after Caesarean (TOLAC): Labor allowed to commence after a previous Caesarean birth in the hope of a vaginal birth.

Trizygotic: Formed from three separate zygotes (fertilized eggs).

Twin transfusion syndrome: See *feto-fetal transfusion syndrome*.

Twinism: Emphasizing the twinship rather than the individual.

Ultrasound: Technology that uses sound waves to view the fetuses within the uterus (diagnostic use) or to treat muscles and ligaments (therapeutic use).

Umbilical arterial catheter: A catheter inserted in the umbilical artery of a preterm baby to draw blood and to give fluids and medications.

Vaginal birth after Caesarean (VBAC): A vaginal birth that follows a previous Caesarean section.

Vanishing twin: The phenomenon in which one multiple fails to develop beyond the first trimester and is reabsorbed. Now called *spontaneous fetal reduction.*

Velamentous insertion of the cord: Into the membranes instead of the placenta.

Vernix: The creamy white substance (made of layers of dead skin cells) that protects the baby's skin in the fluid-filled uterus.

Vertex presentation: Headfirst birth.

Very preterm birth (VPTB): Prior to 34 weeks.

ZIFT: Zygote-intra-fallopian tube technique whereby the fertilized egg is placed in the tube.

Zygote: Fertilized egg.

Zygosity: The genetic relationship between multiples, such as MZ or DZ.

Resources

Twins

4Twins. http://www.4twins.com

Double Trouble Club. http://clubs.yahoo.com/clubs/doubletroubleclub

Facts About Multiples. http://mypage.direct.ca/c/csamson/multiples.html

Life as a Twin. http://tqjunior.advanced.org/4210/index.html
(Information on twinning, and some lists of famous twin parents.)

Marvelous Multiples, Inc. P.O. Box 381164, Birmingham, AL 35238
Tel: 205-437-3575 Fax: 205-437-3574 E-mail: marvmult@aol.com
http://www.marvelousmultiples.com/

Mothers of Multiples Webring. http://r.webring.com/hub?ring=mom&list

Multiple Births. http://whyfiles.org/053multi_birth/

Parenting of Multiples. http://multiples.about.com

Parenting Twins and a Single. http://pages.prodigy.net/twingles/twins.html

Room for Twins. http://www.mkweb.co.uk/butta/

TLC Twins. http://tlc.discovery.com/tlcpages/twins/twins.html
(Strange, true stories about twins)

Twin.com. http://geocities.com/twindotcom (Support for identical twins)

Twinergy Works. PMB 287, 4735 Clairemont Dr., San Diego, CA 92117
E-mail: twnsipes@san.rr.com http://www.sipestwins.com

TwinsAdvice.com, Inc. P.O. Box 5484 Vernon Hills, IL 60061
E-mail:Julie@twinsadvice.com http://www.twinsadvice.com

Twins Help! http://www.twinshelp.com/

Twins Life Magazine. http://www.geocities.com/Augusta/Links/6708/
cpt203/assignment11/FrontPage.html

Twins Lists. http://www.twinslist.org (National and International Organizations for Parents of Multiples)

TwinMajority.org. http://www.twinmajority.org/ (Explains why evolution predicts that from the year 2127, most babies will be twins)

Twins and More. (Jacksonville, FL) Amy Bustamante and Katheryn Hartigan
Tel: 904-334-5012 E-mail: twinsandmorejax@hotmail.com

Twinship. P.O. Box 311, New Alexandria, PA 15670.
E-mail: twinship@twinship.com http://www.twinship.com/

Twinsight. 1137 Second Street, Suite 109, Santa Monica, CA 90403
Tel: 310-458-1373 Fax: 310-451-8761 E-mail: epearlman@twinsight.com
http://www.twinsight.com/ (A counseling service for families of multiples)

Twinstuff. http://www.twinstuff.com/

Twin-Things. http://www.twin-things.com

Twinsworld. 333 East 89th Street, Suite B, New York, NY 10128
Tel: 800-RU Twins Tel: 212-289-1777 http://www.Twinsworld.com
(PlanetTwins: Debra and Lisa Ganz)

Supertwins

Deschler Quadruplets Website. http://www.geocities.com/leedesch.

Full House Mothers of Multiples (MOMs). http://www.spindesign.com/fullhouse/

Keeping Pace with Multiple Miracles. Tel: 508-697-0504
E-mail: ppacex4@gis.net

More The Merrier. San Diego, CA

Mothers of SuperTwins (MOST). P.O. Box 951, Brentwood, NY 11717-0627
Tel: 877-434-MOST (in NY 631-859-1110) http://www.MOSTonline.org

Multiple Blessings International.
http://www.multipleblessingsinternational.twinstuff.com

Parenting Multiples. http://multiples.about.com/

Triplet Connection. http://www.tripletconnection.org Tel:209-474-0885.

Triplet and Twin Club. http://clubs.yahoo.com/clubs/tripletandtwin

Triplets, Moms, & More (Massachusetts). Tel: 781-449-3261
E-mail: TMANDMORE@aol.com http:// www.tripletsmomsandmore.org
(Support during pregnancy with weekly phone support, home visits, hospital
visits, and meals)

Triplet and Twin Club. http://clubs.yahoo.com/clubs/tripletandtwin

Triplets Quads and Quints. http://www.tqq.com/resources.html
E-mail: stephen@tqq.com

Triplets R US. http://www.tripletsrus.com/triplets/index.html

Triplets UK. http://freespace.virgin.net/andrew.berry/

Professional and Research Organizations for Multiple Pregnancy

Boklage, Charles E., Ph.D., Professor and Director, Laboratory of Behavorial &
Developmental Genetics, East Carolina University, School of Medicine, Depart-
ment of Pediatrics, Greenville, NC 27858-4354 E-mail: boklagec@mail.ecu.edu.
(Research into the third type of twin, using triplets)

Center for the Study of Multiple Birth. 333 E. Superior Street, Suite 476, Chicago, IL 60611 Tel: 312-908-7532 Fax: 312-908-8500 E-mail: lgk395@nwu.edu http://www.multiplebirth.com/

The Centers for Disease Control and Prevention. http://www.cdc.gov/nchs/fastats/multiple.html

Centre for Research on Mothering. Room 726, Atkinson College, York University, 4700 Keele Street, Toronto, ON M3J, 1P3 Canada Tel: 416-736-2100 ext. 60366 E-mail: arm@yorku.ca http://www.yorku.ca/crm

Greer, Jane, Ph.D., 141 East 55th Street, Suite 7G, New York, NY 10022 Tel: 212-688-7020 E-mail: Drjanegreer@aol.com (Twin consultant)

Indiana University Twin Studies. Department of Medical Genetics, 975 West Walnut, IB130, Indianapolis, IN 46202 Tel: 317-274-5743 Fax: 317-274-2387 E-mail:trobins1@iupui.edu

International Twins Association (ITA). Sharleen Dow and Sharon Kilbourne. 4459 Hillside St., Gladwin, MI 48624 Tel: 517-425-1942 E-mail: clarktriplets@intltwins.org http://www.intltwins.org/index.htm.

International Twins Foundation (ITF). P.O. Box 6043, Providence, RI 02904-6043 Tel: 401-729-1000 Fax: 401-751-4642 E-mail: twins@twinsfoundation.com http://www.twinsfoundation.com

Louisville Twin Study. Twin Child Development Unit, Health Sciences Center, University of Louisville, Louisville, KY 40292 Tel: 502-852-5140 E-mail: mlriese@gatekeeper.lts.louisville.edu

Luke, Barbara, ScD, MPH, RD, Professor, Depts. of Epedemiology, Public Health and Obstetrics and Gynecology, University of Miami School of Medicine, 1801 NW 9th Ave., Room 200H, Miami, FL 33136 http://www.drbarbaraluke.com

Malmstrom, Patricia. E-mail: twinservices@juno.com http://www.twinservices.org (Directs Twin Services Consulting for professionals and parents of multiples)

Minnesota Center for Twin and Adoption Research. University of Minnesota, Department of Psychology, 75 E. River Road, Minneapolis, MN 55455 Tel: 612-625-4067

Minnesota Twin Family Study. E-mail: Haroi001@umn.edu

National Organization of Mothers of Twins Clubs, Inc. (NOMOTC). P.O. Box 438 Thompsons Station, TN 37179-0438 Tel: 615-595-0936 E-mail: nomotc@aol.com http://www.nomotc.org

The Triplet Connection. P.O. Box 99571, Stockton, CA 95209 Tel: 209-474-0885 Fax: 209-474-9243 E-mail: webmaster@tripletconnection.org http://www.tripletconnection.com/

Twins Day Committee. 10075 Ravenna Road, Twinsburg, OH 44087 Tel: 216-425-7161 http://www.twinsdays.org

Twins Foundation. P.O. Box 9487, Providence, RI 02940-9487 Tel: 401-274-8946 Fax: 775-245-1480 E-mail: twins@twinsfoundation.com http://www.twinsfoundation.com

Organizations Abroad

4Twins. http://4twins.4anything.com/

Association for Scientific Research in Multiple Births. Kwadenplasstraat 12, B-9070 Destelbergen, Belgium Tel: +329-228-3655 Fax: +329-238-2287 E-mail: twinlokaal@hotmail.com

Asociación Puertorriqueña de Nacimientos Multiples. (Puerto Rican Twins Association, en español) E-mail: melendz8@caribe.net

Association for Improvement in Maternity Services. http://www.aims.org.uk/twins.html

Association d'Entraide des Parents de Naissances Multiples (ANEPNM). 18, avenue des Mazades, 31200 Toulouse, France Tel: 05 61 13 80 32 E-mail: jum31@free.fr http://jum31.free.fr/

Association Jumeaux. (French web site) http://www.jumeaux.com/

Australian Multiple Birth Association, Inc. (AMBA). P.O. Box 105, Coogee, NSW 2034 E-mail: amba_national@yahoo.com.au http://www.amba.org.au/

Australian Twin Registry. 200 Berkeley Street, Carlton, VIC 3053 Tel: 800-037 021; 61 3 9347-2983 Fax: 03-9347 6136 E-mail: twins@gpph.unimelb.edu.au. http://www.twins.org.au

Combined Organization of Multiple Birth Organizations (COMBO). c/o Judi Linney, 27 Woodham Park Road, Woodham, Weybridge, Surrey, UK http://www.twinstuff.com/multorgs.html

Disabled Multiples Parent Registry. See Multiple Births Canada.

L'encyclopédie Pratique et Interactive des Jumeaux. (French website) http://webhome.infonie.fr/paulimc/

East Flanders Prospective Twin Study (EFPTS). c/o R. Vlietinck, Centre of Human Genetics, Catholic University of Leuven, Heurestraat 49, B-3000 Leuven, Belgium

European Triplet Association. Bethlehemstr. 8 D-30451 Hannover, Germany Tel: 0511- 2151945 Fax: 0511- 2101431 E-mail: abc-club@t-online.de http://www.abc-club.de/

European Twins Festival. http://www.europeantwins.com/link.htm

Fédération Française Des Parents De Jumeaux et Multiples. (French Web site) http://www. jumeaux-et-plus.asso.fr

Finnish Multiple Families Association. Kauppakatu 18 C 34 40100 Jyväskylä, Finland Tel: 358-14 211 277 Fax: 358-14 374 2100 http://www.suomenmonikkoperheet.fi

Finnish Twin Cohort Registry. Department of Public Health, University of Helsinki, P.O. Box 41, Mannerheimintie 172 00014 University of Helsinki, Finland Tel: +358-9-191 27 595 or +358-9-191 27 596 Fax: +358-9-191 27 600 http://kate.pc.helsinki.Fi/twin/twinhome.html

Freja. http://www.flerlinger.dk/(Danish web site, has English page.)

Gémelos México. http://www.gemelos.org.mx/

Ghana Twins Foundation. http://www.ghanatwinsfoundation.com/

Gregor Mendel Institute of Medical Genetics and Twin Studies. Piazza Galeno 5, 00161 Rome, Italy

Hong Kong Twin Club. (In Chinese) http://twinclub.com.hk/

International Society for Prenatal Psychology and Medicine. Friedhofweg 8, D - 69118 Heidelberg, Germany Tel: +49 6221 892729 Fax: +49 6221 892730 E-mail: secretary@isppm.de http://www.isppm.de/index_e.html

International Society for Twin Studies (ISTS). Queensland Institute of Medical Research, Post Office, Royal Brisbane Hospital, Brisbane, QLD 4029 Australia Tel: 617-3362-0278 Fax: 617-3362-0101 http://www.ists.qimr.edu.au

Japanese Association of Twins Mothers. c/o Hukiko Amua, 5-20 Minami Aoyama, Minatoku, Tokyo, Japan

Jumeaux Infos. (French Web site) http://www.jumeaux-infos.com/

Jumeaux et Plus Zone 51. (French Web site) http://www.jumeaux-51.org

Luigi Gedda Institute. Rome, Italy. http://www.luigigedda.it/

Multifamilias. (Argentinian Web site) http://www.multifamilias.org.ar/

Multiple Births Canada. P.O. Box 234, Gormley, ON L0H 1G0, Canada Tel: 905-888-0725 Fax: 905-888-0727, 800-228-8824 E-mail: office@mulitplebirthscanada.org http://www.multiplebirthscanada.org

Multiple Births Foundation. Hammersmith House, Level 4, Queen Charlotte's & Chelsea Hospital, Du Cane Road, London W12 0HS, England Tel: 0208–383-3519 Fax: 0208 383 3401 E-mail: mbf@ic.ac.uk http://www. multiplebirths.org.uk

Multiples in France. http://www.multiples.free.fr

National Twin Registry of Sri Lanka. Department of Medicine, Faculty of Medical Sciences, Sri Jayewardenepura University, Gangodawila, Nugegoda, Sri Lanka Tel: +94(1) 852696 ext. 316 Fax: +94(1)578336 E-mail: ssiribaddana@hotmail.com http://infolanka.com/org/twin-registry/

Parents of Multiples Across Canada. 1023 Avignon Court, Orleans, Ontario, K1C 2N4, Canada E-mail: sahmiam@mom2many.com http://Mom2Many.com/

New Zealand Multiple Birth Association. Lee Thornburn, 29 Nelson Street, Greymouth, New Zealand http://www.nzmba.org

Romande Association of Help, Exchanges and Information concerning Twins, Triplets and More. c/o Sabine Herbener, ch. De Ballalaz 18, CH-1820 Montreux, Switzerland Tel/Fax: 41-(0)21 963-10-21 CH66 1QQ. 0151-358-0020 Fax: 0151-348-0765

South African Multiple Birth Association (SAMBA). P.O. Box 72260, Lynwood Ridge 0040, Republic of South Africa Tel: 0861-432-432 Liesl@icon.co.za

Swedish Twins Clubs. Valhallavägen 106, 114 Stockholm, Sweden Tel: 08-662-12-22 Fax 08-662-12-03 E-mail: svenska@tvillingklubben.se http://www.tvillingklubben.se/

Swedish Twin Registry. Department of Medical Epidemiology, Box 281, Karolinska Institutet, Se-171 77 Stockholm, Sweden Tel: +46-8-728-74-73 Fax: +46-8-314 –975 E-mail: Twins@Mep.Ki.Se

Twin Research. St. Thomas Hospital, London, UK http://www.twin-research.ac.uk/

Twins and Multiples Education. Perth, Australia http://www.curtin.edu.au/corporate/multiplebirths

Twins (in Switzerland). http://www.zwillinge.ch/

Twins Clubs UK. Pip Humphrey Tel: 01582 833683 http://www.twinsclub.co.uk/ E-mail: pktc@theellams.org.uk

Twins and Multiple Birth Association (TAMBA). 2, The Willows, Gardner Road, Guildford, Surrey GU1 4PG, England Tel: 00 44 1483 304442 Fax: 0870 770 3303 E-mail: enquiries@tamba.org.uk. http://www.tamba.org.uk

TAMBA Triplets and Higher Multiples. c/o Wendy Varley, 95 Calvert Road, Greenwich, London SE10 ODG, England

TAMBA Single Parent Families. 41 Fortuna Way, Aylesby Park, Grimsby, South Humberside DN37 9SJ England; 1 Victoria Place, Stirling FK8 2QX, Scotland, UK

Twins Foundation. Nakula-Sadewa, c/o Seto Mulyadi.Jl. Teuku Cik Ditiro 32, Jakarta 10310, Indonesia Tel: (021) 769-4299, 310-6177

UK National Study of Triplet and Higher Order Births. National Perinatal Epidemiology Unit, Radcliffe Infirmary, Oxford 0X2 6HE, UK

Volunteer Twin Register. Alison McDonald, Room 147, Institute of Psychiatry, De Cresigny Paris, London SE5 8AF, England

General Resources

Blue Ribbon Baby. http://www.blueribbonbaby.org (Web site of Dr. Tom Brewer with free counseling)

Calculation of Nutrients in Food. http://www.ntwrks.com/

Center for Nutrition Policy and Promotion. http://www.usda.gov/cnpp/

Council for Responsible Nutrition. 1875 Eye Street, N.W., Suite 400, Washington, D.C. 20006 Tel: 202-872-1488 Fax: 202-872-1488 E-mail: webmaster@crnusa.org http://www.crnusa.org

Dairy Education Board. 325 Sylvan Avenue, Englewood Cliffs, NJ 07632 Tel: 201-871-5871 Fax: 201-871-9304 E-mail: i4crob@earthlink.net http://www.notmilk.com

Diamond Organics. 800-ORGANIC www.diamondorganics.com (Organic produce shipped anywhere)

Division of the Food and Nutrition Service. USDA, 3010 Park Center Drive, Alexandria, VA 22303 Tel: 703-756-3730 (Supplemental food programs)

European Vegetarian Organization. http://www.european-vegetarian.org.

Focus on Nutrition. http://www.nutritionfocus.com

Good Medicine. Physicians Committee for Responsible Medicine, 5100 Wisconsin Ave, NW, Suite 404, Washington, D.C. 20016 Tel: 202-686-2210 Fax: 202-686-2216 http://www.pcrm.org. Bookstore Tel: 800-695-2241

Guide to Ultrasound in Pregnancy. Suite 935 East, 845 North Michigan Avenue, Chicago, IL 60611-2252 Tel: 3123-37-0732 http://www.drapplebaum.com/pregnancy.html

Healthworld. http://www.healthy.net/cmbm

Home Health Products. 949 Seahawk Circle, Virginia Beach, VA 23452 (Castor oil packs)

The Internet Drug Index. http://www.rxlist.com

Living Foods. http://www.living-foods.com/

Life's Vigor Health & Beauty Care. 13916 Searspoint Ave., Bakersfield, CA 93312 Tel: 661-589-1818 Fax: 661-587-7227 E-mail: service@lifesvigor.com http://www.lifesvigor.com/Home-Health.html (Castor oil)

Manik Hiranandani, M.D. http://www.drmanik.com

Medline. http://www.nlm.nih.gov/databases/freemedl.html

Obstetric Ultrasound. http://www.ob-ultrasound.net

OTT-LITE®. 1214 West Cass Street, Tampa, FL 33606 Tel: 800-842-8848, 813-621-0058 Fax: 813-626-8790 http://www.ott-lite.com/ (Full spectrum lights)

Vegetarian Resource Groups (VRG). P.O. Box 1463, Baltimore, MD 21203 Tel: 410-366-8343 http://www.vrg.org

Pregnancy Planning, Diaries, Names

LifeServ Corporation. 1440 North Dayton Street, Suite 100, Chicago, IL 60622 Tel: 312-573-0343 E-mail: advisors@lifeserv.com http://www.babyserv.com

Day-by-day Calendar. http://www.momdays.com

Pregnancy Diaries. http://www.pregnancydiaries.com

Birth Diaries. http://www.birthdiaries.com

Create Your Own Website. http://www.thebabycorner.com/sites

Names. http://www.babynamecentral.com

Maternity Clothing

Adidas Maternity. http://www.thepoweroftwo.net

Before Baby. 399 Newtown Road, Greenwood, VA 22943-1701
Tel: 877-566-4969 E-mail:info@beforebaby.com http://www.beforebaby.com

Enea Maternity Clothes. http://www.eneamaternity.com

Expecting In Style. 27970 Chagrin Blvd, Suite E203A, Beachwood, Ohio 44122
Tel: 866-4expect, 866-439-7328, 216-464-9020 Fax: 216-464-9108
E-mail: info@maternity-clothing-fashions.com
http://www.expectinginstyle.com

Great Beginnings. E-mail: lbprice@gbmaternity.com
http://www.gbmaternity.com

Imaternity. http://www.imaternity.com

Leased Clothing. http://www.maternityoutfitters.com

Liz Lange Maternity Collection. 958 Madison Avenue, New York, NY 10021
212-879-2191; 346 N. Beverly Drive, Beverly Hills, CA 90210 Tel: 310-273-0099
http://www.lizlange.com

Maternity Mall. http://MaternityMall.com

Maternity Outfitters. P.O. Box 1985, Houston, Texas 77251
E-mail: info@maternityoutfitters.com

Maternity Stop. 103 2nd Ave SW. Cullman, AL 35055 Tel: 877-415-9551
http://www.maternitystop.com

Mom's Maternity online store. Tel: 800-553-1862
http://www.momsmaternity.com/

Motherhood Plus. http://www.motherhoodplus.com

Online Maternity Mall. http://www.onlinematernitymall.com

Pea in the Pod Collection. http://www.apeainthepod.com

Pickles & Ice Cream Retail, Inc. 203 Main Street, Thomson, GA 30824
Tel: 706-595-9779 http://www.picklesmaternity.com

Maternity Comfort and Support

Cascade Health Care Products. 141 Commercial St. NE, Salem, OR 97301
Tel: 800-443-9942, 503-371-4445 Fax: 503-371-5395

E-mail: onecascade@worldnet.att.net
http://www.1cascade.com/ (birth and health books/supplies)

Belly Basics. Tel: 877-ESTYLES (378-9537) E-mail: custcare@babystyle.com
http://www.bellybasics.com

BabyHugger, Lil'Lift, Trennaventions. 113 Ridgeview Park, Derry, PA 15627
Tel: 888-770-0044, 724-694-0711 Fax: 724-694-5081
E-mail: info@babyhugger.com. http://www.babyhugger.com

Baby Style. http://www.babystyle.com

Bailey Manufacturing. P.O. Box 130, Lodi, OH 44254
Tel: 800-321-8372 Fax: 800-224-5390
http://www.baileymfg.com/products/positioningpillows/index.htm
(Positioning wedges, incline mats and bolsters)

BellyBra. http://www.bellybra.com E-mail: sales@bellybra.com

Body Support Systems, Inc. P.O. Box 337, Ashland, OR 97520
Tel: 800-448-2400, 503-488-1172 http://www.bodysupport.com/
(Use the BodyCushion™ to lie on your front in pregnancy and other
positions)

D-Med, Inc. P.O. Box 700, Highland Park, IL 60035 Tel: 800-872-3633
Fax: 847-433-1565 E-mail: Info@d-med.com http://www.d-med.com/
(Customizable arch supports for feet)

Glass Rainbow. 10022 Winzag, Cincinnati, OH 45242 (Double rocker)

Gottfried Medical. P.O. Box 8996, Toledo, OH 43623 Tel: 800-537-1968/328-5216
http://www.gottfriedmedical.com
E-mail:customerservice@gottfriedmedical.com (Vascular support hose)

IEM Orthopedics. P.O. Box 592, Ravenna, OH 44266 Tel: 800-992-6584 and
Canada: 800-243-6594 (Maternity support belt)

Jobst Support Hose. Box 653, Toledo, OH 43694 Tel: 800-537-1063
http://www.jobst.com

Kare Products. Tel: 800-927-KARE (5273) or 303-443-4243 Fax: 303-443-2522
http://www.kareproducts.com (Wedge and other ergonomic products)

Pelvic Muscle Therapy Program. Colonial Medical Supply Tel: 888 444 PMTX
http://www.kegelme.com (Vaginal weights and biofeedback equipment for
weak pelvic floor muscles, incontinence)

Medi Support Hose. 76 W. Seegers Road, Arlington Heights, IL 60005
Tel: 800-633-6334

Prenatal Cradle. http://www.maternaloutreach.com/boutique/prenatal.htm

SacroWedgy. 5647 Hwy 90 West Suite A, Theodore, AL 36582
Tel: 800-737-9295, ext. 12 Fax: 251-653-5845 E-mail: sales@sacrowedgy.com
http://www.sacrowedgy.com/

Self-Care. 5850 Shellmound Street, Emeryville, CA 94608-1901
Tel: 800-345-3371 Fax: 800-345-4021 (Exercise equipment, inversion devices, body pillow)

Skin irritation cream. 1-800-314-BACH

Fitness Equipment

Ball Dynamics International Inc. 14215 Mead Street, Longmont, CO 80504
Tel: 800-752-2255 Fax: 877-223-2962
E-mail: sandi@balldynamics.com http://www.balldynamics.com/

Body Trends. 6385-B Rose Lane, Carpinteria, CA 93013 Tel: 800-549-1667
http://newmoms.bodytrends.com/newmoms

Elgin Exercise Equipment Corp. 270 Eisenhower Lane N, Suite 4A, Lombard,
IL 60148 Tel: 630-268-1000, 800-279-3762 Fax: 630-268-1007
E-mail: elginex@aol.com (Weights, Theraband® etc.)

Gym Balls. New Life Images, 448 Pleasant Lake Avenue, Harwich, MA 02645
Tel: 508-432-8040 E-mail: info@elizabethnoble.com
http://www.elizabethnoble.com

Intellbell, Inc. 1819 South Cedar Avenue, Owatonna, MN 55060
Tel: 800-446-5215 (Simple, comprehensive home weights)

Mothers in Motion, Inc. 2051 Crabapple Cove, Round Rock, TX 78681
Tel: 877-512-8800, 512-246-7756 Fax: 512-238-7642
E-mail: custsvc@mothers-in-motion.com http://www.mothers-in-motion.com

Fathers

National Online Fathers of Twins Club. http://www.nofotc.org/

Fathering Magazine. http://www.Fathermag.com

Just for Fathers. http://www.fathersdirect.com

Birth Partners. http://www.birthpartners.com

John Robinson's Twin's Resource Page. http://www.bovabunch.com

Single Parents

Parents Without Partners, Inc. 1650 South Dixie Highway, Suite 510, Boca
Raton, FL 33432 Tel: 561-391-8833 Fax: 561-395-8557 E-mail: pwp@jti.net
http://www.parentswithoutpartners.org

Single Parent Support Kit. See Multiple Births Canada and NOMTC.

Single Triplet Moms Network. Linda Willis, 408 Holden Avenue, Lafayette,
LA 70506 Tel: 318-235-7697; Diana Vincelli, 809 Westover Hills Blvd., Richmond, VA 23225 Tel: 804-233-0099 www.twinslist.org/resparentorgs.html

Novelties and Gifts

Mainly Multiples. 411 3663 Lee Road, Jefferson Valley, NY 10535
Tel/Fax: 800-567-9559 E-mail:webmster@multipletrends.com
http://www.multipletrends.com (T-shirts, bumper stickers, gifts)

Sets o' Twins. http://www.visi.com/~johnr/twins/link.html (Links to Web
pages of twins around the world)

Twice Blessed. PMB 250, 270 Sparta Ave., Suite 104, Sparta, NJ 07871
Tel: 973-729-9063; 800-972-TWIN (8946) E-mail: nancy@twiceblessed.com
http://www.twiceblessed.com

Multiple.8k. http://multiple.8k.com/t-shirts/ (T-shirts)

Twice as Nice. 155 Bedel Court, San Diego, California 92129 Tel: 858-538-8902
http://www.twice-as-nice-shop.com/

Jan's Custom Knits. P.O. Box 1197, Hollister, CA 95024 Tel: 831-637-3269 (Baby
blankets with names in most languages)

Pregnancy and Birth Information

Alterna Moms Unite. http://www.alternamoms.com

Association Of Labor Assistants And Childbirth Educators (ALACE).
P.O. Box 390436, Cambridge, MA 02139 Tel: 617-441-2500
E-mail: alacehq@aol.com http://www.alace.org

Association for Pre and Perinatal Psychology and Health (APPPAH).
340 Colony Road, Box 994, Geyserville, CA 95441-0994
E-mail: apppah@aol.com http://www.birthpsychology.com

Association of Radical Midwives. 62 Greetby Hill, Ormskirk, Lancashire, L39
2DT, England Tel/Fax: 01695 572776 E-mail: arm@radmid.demon.co.uk
http://www.radmid.demon.co.uk/twins.htm (Normal twin births)

Birth Balance. 309 W. 109th Street, #6D, New York, NY 10025-2136
Tel: 212-222-4349, Fax: 212-222-9308 E-mail: watrbaybee@earthlink.net (Birth
documentarian, counselor, waterbirth resources, tub rental)

BirthLove. http://www.birthlove.com http://www.birthpartners.com/

Birth Works®, Inc. P.O. Box 2045, Medford, NJ 08055 Tel: 888-TO-BIRTH
(862-4784) E-mail: mailroom@birthworks.org http://www.birthworks.org

Bloom! The Maternity Wellness Program. SpaFinder, 91 Fifth Avenue, New
York, NY 10003 Tel: 212-924-6800, 518-678-5555 http://www.spafinder.com
(Nurses, midwives, physical therapists and other certified professionals inter-
ested in participating may contact Gail S. Krebs, The Dutch Barn at Kaaterskill
Creek, 424 High Falls Road Extension, Catskill, NY 12414 Tel: 518-678-5555)

Bradley Method®. American Academy of Husband-Coached Childbirth®
Box 5224 Sherman Oaks, CA 91413-5224 Tel: 1-800-4-A-BIRTH 818-788-6662
http://www.bradleybirth.com/

Center for Humane Options in Childbirth Experiences (CHOICE).
3474 N. High Street, Columbus, OH 43214 Tel: 614-263-BABY (2229)
E-mail: shortstork@aol.com http://choicemidwives.org/options.htm

Childbirth and Postpartum Professionals Association. Tel: 888-548-3672
E-mail: info@cappa.net http://www.childbirthprofessional.com

Childbirth Solutions. P.O. Box 2220, Middleburg, VA 20118 Tel: 540-364-9023
Fax: 540-364-0481 E-mail: inquiries@childbirthsolutions.com
http://www.childbirthsolutions.com

Childbirth Without Pain Education Association. 20134 Snowden Street, Detroit, MI 48235 Tel: 313-341-3876

Citizens for Midwifery. http://www.cfmidwifery.org/

Cot Life 2000 in New Zealand. E-mail: sprott@iconz.co.nz
http://www.cotlife2000.co.nz (Prevention of crib death)

Cot Life Society UK. http://www.geocities.com/cotlife/
http://www.criblife2000.com/index.htm (Both sites seek to eliminate the exposure of all babies and children to the toxins in mattresses that causes crib death.)

Depression after Delivery (DAD). Tel: 800-944-4773
http://www.depressionafterdelivery.com

Doulas of North America. P.O. Box 626, Jasper, IN 47547 Tel: 888-788-DONA
Fax: 812-634-1491 E-mail: Webmistress@DONA.org http://www.dona.com

Everything Pregnancy. http://www.epregnancy.com

Family Life and Maternity Education (FLPME). Tel: 800-776-9248,
703-276-9248

Informed Homebirth — Informed Birth & Parenting (IH/IBP).
P.O. Box 3675, Ann Arbor, MI 48106 Tel: 313-662-6857
http://pub8.ezboard.com/fmommyguidehomebirths.showMessage?topicID=9.topic

International Cesarean Awareness Network (ICAN). 1304 Kingsdale Avenue,
Redondo Beach, CA 90278 Tel: 310-542-6400 Fax: 310-542-5368
E-mail: info@ican-online.org http://www.ican-online.org

International Childbirth Education Association (ICEA). P.O. Box 20048, Minneapolis, MN 55420 Tel: 612-854-8660 http://www.icea.org

Ivillage. (The Woman's Network) http://www.iVillage.com

Kitzinger, Sheila. http://www.sheilakitzinger.com

Lamaze™ International. 2025 M Street, Suite 800, Washington, D.C.
20036-3309 Tel: 202-367-1128, 800-368-4404 Fax: 202-367-2128
http://www.lamaze-childbirth.com

March of Dimes Birth Defects Foundation. 1275 Mamaroneck Avenue, White Plains, NY 10605 Tel: 888-MODIMES (663-4637) http://www.modimes.com

Marilyn's Midwifery Page. http://www.midwifery2000.com/lynx.htm (Large listing of many sites to do with birth)

Maternity Center Association. 281 Park Avenue South, 5th Floor, New York, NY 10010 Tel: 212-777-5000 Fax: 212-777-9320 E-mail: info@maternitywise.org http://www.maternitywise.org

Mother-Friendly Childbirth. Council for the Improvement in Maternity Services (CIMS), P.O. Box 2346, Ponte Vedra Beach, FL 32004 Tel: 888-282-CIMS, 904-285-1613 Fax: 904-285-2120 http://www.motherfriendly.org

Pregnancy Dictionary. http://www.pregnancydictionary.com

Parents Place. http://www.parentsplace.com

Read Natural Childbirth Foundation. P.O. Box 150956, San Rafael, CA 94915-0956 Tel: 415-456-8462 or 415-456-3143

Waterbirth International. P.O. Box 1400, Wilsonville, Oregon 97070 Tel: 503-673-0026 E-mail: info@waterbirth.org http://www.waterbirth.org

Yoga Therapy Center. http://www.yogatherapycenter.org/links.html (Many links to yoga therapists)

Videos

BabyJoy. Exercises and Activities for Parents and Infants, with Elizabeth Noble and Leo Sorger. New Life Images, 448 Pleasant Lake Avenue, Harwich, MA 02165 E-mail: en@elizabethnoble.com http://www.elizabethnoble.com

Babies Know More Than You Think. Touch the Future, 4350 Lime Avenue, Long Beach, CA 90807 http://www.TTFuture.org/services/

Biology, Development and Care of Twins, Triplets and More. Multiple Births Foundation. (Available in SECAM, NTUSC and PAL)

Channel for a New Life. Elizabeth Noble and Leo Sorger. New Life Images, 448 Pleasant Lake Avenue, Harwich, MA 02165 E-mail: en@elizabethnoble.com. http://www.elizabethnoble.com (Outdoor waterbirth of Carsten Noble Sorger)

The Childbirth Institute. Tel: 877-31-BIRTH E-mail: pdoughman@fuse.net. http://www.childbirthinstitute.com (At Home Childbirth Education Video Series for couples who are unable to attend traditional childbirth classes)

Delivery Self-Attachment. Righard, Lennart and Alade, M. Geddes Productions, 10546 Mcvine Ave., Sunland, CA 91040 (Video of babies finding the nipple after birth without help)

InJoy Videos. 435 Yarmouth, Suite 102, Boulder, Colorado 80304 Tel: 800-326-2082, 303-447-2082 Fax: 303-449-8788 http://www.injoyvideos.com/

National Library of Medicine. http://www.nlm.nih.com (Visible Woman)

New Fathers, New Lives. InJoy Videos (see previous page). (Includes a marketing executive with a toddler and twins)

Preparing for Multiples Pack. videos and slides. Multiple Births Foundation, UK

Whose Body, Whose Rights? Dillon, Lawrence, Dillonwood Productions. http://www.noharmm.org/wbwr.htm (circumcision education)

Periodicals and Catalogs

Compleat Mother. 5703 Hillcrest Richmond, IL 60071 Tel: 815-678-7531 E-mail: greg@rsg.org http://www.compleatmother.com

Double Feature. Multiple Births Canada Quarterly newsletter.

Journal for Living. 22 Elm Street, Albany, NY 12202 Tel: 518-465-0582 Fax: 518-462-6836 E-mail: Jflmag@aol.com

More Than One. Tel: 800-388-8946, 704-844-8984 http://www.morethan1.com/

MOTC Notebook. National Organization of Mothers of Twins Clubs.

Mothering. P.O. Box 1690, Santa Fe, NM 87504 Tel: 800-443-9637, 800-354-8400 in California http://www.mothering.com

Right Start Catalog. Right Start Plaza, 5334 Sterling Center Drive, Westlake Village, CA 91361 Tel: 800-LITTLE-1, 800-48-8531 (Mail order catalog for baby care accessories, childhood safety devices, Tummy Rest pregnancy pillow)

Twins Magazine. 11211 E. Arapahoe Rd., Suite 101, Centennial, CO 80112-3851 Tel: 303 290-8500 Fax: 888-55-TWINS (888-558-9467) E-mail: twins.customer.service@businessword.com http://www.twinsmagazine.com

Triplet Connection Magazine. (see page 505)

Alternative Medicine

Alternative Medicine. http://www.Alternativemedicine.com

Cole, Ronald, M.D., 1311 E. General Cavazos Blvd., Suite 302, Kingsville, TX, 78363 Tel: 361-592-2223 http://www.birthhealingandbeyond.com/ (OB-GYN offering natural birth for multiples)

The Farm. P.O. Box 156, Summertown, TN 38433 E-mail: MidwifeIM@aol.com http://www.thefarm.org (Alternative community offering natural birth for twins)

Helios Homoeopathic Pharmacy. 97 Camden Rd, Tunbridge Wells, Kent TN1 2QR, England Tel: (0)1892 537254 Fax: (0)1892 546850 http://www.helios.co.uk pharmacy@helios.co.uk (original placental extract)

German information on placental extract: http://www.homoeopathieforschung.de/placenta.htm

Homeopathy Home. http://www.homeopathyhome.com/

Rx Homeo. http://www.rxhomeo.com/

Home Health Products, Inc. 1160-A Millers Lane, Virginia Beach, VA 23451
Tel: 800-284-9123 (Natural health products including castor oil)

School for Body-Mind Centering. 189 Pondview Drive, Amherst, MA 01002
Tel: 413-258-8615 Fax: 413-256-8239 E-mail BMCschool@aol.com
www.bodymindcentering.com (For finding a therapist to facilitate infant
motor development)

Showalter, Anita. D.O. Twin Springs Medical Center, P.O. Box 247, Kidron,
Ohio 44636 Home Tel: 330-830-9332; Office Tel: 330-857-5787 (OB-GYN offering
natural birth for multiples)

Hypnosis

American Society of Clinical Hypnosis. 2200 E. Devon Ave., Suite 291,
Des Plaines, IL 60018 Tel: 708-297-3317 Fax: 708-297-7309
E-mail: Clinical_Info@nesch.org

Peterson, Gayle, Ph.D. 1749 Vine Street, Berkeley, CA 94703 Tel: 415-527-6216 E-
mail: gp@askdrgayle.com http://www.askdrgayle.com/ (Social worker offering
individual therapy and professional training in body-centered hypnosis for
preterm labor and other pregnancy complications; telephone hypnosis available)

HypnoBirthing® Institute. June 1–Sept. 15: P.O. Box 810, Epsom, NH 03234
Tel: 603-798-4781 Sept. 15–June 1: 10738 W. Citrus Grove, Avondale, AZ 85323
Tel: 623-772-7738 E-mail: hypnobirthing@hypnobirthing.com
http://www.hypnobirthing.com

Klaus, Phyllis H. Tel: 510-559-8000 Fax: 510-527-1984 (Marriage, family, and child
counselor offering telephone counseling and hypnosis to expectant mothers with
preterm labor and other prenatal complications; telephone hypnosis available)

Zygosity Testing

Affiliated Genetics. P.O. Box 58535, Salt Lake City, UT 84158 Tel: 801-582-4200
Fax: 801-582-8460 E-mail: btanner@burgoyne.com
http://www.affiliatedgenetics.com

Genetic Technologies Corporation. (Australia) P.O. Box 115, Fitzroy VIC 3065,
Australia Tel: 03-9415 7688 Fax: 03-9416 4076 E-mail: genetype@netcore.com.au
http://www.genetictechnologies.com.au (Test for twins costs $A165 [about
$US 90]; payment by credit card accepted; form to order kit can be obtained on
their Web site)

PRO-DNA Diagnostic. (Canada) 5345 boul. de l'Assomption, Bureau 165,
Montréal, Canada H1T 4B3 Tel: 514-253-9998, 877-ADN-6444 Fax: 514-899-9669
E-mail: info@proadn.com http://www.zygositytesting.com

Proactive Genetics, Inc. 2 Goodwin's Court, Suite #1, Marblehead, MA 01945
Tel: 781-639-5126 Fax: 800-701-3109 E-mail: info@proactivegenetics.com
http://www.proactivegenetics.com

Zygosity Testing. http://www.zygositytesting.com (Test costs $125; $140 for proactive zygosity testing)

Circumcision

Attorneys for the Rights of the Child. 2961 Ashby Avenue, Berkeley, CA 94705 Tel/Fax: 510-595-5550 E-mail: arc@post.harvard.edu http://arclaw.org/

Circumcision Information and Resource Pages. http://cirp.org/

Circumvent Circumcision. http://circumvent.org/Circumcisers.htm http://circumvent.org/RefuseToCircumcise.htm

Circumcision Resource Center. P.O. Box 232, Boston, MA 02133 Tel: 617-523-0088 E-mail: crc@circumcision.org http://circumcision.org/

Doctors Opposing Circumcision. George C. Denniston, M.D. Tel: 360-385-1882 E-mail: gcd@u.washington.edu http://faculty.washington.edu/gcd/DOC

Fight Sexual Mutilation WebRing. http://www.webmagician.com/fightcirc/

National Organization of Circumcision Information Resource Centers (NOCIRC). P.O. Box 2512, San Anselmo, CA 94960 Tel: 415-488-9883 E-mail: nocirc@cris.com. http://nocirc.org/

National Organization to Halt the Abuse and Routine Mutilation of Males (NOHARMM). http://www.noharmm.org/

The National Organization of Restoring Men. E-mail: waynerobb@aol.com http://www.norm.org/

Mothers Against Circumcision. http://mothersagainstcirc.org/

Nurses for the Rights of the Child. http://cirp.org/nrc/

Origins of Peace and Violence. http://violence.de/

Stop Infant Circumcision Society. P.O. Box 320233 Cocoa Beach, FL 32932-0233. Tel: 321-83-6383 E-mail: sicsociety@aol.com http://SicSociety.org/

Breast-feeding

Breast-feeding. effects of Circumcision http://www.nocirc.org/statements/breastfeeding_statement2002.html.

Cozie Cuddles Nursing Pillow. Tel: 416- 299-5507 E-mail: Sales@CozyCuddles.com http://www.betterbabysling.freeserve.co.uk/http://www.cozycuddles.com

Four Dee Products. Inc. 6014 Lattimer, Houston, TX 77035 Tel: 800-526-2594 (Nursemate — Special pillow to nurse "twogether")

Geddes Productions. P.O. Box 41761, Los Angeles, CA 90041 http://www.geddesproduction.com (Frantz, Kittie. *Breastfeeding Product Guide*, 1994 and *Breastfeeding Product Guide* Supplement)

International Lactation Consultants Association (ILCA). 200 N. Michigan Ave, Suite 300, Chicago IL 60601 Tel: 312-541-1710 Fax: 312-541-1271 E-mail: ilca@erols.com http://www.breastfeeding.org

Knox Breastfeeding Accessories. http://www.knoxbreastfeeding.com

La Leche League International (LLLI). P.O. Box 4079, Schaumburg, IL 60168-4079 Tel: 847-519-7730 Fax: 847-519-0035 E-mail: llli@llli.org http://www.lalecheleague.org

Maternal Outreach, Inc. 23 Wyman Road, Braintree, MA 02184 Tel: 781-849-3833 Fax: 781-849-0855 http://www.maternaloutreach.com/boutique/medela.html (Medela Breast Pumps)

Medela, Inc. P.O. Box 660, McHenry, IL 60051-0660 Tel: 800-435-8316 E-mail: customer.service@medela.com http://www.medela.com (Breast pumps, nursing aids, video)

Moms4Milk. http://www.moms4milk.org

Motherhood Nursing. 456 N. 5th Street, Philadelphia, PA 19123 Tel: 1-800-4mom2be E-mail: info@MotherhoodNursing.com http://www.motherhoodnursing.com

Motherwear. 320 Riverside Dr. Florence, MA 01062 Tel: 800-950-2500 or 413 800-950-2500 or 413-586-3488 E-mail: customerservice@motherwear.com http://www.motherwear.com (Catalog for the nursing mother)

Mother's Milkmate. Tel: 312-492-7860 E-mail: cary1958@ix.netcom.com http://www.mothersmilkmate.com (for storage)

Nursingwear. P.O. Box 1554, Nipomo, CA 93444 E-mail: info@conursingwear.com http://www.conursingwear.com

Optimal Breastfeeding Practices. 191 Clarksville Road, Princeton Junction, NJ 08550 Tel: 877-836-9947, 609-799-70321 Fax: 609-799-4900 http://www.bfmed.org

Twin Connection, Breastfeeding Support Network, Inc. 2050 W. 9th Ave., Oshkosh, WI 54904 Tel: 800-456-8687 Fax: 920-231-1697 E-mail: toman@momsbugs.com http://www.nurturing mothersboutique.com/twinconnection.htm

White River Breast Pump. 41715 Enterprise Circle North, Suite 204, Temecula, CA 92590 Tel: 909-296-0081 Fax: 909-296-0083 E-mail: custsvc@whiteriver.com http://www.whiteriver.com

Home Help

The Care Team Network. 908 S. 20th Street, Suite 189, Birmingham, AL 35294-2050 Tel: 205-975-8923 or 866-435-1391 E-mail:mmarler@uab.edu http://www.careteam.org

AuPair in America. American Institute of Foreign Study, River Plaza, 9 West Broad Street, Stamford, CT 06902-3788 Tel: 800-727-AIFS (2437) http://www.aupairinamerica.com/

AuPair-Homestay USA. 1015 15th Street, N.W., Suite 750, Washington, D.C. 20005 Tel: 800/479-0907 or 202/408-5380 Fax: 202/408-5397 http://www.interexchange.org/aphome.htm

EF AuPair, EF Foundation. One Education Street, Cambridge, MA 02141 Tel: 800-333-6056 Fax: 617-619-1101 E-mail: aupair@ef.com http://www.efaupair.org/

EurAuPair. http://www.euraupair.fi/ususa.htm (from Finland)

Cribs

Arm's Reach® Concepts, Inc. 2081 N Oxnard Blvd. PMB #187, Oxnard, CA 93030 http://www.armsreach.com

Baby Trilogy. Rt. 1, Box 649-A, Lubbock, TX 79401 Tel: 806-829-2122, 888-874-9596 Fax: 806-829-2107 E-mail: tribed@nts-online.net http://www.babytrilogy.com (Three corner crib)

More than One. Tel: 800-388-8946 http://www.morethan1.com (*Double Delight* crib)

Baby Gear

Burlington Coat Factory. http://www.coat.com/ (Discount for second sets purchased in Baby Depot)

KidSTuff℠ Online Catalog. http://www.kidsstuff.com

Leaps and Bounds. Tel: 800-477-2189

More than One. Tel: 800-388-8946, 704-844-8984 http://www.morethan1.com

One Step Ahead. P.O. Box 517, Lake Bluff, IL 60044-0517 Tel: 800-274-8440 Fax: 847-615-2478 http://www.onestepahead.com (Tykes Alike toy line)

Snibbie. Tel: 704-844-8984 http://www.snibbie.com (Bibs)

ToBuyTwo.com. 12909 N 72 Ave, Peoria, AZ 85381 E-mail: comments@tobuytwo.com http://www.tobuytwo.com (Auction web site for multiples)

Unlimited Additions. http://www.unlimitedadditions.com (Matching and coordinating clothing for multiples)

Child Development

About Babies, Inc. 818 Blue Gill Avenue, Clare, MI 48617 Tel: 800-383-3068 E-mail: contact@aboutbabiesinc.com http://www.aboutbabiesinc.com

Autism Society of America. http://www.autism-society.org

Baby Guide. http://geoparent.com/spotlight/babyguide.htm

Bowen, Caroline. http://members.tripod.com/Caroline_Bowen/mbc.html (Speech therapist for twins)

Growth Spurts. http://www.growthspurts.com

Infant Stimulation Education Association (ISEA). Susan Luddington-Hoe, Ph.D, Director, UCLA Medical Center, Factor 5-942, Los Angeles, CA 90024

International Association of Infant Massage Instructors. P.O. Box 1045, Oak View, CA 93022 Tel: 05-644-8524 E-mail: IAIM4US@aol.com

Language Development. The MIT Twins Study
E-mail: mittwins@psyche.mit.edu http://web.mit.edu/mittwins/www/

Prenatal and Post Development By Week.
http://www.babycenter.com/topic/about.html

Safety

Child Help USA. Tel: 800-4-a-Child http://www.childhelpusa.org (A 24-hour hotline for parents who are losing control and putting their children at risk of danger)

Children's Safety Zone. 2429 W. 12th Street, Suite #6 Tempe, Arizona 85281 Tel: 800-522-3308 or 480-966-2100 E-mail: sos@sosnet.com
http://www.sosnet.com/safety/safety1.html

Consumer Product Safety Commission. Washington, D.C. 20207
Tel: 301-504-0990 Fax: 301-504-0124 http://www.cpsc.gov

Inventive Minds Inc. http://www.maternityseatbelt.com

Keeping Safe in Vehicles. http://www.nhtsa.dot.gov/people/injury/childps

KidCo, Inc. 300 Terrace Drive, Mundelein, IL 60060-3836 Tel: 800-553-5529 E-mail info@kidcoinc.com http://www.kidcoinc.com/

National Center for Complementary and Alternative Medicine.
NCCAM Clearinghouse, P.O. Box 7923, Gaithersburg, MD 20898
Tel: 888-644-6226, 301-519-3153 Fax: 866-464-3616 E-mail: info@nccam.nih.gov http://www.altmed.od.nih.gov http://nccam.nih.gov/

National Clearing House on Child Abuse and Neglect Information.
330 C Street, SW, Washington, D.C. 20447 Tel: 800-94-3366 or 703-385-7565 Fax: 703-385-3206 E-mail: nccanch@calib.com. http://www.calib.com/nccanch/

National Coalition Against Domestic Violence. P.O. Box18749, Denver, CO 80218 Tel: 303-839-1852, ext. 108 E-mail: arandall@ncadv.org
http://www.ncadv.org/

National Council on Child Abuse and Family Violence. 1155 Connective Ave NW #400, Washington, D.C. 20036 Tel: 202-429-6695 http://nccafv.org/

National Domestic Violence Hotline. 1-800-799-7233 or 1-800-787-3244 (TTY) (for support, shelter, or services)

National Vaccine Information Center (NVIC). 421-E Church Street, Vienna, VA 22180 Tel: 800-909-SHOT (909-7468) or 703-938-DPT3 Fax: 703-938-5768 http://www.909shot.com/

National Women's Health Network. 514 10th Street NW, Suite 400, Washington, D.C. 20004 Tel: 202-628-7814 Fax: 202-347-1168 http://www.womenshealthnetwork.org/

Parents Anonymous® Inc. 675 W. Foothill Blvd., Suite 220, Claremont, CA 91711 Tel: 909-621-6184 Fax 909-625-6304 E-mail parentsanonymous@parentsanonymous.org http://www.parentsanonymous.org/

Perfectly Safe. Tel: 800-898-3696 Fax: 330-649-5702 E-mail: psafe@kidsstuff.net http://www.perfectlysafe.com/

Rev-A-Shelf. E-mail: mis@rev-a-shelf.com http://www.rev-a-shelf.com/ (Cabinet safety)

Transport of Multiples

Better Baby Sling. 47 Brighton Road, Watford, Hertfordshire, WD24 5HN, England, UK http://www.betterbabysling.freeserve.co.uk/ (Can carry twins in different positions)

Baby Cyberstore. www.babycyberstore.com

Burley Lite. 4020 Stewart Road, Eugene, Oregon 97402 Tel: 800-311-5294 or 541-687-1644 Fax: 541-687-0436 E-mail: burley@burley.com (Trailer holds two or three children when biking)

Cuddle Carriers. 21 Potsdam Road, Unit 61, Downsview, Ontario MSN 1N3, Canada Tel: 416-663-7143 or 877-283-3535 / E-mail: cuddlekarrier@canada.com http://www.cuddlekarrier.com/

L.O.V.E.S. (Lots Of Very Energetic Sets). Michelle Cuttler. Tel: 315-487-9170 E-mail: kmc495@a-znet.com

National Passenger Safety Association. 1050 17th Street, NW, Suite 770, Washington, D.C. 20036 http://www.nhtsa.dot.gov/people/injury/childps/Training/CPSBrochure/ (Information about infant car seats, regional training programs)

Perego Twin and Triplet Strollers. P.O. Box 99571, Stockton, CA 95209 Tel: 209-474-0885 Fax: 209-474-9243 http://www.tripletconnection.com

Premature Infants and Car Seats. http://www.umanitoba.ca/womens_health/carseat.htm http://www2.medsch.wisc.edu/childrenshosp/parents_of_preemies/carseat.html

Racing Strollers, Inc. 516 N. Bronx Avenue, Box 16, Yakima, WA 98902 Tel: 800-548-7230 (Twin all-terrain stroller)

Rear-facing Infant Car Seats. http://www.tc.gc.ca/roadsafety/childsafe/cartenv/intro-e.html

Runabout Strollers. 18770 Rigert Rd., Aloha, OR 97007 Tel: 800-832-2376 or 503-649-7922 Fax: 503-591-9435 E-mail: runabout@teleport.com http://www.bergdesign.net/runabout.htm/ (Stroller/jogging cart with up to 5 seats)

Strollers4Less. http://www.strollers4less.com/products.cfm

Twins Carriages. 5935 W. Irving Park Road, Chicago, IL 60634 Tel: 312-794-CRIB http://www.midwiferytoday.com/articles/slings.asp (Slings and carriers)

Wear Your Baby! P.O. Box 21023, Carson City, NV 89721 Tel: 775-887-0447 E-mail: Lisa@LGFJones.com http://www.wear-your-baby.com

Diapers, Toilet Learning

Fuzzibunz Diapers. http://www.fuzzibunz.com

Green Mountain Diapers. 800-330-9905 http://www.greenmountaindiapers.com

Natural Baby Catalog. 5701 Mayfair Road, North Canton, OH 44720 Tel: 800-550-2461, 888-550-2460 Fax: 330-649-5702 http://www.naturalbaby-catalog.com

Natural Baby Company. http://www.naturalbabycompany.com/

Bumkins, BNM, 1945 E. Watkins, Phoenix, AZ 85034 Tel: 800-533-5302 http://www.bumkins.com (Waterproof, washable diapers)

Mother-ease. http://www.mother-ease.com (Cloth diapers)

Ecobaby. Tel: 888-326-2229 http://www.ecobaby.com.

Diaper Pin. http://www.diaperpin.com

Without Diapers. http://groups.yahoo.com/group/eliminationcommunication

Professional Organizations

American Academy of Family Physicians. P.O. Box 11210, Shawnee Mission, KS 66207-1210 Tel: 800-274-2237 or 913-906-6000 E-mail: fp@aafp.org http://www.aafp.org

American Academy of Medical Acupuncture. 4929 Wilshire Boulevard, Suite 428, Los Angeles, CA 90010 Tel: 323-937-5514 E-mail: JDOWDEN@prodigy.net http://www.medicalacupuncture.org/contact/index.html

Acupuncture and Oriental Medicine Alliance. 14637 Starr Road SE, Olalla, WA 98359 Tel: 253-851-6896 Fax: 253-851-6883 http://www.acupuncturealliance.org

American Academy of Pediatrics (AAP). 141 Northwest Point Boulevard, Elk Grove Village, IL 60007-1098 Tel: 847/434-4000 Fax: 847-434-8000 http://www.aap.org/

The American Association of Naturopathic Physicians. 8201 Greensboro Drive, Suite 300, McLean, VA 22102 Tel: 877 969-2267, 703-610-9037 Fax: 703-610-9005 http://www.naturopathic.org/

American Board of Preventive Medicine. 330 South Wells Street, Suite 1018, Chicago, IL 60606-7106 Tel: 312-939-ABPM (2276) Fax: 312-939-2218 E-mail: abpm@abprevmed.org http://abprevmed.org

American Chiropractic Association. 1701 Clarendon Boulevard, Arlington, VA 22209 Tel: 800-986-4636, 703-243 Fax: 703/-43-2593 http://www.americhiro.org

American College of Osteopathic Obstetricians and Gynecologists (ACOOG). 900 Auburn Road, Pontiac, MI 48342-3365 Tel: 248-332-6360 Fax: 248-332-4607 E-mail: acoog@acoog.com http://www. acoog.com

American College of Obstetricians and Gynecologists (ACOG). 409 12th Street, SW, Washington, D.C. 20024-2188 http://www.acog.org

American College of Nurse-Midwives (ACNM). 818 Connecticut Avenue, NW, Suite 900, Washington, D.C. 20006 Tel: 202-728-9860 Fax: 202-728-9897 http://www.midwife.org

American College of Sports Medicine. P.O. Box 1440, Indianapolis, IN 46206-1440 Tel: 317-637-9200 Fax: 317-634-7817 http://www.acsm.org/

American Council on Exercise (ACE). 4851 Paramount Drive, San Diego, CA 92123 Tel: 858-279-8227 or 800-825-3636 Fax: 858-279-8064 http://www.acefitness.org/contactace/index.cfm

American Holistic Medical Association (AHMA). 6728 McLean Village Drive, McLean, VA 22101-8729 Fax: 703-556-8729 E-mail: info@holisticmedicine.org http://www.holisticmedicine.org/

American Holistic Nurses Association (AHNA). P.O. Box 2130, Flagstaff, AZ 86003-2130 Tel: 800-278-2462 http://ahna.org/home/home.html

American Institute of Preventive Medicine. 30445 NW Highway, Suite 350, Farmington Hills, MI 48334 Tel: 800-345-2476, 248-539-1800 Fax: 248-539-1808 E-mail: aipm@healthylife.com http://www.healthylife.com

American Massage Therapy Association. 820 Davis Street, Suite 100 Evanston, IL 60201 Tel: 847-864-0123 Fax: 847/864-1178 http://www.amtamassage.org

American Music Therapy Association. 8455 Colesville Road, Suite 1000, Silver Springs, MD 20910 Tel: 301-589-3300 Fax: 301-589-5175 E-mail: info@musictherapy.org www.musictherapy.org

American Physical Therapy Association. 111 North Fairfax Street, Alexandria, VA 22314-1488 Tel: 800-999-APTA (ext. 3237 for Section on Women's Health) http://www.apta.org

American Polarity Therapy Association. P.O. Box 19858, Boulder, CO 8030 Tel: 303-545-2080 Fax: 303-545-2161 E-mail: hq@polaritytherapy.org http://www.polaritytherapy.org/

American Society for Psychosocial Obstetrics and Gynecology (ASPOG). 409 12th Street SW, Washington, D.C. 20024-2188 Tel: 202-863-1645 Fax: 202-554-0453 E-mail mbrooks@acog.org. http://www.naspog.org/

American Society of Dowsers, Inc. (ASD). P.O. Box 24, Danville, VT 05828 Tel: 800-711-9497 or 802-748-8565 http://dowsers.new-hampshire.net/ (For information unavailable to the conscious mind)

Association for Treatment and Training in the Attachment of Children (ATTACh). P.O. Box 11347, Columbia, SC 29211 Tel: 866-453-8224 Fax: 803-765-0284 E-mail: info@attach.org http://www.attach.org/

Center for Preventive Medicine. Stuart Zoll, OMD, 7015 Bera Casa Way, Boca Raton, FL 33433 Tel: 561-395-2667 Fax: 561-395-2685 E-mail: szollocean@aol.com

Families USA. 334 G Street, NW, Washington, D.C. 20005 Tel: 202-628-3030 Fax: 202-347-2417 E-mail: info@familiesusa.org http://www.familiesusa.org/

Food and Drug Administration (FDA). 5600 Fishers Lane, Rockville, MD 20857-0001 Tel: 1-888-INFO-FDA, 888-463-6332 http://www.fda.gov/

Healthy Mothers, Healthy Babies (HMHB). 21 North Washington St., Suite 300, Alexandria, VA 22314 Tel: 703-836-6110 Fax: 703-836-3470 E-mail: info@hmhb.org http://www.hmhb.org/contact.html

Institute for Women's Policy Research. 1707 L Street, NW, Suite 750, Washington, D.C. 20036 Tel: 202-785-5100 Fax: 202-833-4362 E-mail: iwpr@iwpr.org http://www.iwpr.org/

International Association of Infant Massage Instructors. P.O. Box 298, Peck Slip Station, New York, NY 10272 E-mail: IAIM4US@aol.com http://www.pracsmart.com/VimalaMcClure.html

Midwives of North America (MANA). 4805 Lawrenceville Hwy, Suite 116-279, Lilburn, GA 30047 Tel: 888-923-MANA (6262) Fax: 801-720-3026 E-mail: info@mana.org http://www.mana.org/

National Assoc. for Holistic Aromatherapy. 4509 Interlake Ave N., #233, Seattle, WA 98103-6773 Tel: 888-ASK-NAHA, 206-47-2164 Fax: 206-547-2680 E-mail: info@naha.org http://www.naha.org/

National Center for Homeopathy. 801 North Fairfax Street, Suite 306, Alexandria, VA 22314 Tel: 703-548-7790 Fax: 703-548-7792 E-mail: info@homeopathic.org http://www.homeopathic.org

National Maternal and Child Health Clearinghouse. Health Resources and Services Administration, U.S. Department of Health and Human Services, Parklawn Building, 5600 Fishers Lane, Rockville, MD 20857 E-mail: ask@hrsa.gov http://www.ask.hrsa.gov/

National Society of Genetic Counselors. 233 Canterbury Drive, Wallingford, PA 19086 Tel: 610-872-7608 E-mail: nsgc@nsgc.org http://www.nsgc.org/resourcelink.asp. http://www/nsgc.org

North American Registry of Midwives (NARM). 5257 Rosestone Dr., Lilburn, GA 30047 Tel: 888-842-4784 E-mail: info@narm.org http://www.narm.org/contact.htm

Primal Health Research Centre. Michel Odent, M.D. 72 Savernake Road, London, NW3 2JR UK Fax: 11 (44) 171 267 5123 E-mail: modent@aol.com. http: michelodent.com http://www.birthworks.com/primalhealth

Section on Women's Health. American Physical Therapy Association, 111 North Fairfax, Alexandria, VA 22314 Tel. 800-999-APTA http://www.apta.org (Referrals to physical therapists who specialize in obstetrics and gynecology)

World Health Organization. Maternal and Newborn Health/Safe Motherhood Unit, Family and Reproductive Health, WHO, 1211 Geneva 27, Switzerland Fax: 41 22 791 0746 http://www.who.int (Also WHO Publications, 49 Sheridan Road, Albany, NY 12210 Fax: 518-436-7433)

Complications

Alliance of Genetic Support Groups. 4301 Connecticut Ave NW, Suite 404, Washington, D.C. 2008-2304 Tel: 800-336-4363 Fax: 202-966-8553 http://www.medhelp.org/www/agsg2.htm

Confinement Line. P.O. Box 1609, Springfield, VA 22151 Tel: 703-941-7183 (For mothers on bed rest)

Conjoined Twins International. P.O. Box 10895, Prescott, Arizona 86304-0895 http://www.familyvillage.wisc.edu/lib_conjoined.html

Dignity Group. 1070 East Hillside Road. Naperville, IL 60540 Tel: 630-369-1119 E-mail: dignitygroup@dignitygroup.org http://ezlink.lc.cc.il.us/dignity.html (For establishing a life plan for children with special needs)

Incest Survivors Resource Network International (ISRNI). P.O. Box 7375, La Cruces, NM 88006 Tel: 505-521-4260 Fax: 505-521-3723 E-mail:isrni@zianet.com.http://www.zianet.com/ISRNI

Monoamniotic Monochorionic Twins Support Site. E-mail: momo@monoamniotic.org http://www.monoamniotic.org

Pocket Ranch/STAR Foundation. P.O. Box 516, Geyserville, CA 95441 Tel: 888-857-STAR, 707-857-3359 Fax: 707-857-3764 E-mail: starfoundation@pobox.com http://www.starfound.org (Crisis therapy)

Sidelines High-Risk Pregnancy Support. P.O. Box 1808, Laguna Beach, CA 92652 Tel: 888: 447-4754 (HI-RISK4) Fax: 949-497-5598 E-mail: sidelines@sidelines.org http://www.sidelines.org

Twin-to-Twin Transfusion Syndrome Foundation (TTTS). 411 Long Beach Parkway Bay Village, Ohio 44140 Tel: 440-899-TTTS Fax: 440-899-1184 E-mail:info@tttsfoundation.org http://www.tttsfoundation.org

For Parents of Premies and Low-Birth-Weight Babies

MUMS: National Parent-to-Parent Network. Julie J. Gordon, 150 Custer Court, Green Bay, Wisconsin 54301-1243 Tel: 877-336-5333, 920-336-5333 Fax: 920-339-0995 E-mail: mums@netnet.net http://www.netnet.net/mums/ (To help parents who have a child with any disorder, medical condition, mental or emotional disorder or rare diagnosis make connections with other parents whose children have the same or similar condition. Many state chapters.)

Parents of Preemies.
http://www2.medsch.wisc.edu/childrenshosp/parents_of_preemies/

The Preemie Place. http://www.thepreemieplace.org/

Supplemental Security Income (SSI). Tel: 800-772 1213 (May pay for low-birth-weight babies until they are one year old)

Clothing for Premies

Austprem Inc. (Australia) http://www.austprem.org.au/

For a Special Baby. 682 Roxanna Lane, New Brighton, MN 55112
Tel: 651-631-3128 E-mail: pat@preemie-clothes.com
http://www.preemie-clothes.com/index.html?GTSE=GOOG

Grow-with-Me. E-mail: jgmc28@aol.com
http://hometown.aol.com/jgmc28/myhomepage/business.html

La Petite Baby. 1915 SE 34th Avenue, Portland, OR 97214 Tel: 800-767-9374
Fax: 413-473-2005 E-mail: michele@snuggletown.com
http://www.snuggletown.com/preemie/index.html

Nana's Boutique. http://www.nanas-boutique.com/preemie.shtml

Preemie Clothes. Diana Thorpe, 2802 Winthrop Dr. S.W., Decatur, AL 35603
E-mail: thorpe1980@earthlink.net
http://www.comeunity.com/disability/shop/preemie-clothes.html (Sewing patterns)

Preemie Place. http://www.thepreemieplace.org/

Preemie Store. Tel: 800-O-SO-TINY (676-8469) Fax: 714-434-7510
http://www.preemie.com/

Preemie Twins. E-mail: kim@preemietwins.org
http://www.preemietwins.com/

Pump Station. E-mail: info@pumpstation.com
http://www.pumpstation.com/frmSubCatIndex-1.cfm?SCID=14

Tiny Bundles. Patricia Park, 11468 Ballybunion Square, San Diego, CA 92128
Tel: 858-451-9907 E-mail: info@tinybundles.com http://www.tinybundles.com

Death of a Multiple

Center for Loss in Multiple Birth, Inc. (CLIMB). c/o Jean Kollantai, P.O. Box 91377, Anchorage, AK 99509 Tel: 907-222-5321
E-mail: newsletter@climb-support.org http://www.climb-support.org

eLIMBO. Electronic Loss In Multiple Birth Outreach
http://groups.yahoo.com/group/elimbo

Share: Pregnancy and Infant Loss Support, Inc. St. Joseph Health Center, 300 First Capitol Drive, St. Charles, MO 63301-2893 Tel: 800-821-6819 or 636-947-6164 Fax: 636-947-7486 E-mail: share@nationalshareoffice.com http://www.nationalshareoffice.com

Twin Hope, Inc. 2592 West 14th Street, Cleveland, OH 44113 Tel: 502-243-2110 or 859-879-9120 (24-hour hotline) http://www.twinhope.com

Parenting of Multiples. http://multiples.about.com

Twinless Twins Society of Canada. Tel/Fax 403-469-9121 or 403-463-8582 (phone before faxing) http://bradstwin.tripod.com/

Twinless Twins International. P.O. Box 980481, Ypsilanti, MI 48198-0481 Tel: 888-205-8962 E-mail: contact@twinlesstwins.org. http://www.twinlesstwins.org/

Twins World. 11220 St. Joe Road, Ft. Wayne, IN 46835 http://www.twinsworld.com (Magazine for Twins and Twinless Twins Throughout the World)

The Lone Twin Network. P.O. Box 5653, Birmingham, B29 7JY, UK

Bibliography and Further Reading

Multiple Pregnancy and Birth

Agnew, Connie L. J. D. et al. *Twins! Expert Advice from Two Practicing Physicians on Pregnancy, Birth and the First Year of Life with Twins.* New York: Harper, 1997.

American College of Obstetricians and Gynecologists, *Compendium of Selected Publications.* Washington, DC, 2003.

Birch, Kathleen, and Janet Bleyl. *Exceptional Pregnancies: A Survival Guide for Parents Expecting Twins.* Rhode Island: Elm Street Press, 2000. (See also Resources, The Triplet Connection and a similar book on triplets.)

Bryan, Elizabeth. *Twins, Triplets and More.* London: Multiple Births Foundation, 1995.

Clay, Marie. *Quadruplets and Higher Multiple Births.* London: Mackeith Press, 1989.

Gromada, Karen, and Kerkhoff and Mary Hurlburt. *Keys to Parenting Twins.* Hauppauge, NY: Barron, 2001.

Laut, William and Sheila. *Raising Multiple Birth Children.* Worcester, MA: Chandler House Press, 1999.

Luke, B., and T. Eberlein. *When You Are Expecting Twins, Triplets or Quads.* New York: Harper Perennial, 1999.

Lyons, Suzanne, ed. *Finding Our Way: Life with Triplets, Quads and Quintuplets.* Canada: Triplets, Quads and Quints Association of Canada, 2001.

Moskwinski, Rebecca, ed. *Twins to Quints — The Complete Manual for Parents of Multiple Birth Children.* Brentwood, TN: Harpeth House, 2002.

Novotny, Pamela. *The Joy of Twin and Other Multiple Births: Having, Raising & Loving Babies Who Arrive in Groups.* New York: Crown, 1994.

Rothbart, B. *Multiple Blessings.* New York: Hearst Books, 1994.

Sandbank, Audrey, ed. *Twin and Triplet Psychology.* New York: Routledge, 1999.

Sipes, Nancy J., and Janna S. Sipes. *Dancing Naked in Front of the Fridge: And Other Lessons from Twins.* Massachusetts: Fairwinds Press, 1999.

Zentner, Carola. *Twins: The Parents' Survival Guide.* Edinburgh: McDonald, 1984.

Goal Setting

Grabhorn, Lynn. *Excuse Me, Your Life Is Waiting.* Charlottesville, VA: Hampton Roads Publishing Company Inc., 2000.

Hay, Louise. *You Can Heal Your Life.* Santa Monica, CA: Hay House, 1999.

Hill, Napoleon. *Think and Grow Rich.* Del Rey/Fawcett/Ivy 1960, Ballantine, 1983.

Pert, Candace, and D. Chopra. *Molecules of Emotion: Why You Feel the Way You Feel.* New York: Simon and Schuster, 1999.

Ponder, Catherine. *The Dynamic Laws of Prosperity.* Marina del Rey, CA: DeVorss & Co, 1988.

Nutrition

Barnard, Neal D., M.D. *The Power of Your Plate: A Plan for Better Living.* Summertown, TN: Book Publishing Company, 1995.

Brewer Pregnancy Hotline. Olympia, Washington: Kalico Communications, 2000. http://ebooks.kalico.net/about.html (CD and ebook).

Brewer, T. H. *Metabolic Toxemia of Late Pregnancy.* New Canaan: Keats Publishing, Inc., 1985.

Burke, Bertha et al. "Nutrition Studies During Pregnancy." *American Journal of Obstetrics & Gynecology* 46 (1943): 38.

Campbell, D. M., and I. MacGillivray. "The Importance of Plasma Volume Expansion and Nutrition in Twin Pregnancy." *Acta Geneticae Medicae et Gemellologiae* 33 (1984): 1924.

Chesley, Leon. "Plasma Volume and Red Cell Volume in Pregnancy." *American Journal of Obstetrics & Gynecology* 112 (1972): 440.

Cox, Peter, Linda McCartney, and Neal Barnard. *You Don't Need Meat.* New York: Thomas Dunne Books, 2002.

Critser, Greg. *Fat Land.* Boston: Houghton Mifflin, 2003.

Dobbing, John. "The Later Growth of the Brain and Its Vulnerability." *Pediatrics* 53 (1974): 2.

Dubois, S., C. Dougherty, M. Duquette, J. Hanley, and J. Moutquin. "Twin Pregnancy: The Impact of the Higgins Nutrition Intervention Program on Maternal and Neonatal Outcomes." *American Journal of Clinical Nutrition* 53 (1991): 1397–1403.

Ebbs, John H. et al. "The Influence of Improved Nutrition Upon the Infant." *Canadian Medical Association Journal* 46 (1942): 6.

Erasmus, Udo. *Fats That Heal, Fats That Kill.* Alive Books, 1999.

Ericson, A. et al. "Use of Multivitamins and Folic Acid in Early Pregnancy and Multiple Births in Sweden." *Twin Research* 4, no. 2 (April 2001): 63–66.

Evans, William. *Astrofit.* New York: Free Press, 2002.

Hamlin, R. H. J. "The Prevention of Eclampsia and Pre-Eclampsia." *Lancet* 1 (1952): 64.

Higgins, Agnes C. "Nutritional Status and the Outcome of Pregnancy." *Journal of Canadian Dietetics Association* 37 (1976): 17.

Laross, R. A. "Relation of Vitamin Deficiency to Toxemias of Pregnancy." *South Medical Journal* 28 (1935): 120.

Luke, B. et al. "The Association between Maternal Weight Gain and the Birth Weight of Twins." *Journal of Maternal Fetal Medicine* 1(1992): 267–276.

McConnaughey. *Sea Vegetables Harvesting Guide and Cookbook.* Happy Camp, CA: Naturegraph, 1985.

Mellanby, Edward. "Nutrition and Childbearing." *Lancet* 2 (1933): 1131.

Nutritive Value of Foods Home and Garden Bulletin. 72(HG-72) USDA Nutrient

Data Laboratory, Government Printing Office. http://bookstore.gpo.gov/index.html.

O'Connell, J. M., M. J. Dibley, J. Sierra, B. Wallace, J. S. Marks, R. Yip. "Growth of Vegetarian Children: The Farm Study." *Pediatrics* 84 (1989): 475–481.

Odent, Michel. "Hypothesis: Preeclampsia as a Maternal-Fetal Conflict." *Medgenmed* (September 5, 2001): Medscape, Inc.

Odent, M., L. McMillan, and T. Kimmel. "Prenatal Care and Sea Fish." *European Journal of Obstetrics & Gynecology* 681, no. 2 (1996): 49–51.

Olsen, S. F., and N. J. Secher. "A Possible Preventive Effect of Low-Dose Fish Oil on Early Delivery and Pre-Eclampsia: Indications From a 50-Year-Old Controlled Trial." *British Journal of Nutrition* 64 (1990): 599–609.

Pennington, J. A. T. *J.A.T. Pennington, Bowes and Church's Food Values of Portions Commonly Used.* New York: Harper and Row, 1989.

Robbins, John. *Diet for a New America: How Your Food Choices Affect Your Health, Happiness and Future of Life on Earth.* HJ Kramer, 1987.

Robbins, John, and Dean Ornish. *The Food Revolution: How Your Diet Can Help Save Your Life and Our World.* Berkeley, CA: Conari, 2001.

Schlosser, Eric. *Fast Food Nation.* Boston: Houghton Mifflin, 2001.

Spillman, J. "The Role of Birthweight in Maternal-Twin Relationships." MSc thesis, Cranfield Institute of Technology, 1984.

Tompkins, Winslow. "The Significance of Nutritional Deficiency on Pregnancy." *International College of Surgeons* 4 (1941): 147.

Williams, R. *Nutrition Against Disease.* New York: Bantam, 1973.

Worthington-Roberts, B. "Weight Gain Patterns in Twin Pregnancies with Desirable Outcomes." *Clinical Nutrition* 7, no. 5 (1988): 191–196.

Yntema, Sharon K. *New Vegetarian Baby.* rev. ed. Ithaca, NY: McBooks, 1999.

Young, V. R., and P. L. Pellett. "Plant Proteins in Relation to Human Protein and Amino Acid Nutrition." *Am J Clin Nutr.* 59 (no. 5) (1994): 1203S–1212S.

Hazards of Dairy Products

Cohen, Robert. *Milk: The Deadly Poison.* Englewood Cliffs, NJ: Argus, 1997.
———. *Milk: A-Z,* Englewood Cliffs, NJ: Argus, 2001.

Hulse, Vurgil, M.D. *Mad Cows and Milk Gate.* Marble Mountain Publishing, 1966.

Kradjian, Robert M., M.D. "The Milk Letter: A Message to My Patients." *New York Times Magazine*, October 6, 2002 (or download from www.notmilk.com).

Madison, Deborah. *Vegetarian Cooking for Everyone.* New York: Broadway Books, 1997.

Oski, Frank, M.D. *Don't Drink Your Milk.* Brushton, NY: TEACH Services, Inc., 1996. (Oski was chief of pediatrics at Johns Hopkins School of Medicine.)

Twogood, Daniel A. *No Milk.* Victorville, CA: Wilhelmina Books, 1991.

Prenatal Care

Beech, B. L. "Ultrasound — Weighing the Propaganda against the Facts." *Midwifery Today* (Autumn 1999).

Blickstein, I. R., D. Goldman, M. Smith-Levitin, M. Greenberg, D. Sherman, and H. Rydhstroem. "The Relation Between Inter-Twin Birth Weight Discordance and Total Twin Birth Weight." *Journal of Obstetrics and Gynecology* 93 (1999): 113–116.

Bricker, L., and J. P. Neilson. "Routine Ultrasound in Late Pregnancy." (2001). *The Cochrane Library Online.* http://www.update-software.com/cochrane/cochrane-frame/html.

Brown, J. E., and P. T. Scholesser. "Prepregnancy Weight Status, Prenatal Weight Gain, and the Outcome of Term Twin Gestations." *American Journal of Obstetrics and Gynecology* 162 (1990): 182–186.

Dallapiccola, B. et al. "Discordant Sex in One of Three Monozygotic Triplets." *Journal of Medical Genetics* 22 (1985): 6–11.

Derom, C. et al. "Increased Monozygotic Twinning Rate After Ovulation Induction." *Lancet* 1 (1987): 1236.

Dickey, R. P. et al. "The Probability of Multiple Births When Multiple Gestational Assessed Sacs or Viable Embryos Are Diagnosed at First Trimester Ultrasound." *Human Reproduction* 3: 880–882.

Edmunds, L. "Multiple Births, Twin Pregnancy: Exercising Your Options." *Midwifery Today* 39 (1996): 18–19.

El Halta, V. "A Study Outline on Twin Pregnancy, Labour and Delivery." *Midwifery Today* 39 (1996): 25–26.

Ellings, J. M., R. B. Newman, T. Hulsey, H. A. Bivins, and A. Keenan. "Reduction in Very Low Birth Weight Deliveries and Perinatal Mortality in a Specialized, Multidisciplinary Twin Clinic." *American Journal of Obstetrics & Gynecology* 81, no. 3 (1993): 387–391.

Katz, V. L. et al. "A Comparison of Bed Rest and Immersion for Treating the Edema of Pregnancy." *Obstetrics and Gynecology* 75, no. 2 (February 1990): 147–151.

Keith, L., E. Papiernik, D. Keith, and B. Luke, eds. *Multiple Pregnancy: Epidemiology, Gestation & Perinatal Outcome.* New York: Parthenon Publishing Group, 1995.

Luke, B., J. Minogue, F. Witter, L. Keith, and T. Johnson. "The Ideal Twin Pregnancy: Patterns of Weight Gain, Discordancy, and Length of Gestation." *American Journal of Obstetrics and Gynecology* 169, no. 3 (1993): 588–597.

Newnham, J. P., S. F. Evans, C. A. Michael, F. J. Stanley, and L. I. Landau. "Effects of Frequent Ultrasound During Pregnancy: A Randomised Controlled Trial." *Lancet* (October 9, 1993): 342.

O'Grady, J. P. "Clinical Management of Twins." *Contemporary OB/GYN* 29 (April 1987): 126–142.

Renzo, G. C., R. Luzietti, S. Gerli, and G. Clerici. "The Ten Commandments in Multiple Pregnancies." *Twin Resources* 4 (2): 159–164.

Samueloff, A. et al. "Fetal Movements in Multiple Pregnancy." *American Journal of Obstetrics and Gynecology* 146 (1983): 789–792.

Birth

Capacchione, Lucia, and Sandra Bardsley. *Creating a Joyful Birth Experience.* New York: Fireside/Simon & Schuster, 1994.

Carman, E. and N. J. *Cosmic Cradle: Souls Waiting in the Wings for Birth.* Fairfield, IA: Sunstar, 2000. http://www.cosmiccradle.com

Chamberlain, David. *The Mind of Your Newborn Baby.* 3rd ed. Berkeley: North Atlantic Books, 1998.

England, Pam. *Birthing From Within.* Albuquerque, NM: Partera, 1998.

Enkin, M., M. Keirse, J. Neilson, C. Crowther, et al. *A Guide to Effective Care in Pregnancy and Childbirth.* 3rd ed. Oxford: Oxford University Press, 2000.

Goer, H. *The Thinking Woman's Guide to a Better Birth.* New York: Perigee Books, 1999.

Golay, Jane, Saraswathi Vedum, and Leo Sorger. "The Squatting Position for the Second Stage of Labor: Effects on Labor and on Maternal and Fetal Well-Being." *Birth* 20, no. 2 (1993): 73–78.

Noble, Elizabeth. *Childbirth with Insight.* Boston: Houghton Mifflin, 1983.

———. *Essential Exercises for the Childbearing Year.* 4th edition, revised. Harwich, MA: New Life Images, 2003.

———. *Primal Connections.* Simon and Schuster, 1991.

(Available from New Life Images, 448 Pleasant Lake Avenue, Harwich, MA 02645.)

Odent, M. *The Farmer and the Obstetrician.* London: Free Association Books, 2002.

Olofsson, R., and H. J. Rydhstrom. "Twin Delivery: How Should the Second Twin Be Delivered?" *American Journal of Obstetrics and Gynecology* 153 (1985): 479.

Peterson, Gayle. *An Easier Childbirth: A Mother's Workbook for Health and Emotional Well-Being During Pregnancy and Delivery.* Los Angeles: Jeremy Tarcher, 1991.

Taylor, Catherine. *Giving Birth.* New York: Perigee, 2002.

Tsiaras, A. and Barry Werth. *From Conception to Birth: A Life Unfolds.* New York: Doubleday, 2002.

Verny, Thomas. *Tomorrow's Baby.* New York: Simon and Schuster, 2002.

Vincent, Peggy. *The Baby Catcher.* New York: Scribner, 2002.

Placenta

Biggs, Kathy, and Linda Gwillim. *Placenta Humanum.* The Welsh School of Homœopathy, Lys-y-Coed, Lanwrtyd Wells, Powys, LD5 4SA, UK 01591 610787 http://www.jkeates.freeserve.co.uk

McFarland, R. B. "Indian Medicine Wheels and Placentas: How the Tree of Life and the Circle of Life Are Related." *Journal of Psychohistory* 20 (1993): 454–464.

McFarland, R. B., and W. Schalaben. "Placentas and Prehistoric Art." *Journal of Psychohistory* 23, no. 1 (Summer 1995): 41–50.

Shivam, Rachan. *A Lotus Birth.* Steels Creek, Australia: Greenwood Press, 2000.

Circumcision

Douglas, Gairdner, D.M., M.R.C.P. "The Fate of the Foreskin." *British Medical Journal* 2 (December 24, 1949): 1433–1437.

Fleiss, Paul M., and Frederick M. Hodges. *What Your Doctor May Not Tell You*

About Circumcision: Untold Facts on America's Most Widely Performed and Most Unnecessary Surgery. New York: Warner Books, 2002.

Goldman, Ronald. *Circumcision: The Hidden Trauma.* Boston: Vanguard, 1997.

———. *Questioning Circumcision: A Jewish Dilemma.* Boston: Vanguard, 2000.

Hammond, Tim. *Awakenings: A Preliminary Poll of Circumcised Men: Revealing the Harm and Healing the Wounds of Infant Circumcision.* 1994. (NOHARMM, see Resources.)

Noble, Elizabeth, and Leo Sorger. *The Joy of Being a Boy.* Harwich: New Life Images, 1993.

Ritter, Thomas, M.D., and George Denniston, M.D. *Doctors Re-Examine Circumcision.* Seattle, WA: Third Millenium Publications, 2002.

Taylor, J. R. et al. "The Prepuce: Specialized Mucosa of the Penis and Its Loss to Circumcision." *British Journal of Urology* 77 (1996): 291–295.

Birth of Multiples

Acker, D. et al. "Delivery of the Second Twin." *Obstetrics and Gynecology* 59 (1982): 710.

Adam, C., A. C. Allen, and T. F. Baskett. "Twin Delivery Influence of the Presentation and Method of Delivery of the Second Twin." *American Journal of Obstetrics and Gynecology* 165, no. 1 (1991): 23–27.

Bartnicki, J., M. Meyenburg, and E. Saling. "Time Interval in Twin Delivery — The Second Twin Need Not Always Be Born Shortly After the First." *Gynaecologic Obstetric Investigation* 33, no. 1 (1992): 19–20.

Blickstein, I., A. Weissman, H. Ben-Hur, R. Borenstein, and V. Insler. "Vaginal Delivery for Breech-Vertex Twins." 38 (1993): 879–882.

Blickstein, I, R. D. Goldman, and M. Kuperminc. "Delivery of Breech-First Twins: A Multicenter Retrospective Study." *American Journal of Obstetrics & Gynecology* (1999).

Cardwell, M. S. et al. "Triplet Pregnancy with Delivery on Three Separate Days. Part 2." *Obstetrics and Gynecology* 71, no. 3 (March 1988): 448–449.

———. "Intrapartum External Version of the Second Twin." *Obstetrics and Gynecology* 62 (1983): 160.

Chauhan, S. P., W. E. Roberts, P. A. McLaren et al. "Delivery of the Non Vertex Second Twin Breech Extraction Versus External Cephalic Version." *American Journal of Obstetrics and Gynecology* 4 (1995): 1015–1020.

Feng, T. I., R. E. Swindle, and J. F. Huddleston. "A Lack of Adverse Effect of Prolonged Delivery Interval Between Twins." *Journal of Maternal-Foetal Investigation* 5, no. 4 (1995): 222–225.

Evans, Jane. "Can a Twin Birth Be a Positive Experience?" *Midwifery Matters* (Autumn 1997): 74.

Fishman, A., D. K. Grubb, and B. W. Kovacs. "Vaginal Delivery of the Non-Vertex Second Twin." *American Journal of Obstetrics and Gynecology* 168 (1993): 861–864.

Fisk, N. M., and E. M. Bryan. "Routine Prenatal Determination of Chorionicity in Multiple Gestation: A Plea to the Obstetrician." *British Journal of Obstetrics & Gynaecology* 100 (1993): 975–977.

Gaskin, I. M. "On Breeches and Twins at Home." *Mothering* 64 (1992): 92–95.

Gocke, S. E., M. P. Nageotte, T. Garite, C. V. Towers, and W. Dorcester. "Management of the Non-Vertex Second Twin: Primary Caesarean Section, External Version, or Primary Breech Extraction." *American Journal of Obstetrics and Gynecology* 161, no. 1 (1989): 111–114.

Greig, P. C., J. C. Veille, and T. Morgan et al. "The Effect of Presentation and Mode of Delivery on Neonatal Outcome in the Second Twin." *American Journal of Obstetrics and Gynecology* 167, no. 4 (1992): 901–906.

Gowdey, A. C. "Notes on a Case of Quadruplets." *Lancet* 2 (1904): 1020–1021.

Ogbonna, B., and E. Daw. "Epidural Analgesia and the Length of Labour for Vaginal Twin Delivery." *Journal of Obstetrics and Gynecology* 6 (1986): 166–168.

Robertson, F. "A Case of Quadruplet Birth." *Australasian Medical Gazette* 8 (1889): 208–209.

Smith, S. "Homebirth Twins." *Midwifery Today* 39 (1996): 22–25.

Sullivan, C.A. et al. "Cesarean Delivery for the Second Twin." *South Medical Journal* 91, no. 2 (February 1998): 155–159.

Tchabo, J. G., and T. Tomau. "Selected Intrapartum External Cephalic Version of the Second Twin." *Obstetrics and Gynecology* 79, no. 3 (1992): 421–423.

Thiery, M., G. Kermans, and R. Derom. "Triplet and Higher Order Births: What Is the Optimal Delivery Route?" *Acta Geneticae Medicae et Gemellologiae* 37 (1988): 89–98.

Woolfson, J. et al. "Twins with 54 Days Between Deliveries: Case Report." *British Journal of Obstetrics and Gynaecology* 90, no. 7 (July 1983): 685–686.

Caesarean Section and VBAC for Mothers of Twins

Cohen, N. W., and L. Estner. *Silent Knife: Cesarean Prevention and Vaginal Birth After Cesarean.* South Hadley, MA: Bergin and Garvey, 1983.

Crowther, C. A. "Effect of Caesarean Delivery of the Second Twin. Cochrane Database of Systematic Reviews." *Cochrane Library* (1997).

English, Jane. *Different Doorway: Adventures of a Cesarean Born.* Earth Heart, Box 7, Mt. Shasta, CA 96067, 1985.

Gocke, S. E. "Management of the Nonvertex Second Twin: Primary Cesarean Section, External Version, or Primary Breech Extraction." *American Journal of Obstetrics and Gynecology* 161, no. 1 (July 1989): 29.

Laros, R. K., Jr., and B. J. Dattel. "Management of Twin Pregnancy: The Vaginal Route Is Still Safe. Part 1." *American Journal of Obstetrics and Gynecology* 158 (June 1988): 1330–1338.

Miller D.A., P. Mullin, D. Hou, and R. H. Paul. "Vaginal Birth after Cesarean Section in Twin Gestation." *American Journal of Obstetrics and Gynecology* 175, no. 1 (July 1996): 194–198.

Myles, T. "Vaginal Birth of Twins After a Previous Cesarean Section." *Journal of Maternal Fetal Medicine* 10, no. 3 (June 2001): 171–174.

Odeh M., L. Tarazova, M. Wolfson, and M. Oettinger. "Evidence that Women with a History of Cesarean Section Can Deliver Twins Safely." *Acta Obstetrics & Gynecology Scand* 76, no. 7 (August 199?): 663–666.

Strong, T. H., Jr., et al. "Vaginal Birth After Cesarean Section in the Twin Gestation." *American Journal of Obstetrics and Gynecology* 161, no. 1 (July 1989): 25.

Wax, J. R., C. Philput, J. Mather, J. D. Steinfeld, and C. J. Ingardia. "Twin Vaginal Birth After Cesarean." *Conn Medicine* 64, no. 4 (April 2000): 205–208.

Feeding of Multiples

Driscoll, Jeanne, and Marsha Walker. *Breastfeeding Your Premature or Special Care Baby: A Practical Guide for Nursing the Tiny Baby.* Lansing, MI: Leaven, 2000.

Hattori, R., and H. Hattori. "Breastfeeding Twins: Guidelines For Success." *Birth* 26 (1999): 37–42.

Irvine, C. et al. "The Potential Adverse Effects of Soybean Phytoestrogens in Infant Feeding." *New Zealand Medical Journal* (May 24, 1995): 318.

Kitzinger, Sheila. *Breastfeeding Your Baby.* New York: Knopf, 1989.

La Leche League. *The Womanly Art of Breastfeeding.* (See Resources.)

Luke, B., M. J. O'Sullivan, D. Martin, C. Nugent, F. R. Witter, R. B. Newman. "Outcomes in Quadruplet Pregnancies: Role of Maternal Nutrition." Society for Maternal-Fetal Medicine, New Orleans, Louisiana, January 14–19, 2002. *Am J Obstet Gynecol* 185 (2001): S105.

Minchin, Maureen. "Infant Formula: A Mass, Uncontrolled Trial in Perinatal Care." *Birth* 14 (March 1987): 1.

Newman, Jack, and Teresa Pitman. *The Ultimate Breastfeeding Book of Answers.* Roseville, CA: Prima, 2000.

Renfrew, Mary, Chloe Fisher, and Suzanne Arms. *Bestfeeding: Getting Breastfeeding Right for You.* Berkeley, CA: Celestial Arts, 2000.

Sears, William and Martha. *The Breastfeeding Book: Everything You Need to Know About Nursing Your Child From Birth Through Weaning.* Boston: Little Brown, 2000.

Setchell, K. D. et al. "Isoflavone Content of Infant Formulas and the Metabolic Fate of These Early Phytoestrogens in Early Life." *American Journal of Clinical Nutrition.* (December 1998): Supplement, 1453S–1461S.

Sollid, D., B. Evans, S. McClowry, and A. Garrett. "Breastfeeding Multiples." *Journal of Perinatal and Neonatal Nursing* (July 1989): 47–85.

Complications in Pregnancy

Curtis, S. et al. "Pregnancy Effects of Non-proteinuric Gestational Hypertension." SPO abstracts, *American Journal of Obstetrics & Gynecology* 418 (January 1995): 376.

Jarrett, R. J. "Gestational Diabetes; A Non-entity?" *British Med Journal* 306 (1993): 37–38.

Lachmeijer, A. M., J. G. Aarnoudse, L. P. Ten Kate, G. Pals, and G. A. Dekker. "Concordance for Pre-Eclampsia in Monozygous Twins." *British Journal of Obstetrics & Gynaecology* 105, no. 12 (December 1998): 1315–1317.

Malone, F. D., G. E. Kaufman, D. Chelmow, A. Athanassiou, J. A. Nores, and M. E. Dalton. "Maternal Morbidity Associated with Triplet Pregnancy." *American Journal of Perinatology* 1, no. 1 (January 1998): 3–7.

Mehl-Madrona, Lewis. "Psychosocial Variables Predict Complicated Birth." *Journal of Prenatal and Perinatal Psychology and Health* 17, no. 1 (Fall 2002): 3–28.

Powers, R. W. et al. "Plasma Homocysteine Is Increased in Preeclampsia and Is Associated with Evidence of Endothelial Activation." *American Journal of Obstetrics and Gynecology* 179 (1998): 1605–1611.

Rich, Laurie A. *When Pregnancy Isn't Perfect: A Layperson's Guide to Complications in Pregnancy*. Larata Press, 1996.

Santema J. G., I. Koppelaar, and H. C. Wallenburg. "Hypertensive Disorders in Twin Pregnancy." *European Journal of Obstetrics, Gynecology, & Reproductive Biology* 58 (1) (January 1995): 9–13.

Sarhanis, P., and Pugh Dho. "Resolution of Pre-Eclampsia Following Intrauterine Death of One Twin." *British Journal of Obstetrics & Gynaecology*.[dates missing]

Sibai, B. M. et al. "Hypertensive Disorders in Twin Versus Singleton Gestations. National Institute of Child Health and Human Development Network of Maternal-Fetal Medicine Units." *American Journal of Obstetrics & Gynecology* 184, no. 4 (April 2000): 938–942.

Tilstra, J. H. et al. "Hypertensive Disorders in Twin Versus Singleton Gestations." *American Journal of Obstetrics & Gynecology* 182, no. 4 (April 2000): 938–942.

———. "Two Patients with Postpartum HELLP Syndrome After a Normotensive Twin Pregnancy." *International Journal of Gynaecology & Obstetrics* 47, no. 1 (October 1994): 49–51.

Wang, Y. et al. "Decreased Levels of Polyunsaturated Fatty Acids in Preeclampsia." *American Journal of Obstetrics and Gynecology* 164 (1994): 812–818.

Williams, M. A. et al. "Risk of Pre-eclampsia in Relation to Elaidic Acid Transfatty Acids in Maternal Erthyrocytes." SPO Abstracts. *American Journal of Obstetrics and Gynecology* 80 (January 1995): 436.

Bed Rest

"Bed Rest in Obstetrics." Editorial. *Lancet* 1 (1981): 1137–1138.

Chalmers, I., M. Enkin, and M. J. N. C. Keirse. *Effective Care in Pregnancy and Childbirth*. Oxford: Oxford University Press, 1989, pp. 625–631.

Crowther, C. A. "Hospitalisation and Bed Rest for Multiple Pregnancy." *Cochrane Database*. (2001): Systems Review.

———. "Commentary on Bed Rest for Women with Pregnancy Problems: Evidence for Efficacy Is Lacking." *Birth* 22, no. 1 (1995): 13–14.

Enkin, M., M. J. N. C. Keirse, M. Renfrew, and J. Neilson. *A Guide to Effective Care in Pregnancy and Childbirth*. 2nd ed. Oxford: Oxford University Press, 1995, p. 106.

Gordin, P., and B. Johnson. "Technology and Family-Centered Perinatal Care: Conflict or Synergy?" *Journal of Obstetric, Gynecologic and Neonatal Nursing*. 28, no. 4 (1999): 401–408.

Gupton, A., M. Heaman, and T. Ashcroft. "Bed Rest from the Perspective of the High-Risk Woman." *Journal of Obstetric, Gynecologic and Neonatal Nursing* 26, no. 4 (1997): 423–430.

Johnston, Susan, H. M. S. W. and Deborah A. Kraut. *Pregnancy Bedrest: A Guide for the Pregnant Woman and Her Family.* New York: Holt, 1990.

Josten, L., K. Savik, S. Mullett, R. Campbell, and P. Vincent. "Bed Rest Compliance for Women with Pregnancy Problems." *Birth* 22, no. 1 (1995): 1–12.

Katz, V. L. et al. "A Comparison of Bed Rest and Immersion for Treating the Edema of Pregnancy." *Obstetrics and Gynecology* 75, no. 2 (February 1990): 147–151.

Kovacevich, G. J., S. A. Gaich, J. P. Lavin, M. P. Hopkins, S. S. Crane, J. Stewart, D. Nelson, and L. M. Lavin. "The Prevalence of Thromboembolic Events Among Women with Extended Bed Rest Prescribed as Part of the Treatment for Premature Labor or Preterm Premature Rupture of Membranes." *American Journal of Obstetrics & Gynecology* 182, no. 5 (May 2000): 1089–1092.

Maloni, J. "Bed Rest and High-Risk Pregnancy." *Nursing Clinics of North America* 31, no. 2 (1996): 313–325.

Maloni, J. A., J. E. Brezinski-Tomasi, and L. A. Johnson. "Antepartum Bed Rest: Effect Upon the Family." *Journal of Obstetric and Gynecological Neonatal Nurses.* 30, no. 2 (Mar-Apr 2001): 165–173.

Maloni, J., B. Chance, C. Zhang, A. Cohen, D. Betts, and S. Gange. "Physical and Psychological Side Effects of Antepartum Bed Rest." *Nursing Research* 42, no. 4 (1993): 197–203.

——— and C. Kasper. "Physical and Psychosocial Effects of Bed Rest: A Review of the Literature." *Image: Journal of Nursing Scholarship* 23, no. 3 (1993): 187–192.

——— and B. Ponder. "Father's Experience of Their Partner's Antepartum Bed Rest." *Image: Journal Scholarship* 29, no. 2 (1997): 183–187.

McFee, J. G. et al. "Multiple Gestations of High Fetal Number." *American Journal of Obstetrics & Gynecology* 44 (1974): 99–106. (Lists neuroses from bed rest)

McLennan, A. H. et al. "Routine Hospital Admission in Twin Pregnancy between 26 and 30 Weeks Gestation." *Lancet* 335 (1990): 267–269.

Odent, M. "Et le systeme vestibulaire?" In *L'aube des sens*, edited by E. Herbinet and M. C. Busnel. *Les Cahiers du Nouveau Né.* Paris: Stock, 1981, pp. 295–299.

——— . Research Letter, "Long-Term Effects on the Offspring of Mothers Placed on Bed Rest During Pregnancy." (to be published)

Rydhstrom, H. et al. "Routine Hospital Care Does Not Improve Prognosis in Twin Gestation." *Acta Obstetrica and Gynecologica Scandinavica* 66, no. 4 (1987): 361–364.

Sather, S., and E. Zwelling. "A View from the Other Side of the Bed." *Journal of Obstetric, Gynecologic and Neonatal Nursing* 27, no. 3 (1998): 322–328.

Saunders, M. C. et al. "The Effects of Hospital Admission for Bedrest on the Duration of a Twin Pregnancy." *Lancet* 2, no. 8495 (1985): 73–75, 793–795.

Schroeder, C. "Bed Rest in Complicated Pregnancy: A Critical Analysis." *Maternal Child Nursing* 23 (January/February, 1998): 45–49.

Van Der Pol, J. G. et al. "Clinical Bed Rest in Twin Pregnancies." *Biology* 14 (1982): 75–80.

Warner, J. A., C. A. Jones, A. C. Jones, and J. O. Warner. "Prenatal Origins of Allergic Disease." *Journal of Allergy & Clinical Immunology* 105, no. 2 (2000): Part 2, S493.

Preterm Labor and Birth

Albrecht, J. L., and P. G. Tomich. "The Maternal and Neonatal Outcome of Triplet Gestations." *American Journal of Obstetrics & Gynecology* 174, no. 5 (May, 1996): 1551–1556.

Al-Najashi, S., and A. Al-Mulhim. "Prolongation of Pregnancy in Multiple Pregnancy." *International Journal of Gynaecology & Obstetrics* 54, no. 2 (August 1996): 131.

Cole, F. S. "Extremely Preterm Birth — Defining the Limits of Hope." Editorial. *New England Journal of Medicine* (August 10, 2000): 343.

Dellaporta, K., D. Aforismo, and M. Butler-O'Hara. "Co-Bedding of Twins in the Neonatal Intensive Care Unit." *Pediatric Nursing* 24 (1998): 529–531.

Goldenburg, R. L. "The Management of Preterm Labor." *Obstetrics and Gynecology* 100 (2002): 1020–1037.

Gyetvi, K. et al. "Tocolytics for Preterm Labor: A Systematic Review." *American Journal of Obstetrics & Gynecology* 94, no. 5 (1999): Part 2, 869–877.

Huttenen, M. et al. "Prenatal Loss of Father and Psychiatric Disorders." *Arch. General Psychiatry* 35 (1978): 429–431.

Keith, L. G., E. Papiernik, D. M. Keith, and B. Luke, eds. *Multiple Pregnancy: Epidemiology, Gestation and Perinatal Outcome.* Carnforth: Parthenon, 1995.

Kh, Nyqvist, and L. M. Lutes. "Co-Bedding Twins: A Developmentally Supportive Care Strategy." *Journal of Obstetric, Gynecology & Neonatal Nursing* 27 (1998): 450–456.

Kilpatrick, S. et al. "Unlike Preeclampsia, Gestational Hypertension Is Not Associated with Increased Neonatal and Maternal Morbidity Except Abruption." SPO Abstracts, *American Journal of Obstetrics & Gynecology* 419 (January 1995): 376.

Luke, B., and L. B. Keith. "The Contribution of Singletons, Twins and Triplets to Low Birth Weight, Infant Mortality and Handicaps." *Journal of Reproductive Medicine* 37 (1992): 661–666.

Morales, W. J., W. F. O'Brien, and R. A. Knuppel et al. "The Effect of Mode of Delivery on the Risk of Intraventricular Haemorrhage in Non-Discordant Twin Gestation Under 1500 gm." *Obstetrics and Gynecology* 73, no. 1 (1989): 107–110.

Murray, L., and P. J. Cooper. "Effects of Postnatal Depression on Infant Development." *Arch Disabled Child* 17 (1997): 99–101.

Odent, M. *Primal Health Research* 2 (1995): 4.

Olatunbosun, O. A., R. W. Turnell, K. Sankaran, and A. Ninan. "Delayed Interval Delivery in Quadruplets." *International Journal of Gynaecology & Obstetrics.* 50, no. 3 (September 1995): 287–290.

Olsen, S., and N. J. Secher. "Low Consumption of Seafood in Early Pregnancy as a Risk Factor for Preterm Delivery: Prospective Cohort Study." *BMJ* 324 (Feb. 23, 2002): 447.

Platt, J. A., and C. L. Rosa. "Delayed Intervals." *International Journal of Gynaecology & Obstetrics* 50, no. 3 (September 1995): 287–290.

Rydhstrom, H. "Factors Influencing Twin Perinatal Mortality." Ph.D. Dissertation, University Hospital of Lund, Sweden, 1990.

Salat-Baroux J., and J. M. Antoine. "Multiple Pregnancies: The Price to Pay." *European Journal of Obstetrics, Gynecology & Reproductive Biology* 65 (April 1996): Supplement S17.

Slattery, M. M., and J. J. Morrison. "Preterm Delivery." *Lancet* 360 (2002): 1489–1497.

Stanley, F., and B. Petterson. "Cerebral Palsy in Multiple Births." In *The Changing Epidemiological Patterns in Multiple Pregnancy*, edited by R. H. Ward and M. Whittle. London: Royal College of Obstetricians and Gynaecologists, 1995, 309–325.

Child Care and Development

Allen, M. G. et al. "Parental Birth and Infancy Factors in Infant Twin Development." *American Journal of Psychiatry* 127 (2000): 1597–1604.

Anderson, A., and B. Anderson. "Mothers' Beginning Relationship with Twins." *Birth* 14, no. 2 (June 1987): 94–98.

Bernabei, R., and G. Levi. "Psychopathologic Problems in Twins During Childhood." *Acta Geneticae Mediate et Gemellologiae*, 1976.

Faber, Adele, and Elaine Mazlish. *How to Talk So Kids Will Listen and Listen So Kids Will Talk.* New York: Avon, 1999.

———— *Siblings Without Rivalry.* New York: Avon, 1998.

Fleiss, Paul, and F. Hodges. *Sweet Dreams: A Pediatrician's Secret for a Good Night's Sleep.* Contemporary Books, 2000.

Goshen-Gottstein, E. R. "The Mothering of Twins, Triplets, and Quadruplets." *Psychiatry* 43 (1980): 189–204.

Gringas, P. "Identical Differences — Monozygotic Twins with Different Hair Color." *Lancet* 353 (1999): 562.

Groothius, J. R., W. A. Altemeier, and J. P. Robarge et al. "Increased Child Abuse in Families with Twins." *Pediatrics* 70 (1982): 769.

Growing Without Schooling, 2269 Massachusetts Avenue, Cambridge, MA 02140. Tel: 617-864-3100. (Periodical from support group, bookstore, etc.)

Hay, D. A. "The Older Sibling of Twins." *Australian Journal of Early Childhood* 13 (1988): 25–28.

Klaus, Marshall H., John H. Kennell (Contributor), and Phyllis H. Klaus. *Bonding: Building the Foundations of Secure Attachment and Independence.* New York: Perseus, 1996.

Leonard, L. "Postpartum Depression in Mothers of Twins." *Maternal Child Nursing* 10 (1981): 99–109.

Levy, F., D. Hay, M. McLaughlin, C. Wood, and I. Waldman. "Twin Sibling Differences in Parental Reports of ADHD, Speech, Reading and Behavior Problems." *Journal of Child Psychology & Psychiatry* 37 (1996): 569–578.

Liedloff, Jean. *The Continuum Concept.* Cambridge, MA: Perseus, 1986.

McMahon, S., and B. Dodd. "A Comparison of the Expressive Communication Skills of Triplets, Twin and Singleton Children." *Eur J Disorders Communication* 32 (1997): 328–345.

Mendelsohn, R. *How to Raise a Healthy Child In Spite of Your Doctor.* New York: Ballantine, 1990.

Montagu, A. *Touching: The Human Significance of the Skin.* New York: Harper and Row, 1986.

O'Brien, Diane. "The Twins Who Made Their Own Language." *Family Health/Today's Health*, September 1978.

Pearce, J. C. *The Biology of Transcendence: A Blueprint for the Human Spirit.* Inner Traditions International, 2002.

Pedersen, I. K. et al. "Monozygotic Twins with Dissimilar Phenotypes and Chromosome Complements." *Acta Obstetrica and Gynecologica Scandinavica* 59, no. 5 (1980): 459–462.

Richardson, Barry. "Sudden Infant Death Syndrome: A Possible Primary Cause." *Journal of the Forensic Science Society* 34, no. 3 (1994): 199–204.

Riese, M. L. "Neonatal Temperament in Full-Term Pairs Discordant for Birth Weight." *Journal of Developmental & Behavorial Pediatrics* 15 (1994): 342–347.

————. "Discordant and Nondiscordant Twins: Comparative Multimethod Risk Assessment in the Neonatal Period." *Journal of Developmental and Behavioral Pediatrics* 22 (2001): 102–112.

Rowland, C. "Family Relationships." In *The Stress of Multiple Births*, edited by D. Harvey and E. Bryan. London: Multiple Births Foundation, 1991, pp. 59–67.

Sandbank, A. C. "The Effect of Twins on Family Relationships." *Acta Genetics* 37, no. 2 (1998): 161–172.

Segal, Nancy. "Cooperation, Competition, and Altruism Within Twin Sets: A Reappraisal." *Ethology and Sociobiology* 5 (1984): 153–177.

Solter, Aletha. *The Aware Baby: A New Approach to Parenting.* P.O. Box 206, Goleta, CA: Shining Star Press, 1990.

Taylor, E. M., and J. L. Emery. "Maternal Stress, Family and Health Care of Twins." *Children and Society* 4 (2000): 351–366.

Terasaki, P. et al. "Twins with Two Different Fathers Identified by HLA." *New England Journal of Medicine* 299 (September 1978): 11–14.

Tsujino, J. et al. "Specificity of a Mother's Attachment to Her Child Using the Attachment Inventory and Factors Related to Attachment: Longitudinal Research from Prenatal to Age 3." *Journal of Prenatal and Perinatal Psychology and Health* 17, no. 1 (Fall 2002): 63-84.

Tymms, P., and P. Preedy. "The Attainment and Progress of Twins at the Start of School." *Educational Research* 40 (1998): 244–249.

Zazzo, R. "The Twin Condition and the Couple Effect on Personality Development." *Acta Genet Med Gemellog* 25 (1979): 343–352.

Children with Disabilities

Biale, R. "Counseling Families of Disabled Twins." *Social Work* 34, no. 6 (1989): 531–536.

Hay, David, and Florence Levy. *Attention, Genes and ADHD.* New York: Bruner Routledge, 2001.

McDonald, Linda. *These Are Our Children: Twins, Triplets and Down Syndrome.* 4 Sugar Gum Drive, Mooloolah, Queensland 7147, Australia.

Wood, N. S., N. Marlow, K. Costeloe, A. T. Gibson, and A. R. Wilkinson. "The EPICure Study Group. Neurologic and Developmental Disability After Extremely Preterm Birth." *New England Journal of Medicine* 343 (August 10, 2000): 378–384.

Books and Articles about Twins

Abbe, Kathryn McLaughlin, and Frances McLaughlin Gill. *Twins on Twins.* New York: Clarkson Potter, 1980.

Ainslie, Ricardo. *The Psychology of Twinship.* Northvale, NJ: Jason Aronson, 1997.

Amis, Martin, *Success.* London: Vintage, 1978.

Anderson, K., and J. Robinson. *Full House: The Story of the Anderson Quintuplets.* Boston: Little, Brown, 1986.

Case, Betty Jean. *Exploring Twin Relationships: Is Being a Twin Always Fun?* Portland, OR: Tibbutt, 1996.

———. *We Are Twins, But Who Am I?* Portland, OR: Tibbutt. 1991.

Clegg, Avril, and Anne Woollett. *Twins from Conception to Five Years.* London: Century, 1988.

Duff, Kat. "Gemini and the Path of Paradox." *Parabola: The Magazine of Myth and Tradition.* XIX (Summer, 1994): 2. (http://www.parabola.org)

Elniski, James. "Finding One's Twin." *Parabola: The Magazine of Myth and Tradition.* XIX (Summer, 1994): 2. (http://www.parabola.org)

Enright, Anne. *What Are You Like?* London: Vintage, 2001.

Farmer, Penelope. *Two: The Book of Twins & Doubles.* London: Virago, 1996.

Gantz, Debra and Lisa. *The Book of Twins.* New York: Delacorte, 1998.

Pottker, J., and B. Speziale. *Dear Ann, Dear Abby.* New York: Paperjacks, 1988.

Rosenberg, Maxine B. *Being a Twin, Having a Twin.* New York: Lothrop, Lee, and Shepherd, 1985.

Sandbank, A., ed. *Twin and Triplet Psychology: A Professional Guide to Working with Multiples.* London: Routledge, 1999.

Scheinfeld, Amram. *Twins and Supertwins.* Baltimore: Penguin, 1973.

Segal, Nancy. *Entwined Lives: Twins and What They Tell Us About Human Behavior.* New York: Penguin Putnam, 1999.

Sheldon, Sidney. *Master of the Game.* New York, Warner, 1998.

Singh, Amrit, and K. D. Kaur Rabindra. *Twins Perspectives.* United Kingdom: Twin Studio, 1999. Tel/Fax 0151-653-0783.

Stewart, Elizabeth A. *Exploring Twins: Towards a Social Analysis of Twinship.* London: MacMillan, 2000.

Wallace, Majorie. *The Silent Twins.* London: Vintage, 1996.

Winnicott, D. W. "Twins." *The Child, the Family and the Outside World.* United Kingdom: Penguin, 1964.

Wolnewr, T., and H. Stein. *Parallels: A Look at Twins.* New York: Dutton, 1978.

Wright, Lawrence. *Twins: Genes, Environment and the Mystery of Identity.* Phoenix: Trafalgar Square, 1997.

Children's Books about Twins

Abolafia, Yossi. *My Three Uncles*. New York: Greenwillow, 1984.

Adalpe, Virginia T. *David, Donny and Darren: A Book About Identical Triplets*. Minneapolis: Lerner, 1997.

Chatwin, Bruce. *On the Black Hill*. London: Jonathan Cape, 1982.

Cleary, Beverly. *Two Dog Biscuits*. New York: Dell, 1987.

———. *The Real Hole*. New York: Dell, 1980.

———. *Mitch and Amy*. New York: Avon, 2000. (Beverly Cleary is a mother of twins).

Cole, J., and Edmondson, M. *Twins: The Story of Multiple Birth*. New York: Morrow, 1972.

Dadey, Debbie, and Marcia Thornton-Jones. *Triplet Trouble* series. New York: Scholastic, 1997.

DeClements, Barthe, and Christopher Grimes. *Double Trouble*. New York: Penguin, 1987.

DePaola, T. *Too Many Napkins*. New York: Putnam, 1989.

Firer, B. *Twins*. Spring Valley, NY: Feldheim, 1983.

Frechtman, Patricia, and Richard Harbin. *The Browne Series*. Twin Pleasures Publishing Corporation, P.O. Box 36097, Indianapolis, IN 46236, Tel: 800-TWIN-BKS, 1-800-894-6257 Fax: 317-823-7642 TwinGma@BrowneTwins.com.

Hill, Alan. *The Bedsers Twinning Triumphs*. London: Mainstream, 2001.

Lacoe, Addie. *Just Not the Same*. Boston: Houghton Mifflin, 1992.

Lindman, Maj. *Flicka, Ricka, Dicka* series. New York: Whitman, 1994.

———. *Snipp, Snapp, Snurr* series New York: Whitman, 1994.

Neasi, Barbara J. *Just Like Me*. New York: Children's Press, 2002.

Pascal, Francine. *Sweet Valley High Series*, New York: Bantam. http://www.randomhouse.com/sweetvalley/

Paterson, Katherine. *Jacob Have I Loved*. Caedmon Audio Cassette, October 1995.

Pirani, Felix. *Triplets*. New York: Viking, 1991.

Rogers, Fred. *The New Baby*.

Rotner, Shelley. *About Twins*. New York: Dorling Kindersley Publishing, 1999.

Seuling, Barbara. *The Triplets*. Boston: Houghton Mifflin, 1980.

Vogel, Ilse-Margaret. *My Twin Sister Erika*. New York: Harper and Row, 1976.

(The *Bobsey Twins* series, the series *Flicka, Ricka, Dicka* . . . as well as *Snip, Snap, Snurr* … are out of print but available from used books stores, libraries, or online searches.)

Books for Children about Preterm Birth

Hawkins-Walsh, Elizabeth. *Katie's Premature Baby Book*. Centering Corporation, Box 3367, Omaha, NE 68103 (coloring book).

Murphy-Melas, Elizabeth. *Watching Bradley Grow — A Story About Premature Birth*. 1996. Available from ICEA BookCenter, PO Box 20048, Minneapolis, MN 55420. Tel: 952-854-8660 or 800-624-4934 Fax: 952-854-8772. Email: info@icea.org.

Oehler, Jerri. *The Frogs Have a Baby, a Very Small Baby.* Route 7, Box 197B, Durham, NC 27707 (coloring book).

Pankow, Valerie. *No Bigger than My Teddy Bear.* 1987. Available from ICEA Book-Center, PO Box 20048, Minneapolis, MN 55420. Tel: 952-854-8660 or 800-624-4934 Email: info@icea.org.

Wilkie, David, and Diane. *Mommy, What Is a Preemie?* 1990. Available from ICEA BookCenter, PO Box 20048, Minneapolis, MN 55420. Tel: 952-854-8660 or 800-624-4934 Email: info@icea.org.

Death of a Twin

Benirschke, K. "Intrauterine Death of a Twin: Mechanisms, Implications for Surviving Twin, and Placental Pathology." *Semin Diagn Pathol* 10, no. 3 (August 1993): 222–231.

Case, Betty Jean. *Living Without Your Twin.* Portland, OR: Tibbutt, 2001.

Cuisinier, M. C. et al. "Grief Following the Loss of a Newborn Twin Compared to a Singleton." *Acta Paed* 85 (1996): 339–343.

Davis, Kellie. *Forever Silent, Forever Changed: The Loss of a Baby in Miscarriage, Stillbirth, Early Infancy. A Mother's Experience and Your Personal Journal.* Booklocker.com. June 1, 2001.

Landy, H. J., and L. G. Keith. "The Vanishing Twin: A Review." *Human Reproduction Update* 4, no. 2 (March/April 1998): 177–183.

Phol, P., and K. Geith. *I Miss You, I Miss You!* Roscoe, IL: R & S, 1999. (The sudden death of a teenage twin.)

Wegner-Hay, Martha. *How Can I Help? Suggestions for People Who Care About Someone Whose Baby Died Before Birth.* Abilene, TX: Hillcrest, 1999. (The grief and healing following the death of an infant twin)

Woodward, J. *The Lone Twin: Understanding Twin Bereavement and Loss.* London: Free Association Books Ltd, 1998.

Assisted Reproductive Technologies (ART)

Abdalla, H. I., C. Gearon, and M. Wren. "Swedish In Vitro Fertilisation Study." Letter to the Editor, *Lancet* 355, no. 9206 (2000): 844–845.

Angel, J. et al. "Aggressive Perinatal Care for High-Order Multiple Gestations: Does Good Perinatal Outcome Justify Aggressive Assisted Reproductive Techniques?" *American Journal of Obstetrics and Gynecology* 181 (August 1, 1999): 253–259.

Bergh, T. et al. "Deliveries and Children Born After In Vitro Fertilization in Sweden 1982–95: A Retrospective Cohort Study." *Lancet* 354, no. 9190 (1999): 1579–1585.

Bryan, E., R. Higgins, and D. Harvey. "Ethical Dilemmas." In *The Stress of Multiple Birth,* edited by D. Harvey and E. Bryan. London: Multiple Births Foundation, 1991.

Callahan, T. L. et al. "The Economic Impact of Multiple Gestation Pregnancies and the Contribution of Assisted Reproduction Techniques to their Incidence." *New England Journal of Medicine* 331 (1994): 244–249.

Fisk, N. M., and G. Trew. "Two's Company, Three's a Crowd for Embryo Transfer." Commentary, *Lancet* 354, no. 9190 (1999): 1572–1573.

Human Fertilization and Embryology Authority. http://Hfea.Gov.Uk/Annrep2000.

Jewell, S. E., and R. Yip. "Increasing Trends in Plural Births in the United States." *American Journal of Obstetrics & Gynecology* 85, no. 2 (1995): 229–232.

Luke, B. "The Changing Pattern of Multiple Births in the United States: Maternal and Infant Characteristics 1973 and 1990." *American Journal of Obstetrics & Gynecology* 84, no. 1 (1994): 101–106.

Melgar, C. A. et al. "Perinatal Outcome After Multifetal Reduction to Twins Compared with Nonreduced Multiple Gestation." *American Journal of Obstetrics & Gynecology* 78 (5) 73-767

Porreco, R. P. et al. "Multifetal Reduction of Triplets and Pregnancy Outcome." *American Journal of Obstetrics & Gynecology* 78, no. 3 (1991): 335–339.

Schreiner-Engel, W. N. et al. "First Trimester Multifetal Pregnancy Reduction: Acute and Persistent Psychological Reactions." *American Journal of Obstetrics & Gynecology* (1995): 172, 541–547.

Wenstrom, K. D. et al. "Increased Risk of Monochorionic Twinning Associated with Assisted Reproduction." *Fertility & Sterility* 60 (1993): 510–513.

Photo Credits

Abel: 95
Suzanne Arms: 255
Artemis/Hartigan: 277, 278
Sherry Bechtel: 364
Nils Bergman: 413 right
Meg Bost: 15 right, 365
Bernadine Brook: 367
Amy Bustamente: 340
Linda Cooper: 415
Alison Coppock: 3 left, 301, 349
Alison Curtis: 262
Lee Deschler: 3 right, 348, 350
Becky Dodds: 309
Elise F. Drake: 312, 326 left
Heather Ewer: 290
Fertility Center of New England: 202 top left/right, 437
Katrina Folkwell: 258
Four-Dee Products: 289 left
Anne Guter: 358, 360
Linda Gwillem: 42
Kay Hoover: 293, 294
Allessandra Hubbell: 28
Carol Ann M. Innbornone: 315
Jeffrey Kelly: 368
Janet Kizzlar, Phd.: 266
Jean Kollantai: 467
Lehigh Valley Hospital: 202 bottom

Wilma Lewis: 420, 426
Mark Masaki: 413 left
Metropolitan Museum of Art: 282
Multiple Births Foundation: 325
Myers: 64
National Center for Health Statistics: 53, 54, 55, 57, 59, 111, 112, 117, 121, 123, 271
Elizabeth Noble: 304
Dorothy Nunemaker: 34
Sharon Greene-O'Kane: 378
E.G. Parrinder: 13
Patti Ramos: 43, 276
Paul Rico: 15 left, 22
Chris Ridge: 326 right
Kimberly Smith: 427
Clinton Stoneking: 292
Tami Strong: 310, 376
Susan Van Lierup: 153
Carlo Verdisi: 9
Jill Werner, M.D.: 308
Cody White: 289 right
Kirsten Winspear: 407, 409
Wintergreen Press: 443

Line Art
Katherine Anderson, Victory Productions, Inc.; and Briar Lee Mitchell

Index